Modern Management Of

OCULAR DISEASES

EDITED BY
THOMAS C. SPOOR, MD

Printed in the United States of America

Library of Congress Catalog Card Number: 84-50588

ISBN: 0-943432-29-4

Published by: SLACK Incorporated
6900 Grove Rd.
Thorofare, NJ 08086

Last digit is print number: 10   9   8   7   6   5   4   3   2   1

DEDICATION

To those who said they would and did . . .
To Deanne for making it possible and Kristen for making it difficult.

CONTRIBUTORS

Richard L. Anderson, M.D.
Professor of Ophthalmology
University of Utah
Salt Lake City, Utah

Clifford Dacso, M.D., M.P.H.
Associate Professor of Medicine
University of South Alabama
Mobile, Alabama

Jonathan J. Dutton, M.D., Ph.D.
Assistant Professor of Ophthalmology
Duke University Eye Center
Durham, North Carolina

Mitchell H. Friedlaender, M.D.
Department of Ophthalmology
Francis I. Proctor Foundation
San Francisco, California

Lawrence H.A. Gold, M.D.
Department of Radiology
University of Minnesota
Minneapolis, Minnesota

M. Gilbert Grand, M.D.
Retinal Associates
Washington University
St. Louis, Missouri

Mark E. Hammer, M.D., M.S.
Associate Professor of Ophthalmology
University of South Carolina
Columbia, South Carolina

Walter E. Hartel, M.D.
Fellow, Neuro-Ophthalmology &
Orbital Service
University of Pittsburgh
Pittsburgh, Pennsylvania

Eugene Helveston, M.D.
Coleman Professor of Ophthalmology
University of Indiana
Indianapolis, Indiana

John S. Kennerdell, M.D.
Professor of Ophthalmology &
Neurology
University of Pittsburgh
Pittsburgh, Pennsylvania

John McCrary, M.D.
Associate Professor of Ophthalmology
& Neurosurgery
Baylor University
Houston, Texas

Bartly J. Mondino, M.D.
Associate Professor of Ophthalmology
Jules Stein Eye Institute - UCLA
Los Angeles, California

Matthew W. Mosteller, M.D.
Resident - Ophthalmology
Ochsner Clinic & Alton Ochsner
Medical Foundation
New Orleans, Louisiana

Edward O'Malley, M.D.
Pediatric Ophthalmologist
Henry Ford Hospital
Detroit, Michigan

Patric E. Nolan
Fellow, Infectious Disease Section
University of South Alabama
Mobile, Alabama

Paul R. Rosenberg, M.D.
Associate. Retina Service
Albert Einstein College of Medicine
Bronx, New York

James Rush
Neuro-ophthalmologist
Tampa, Florida

Thomas C. Spoor, M.D., M.S., FACS
Associate Professor of Ophthalmology
Kresge Eye Institute/Wayne State University
Detroit, Michigan

Thomas Tredici, M.D.
Fellow, Neuro-ophthalmology
Baylor University
Houston, Texas

Joseph B. Walsh, M.D.
Associate Professor of Ophthalmology
Albert Einstein College of Medicine
Bronx, New York

Robert Webb, M.D.
Assistant Professor of Ophthalmology
Albany Medical College
Albany, New York

Jonathan Wirtschafter, M.D.
Professor of Ophthalmology
University of Minnesota
Minneapolis, Minnesota

Paula J. Wynn, M.D.
Ophthalmologist
Greenville, South Carolina

Thom J. Zimmerman, M.D., Ph.D
Professor of Ophthalmology &
Pharmacology
Louisiana State University
& Alton Ochsner Medical Foundation
New Orleans, Louisiana

CONTENTS

Modern
Management Of
OCULAR
DISEASES

PREFACE

I intend this text to serve as a practical guide to common subspecialty problems that present to the practicing ophthalmologist or ophthalmology resident. It is not intended to be an encyclopedic compendium of ophthalmic knowledge. Common office problems such as cataract, refraction, and contact lenses are intentionally neglected.

I have asked physicians with expertise in their sub-specialties to write a practical guide to the manifestations and management of various other ocular disorders they encounter in their practices. We hope to describe how we approach problems in our areas of expertise, updating the subjects covered in a practical fashion and enabling the clinician to recognize, evaluate and appropriately manage these problems. I hope that we accomplish this goal and thank my contributors for their time and effort.

Section I

Adnexal Disorders

ADNEXAL DISORDERS

This section reviews the diagnosis and management of common diseases involving the ocular adnexa. In Chapter 1, Dutton and Anderson review the plethora or disorders presenting on the eyelids. These may be benign "lumps and bumps," aggressive neoplasms or manifestations of an underlying systemic disease. Their numerous illustrations facilitate our ability to recognize and/or treat these disorders.

The next chapter concerns common orbital disorders. A myriad of disease processes may involve the orbit, perplexing even the orbitologist. However, the clinician, armed with a basic knowledge of orbital anatomy, aware of the relationship between the orbit and adjacent structures (sinuses and brain) and cognizant of a few common disease entities affecting the orbit can diagnose, refer or manage many patients presenting with proptosis. Common disorders covered include metastatic tumors, infections, idiopathic orbital inflammation and lacrimal fossa masses.

Dystyroid orbitopathy is so common that an entire chapter has been devoted to it. In this chapter, Hartel and Kennerdell review the pathogenesis, diagnosis and management of this most common cause or orbital dysfunction.

The surgical management of strabismus is familiar to all of us: weakening and/or strengthening the appropriate muscles to straighten the eye. What to do when surgery is not indicated and appropriate pre-operative evaluation and treatment of the strabismus patient may be a bit more complex. The chapter by O'Malley and Helveston clarifies this often murkey area of strabismology and will be especially useful to clinicians lacking orthoptic abilities.

The section concludes with a short chapter discussing the neuro-opthalmologic causes of diplopia and the evaluation and management of these patients.

(Editor)

Chapter 1

Eyelid Disorders

Jonathan J. Dutton, MD, PhD
Richard L. Anderson, MD

EYELID DISORDERS

The eyelids are composed of skin, muscle, tarsus and conjunctiva. Subsequently, they are susceptible to many inflammatory, infectious and neplastic processes, as well as trauma and aging. Understanding eyelid anatomy facilitates the recognition and treatment of these processes. This chapter aims to augment such knowledge by reviewing the eyelid anatomy followed by a discussion of congenital defects, benign cysts and lesions, malignancies, systemic diseases and involutional changes.

(Editor)

Anatomy

Along with the orbital rims, brow, and periorbital soft tissues, the eyelids serve to protect the exposed anterior surfaces of the eye. Their unique anatomic structure, physiology and constant reflex and voluntary movements provide essential defensive and protective mechanisms against glare, foreign matter, dessication, trauma and infection.

The eyelids form the thin outer covering of the orbit extending from the brow above to the cheek below, and from the medial to the lateral orbital rims. Between the lids is the interpalpebral fissure which normally measures from 25 to 28 mm horizontally, and from 7 to 11 mm vertically. Movements of the lids are complex, allowing intimate contact between the conjunctival surfaces of both lids with the cornea in all positions of gaze.[17] Lying medially between the plica and medial canthus is the caruncle, a fleshy protuberance which measures 4 to 5 mm vertically by 3 mm horizontally. This is formed from modified skin, and represents an evolutionary vestige.

The lid margins are formed from modified skin anteriorly and conjunctiva posteriorly, with a mucocutaneous junction separating them. On the anterior edge of the lid margins are several rows of cilia which serve to protect the eye from wind-blown particles. In the posterior one-half of the lid margins are the openings of the meibomian glands which supply the lipid component to the precorneal tear film. The meibomian glands are large sebaceous glands lying within the tarsal plates, and number about 25 in the upper lid and 20 in the lower lid.

Glands of Zeis are microscopic sebaceous glands associated with each eyelash follicle. Moll's glands are modified sweat glands that empty onto the lid margins between the cilia or into the ductules of Zeis glands. Unlike the meibomian glands and Zeis glands which are holocrine glands, Moll's glands are apocrine glands.

The main portion of the eyelid is a thin structure composed of several laminae (Figure 1-1). At a level 3 mm proximal to the lid margin these laminae are from anterior to posterior: 1) skin, 2) subcutaneous areolar tissue, 3) pretarsal orbicularis muscle, 4) postorbicular areolar tissue, 5)

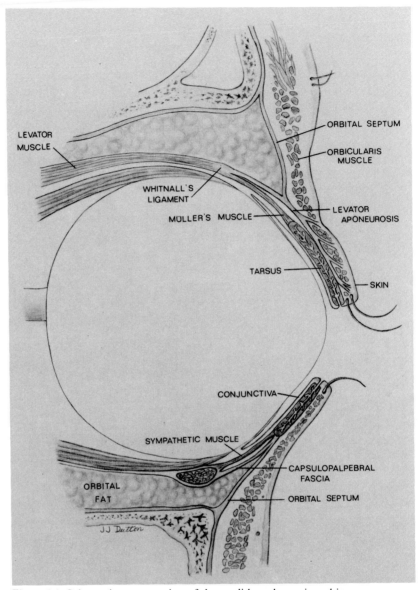

Figure 1-1. Schematic cross-section of the eyelids and anterior orbit.

tarsal plate, and 6) conjunctiva. At a level 15 mm above the upper lid margin, the laminae are as follows: 1) skin, 2) subcutaneous areolar tissue, 3) preseptal orbicularis muscle, 4) postorbicular areolar tissue, 5) orbital septum, 6) preaponeurotic fat pad, 7) levator aponeurosis, 8) Müller's sympathetic muscle, and 9) conjunctiva.

The skin of the eyelids is exceptionally thin and loosely attached to underlying tissues except in the pretarsal portions of the eyelids and at the canthi. This accounts for a number of conditions such as stretched redundant skin (dermatochalasis) in older patients, and the ready accumulation of preseptal subcutaneous edema and hemorrhage.

Beneath the subcutaneous areolar tissue the orbicularis oculi fibers run parallel to the lid margins. The orbicularis muscle is divided anatomically into several portions. The orbital portion arises from the medial orbital rim, fans out above and passes around the periphery of the eyelids to insert near its site of origin at the medial orbital rim. The palpebral portion is confined to the mobile portion of the lids. It arises from the medial canthal tendon, arcs superiorly and inferiorly, and inserts along the lateral horizontal raphe and lateral canthal tendon. It is further subdivided into a pretarsal portion overlying the anterior surface of the tarsal plates, and a preseptal portion which overlies the orbital septum proximal to the tarsal plates. Along the lid margins and forming a delicate band of striated fibers is the muscle of Riolan. The main pretarsal orbicularis fibers pass laterally into the lateral canthal tendon which inserts into the periosteum at the lateral orbital tubercle, and medially into the medially canthal tendon which inserts into the periosteum on the frontal process of the maxillary bone. Small slips of orbicularis, Horner's muscle, pass from the deep medial portion of the pretarsal fibers and from the muscle of Riolan, and insert into the periosteum of the posterior lacrimal crest. They contribute to functioning of the lacrimal pump system by shortening the canaliculus. The orbicularis muscle is innervated by branches of the seventh cranial nerve.

The postorbicular areolar plane is composed of loose connective tissue and contains the seventh cranial nerve fibers that supply the orbicularis muscle.

The orbital septum originates from the arcus marginalis formed by the junction of periorbita and periosteum around the periphery of the orbital rim. In the upper lid the septum blends distally into the fibers of the underlying levator aponeurosis some 4 to 6 mm above the tarsal plate. In the lower lid the septum extends from the arcus marginalis at the lower orbital rim to the lower border of the tarsal plate where it joins the lower lid retractors. Medially the orbital septum of both lids pass behind the lacrimal sac, blending with fibers of the posterior crus of the medial canthal tendon, to insert onto the posterior lacrimal crest. Laterally the septum fuses to and forms the posterior layer of the lateral palpebral raphe. Weak and thin areas in the septum permit herniation of orbital fat into the lids, especially prominent in the elderly. The orbital septum acts as a barrier to the spread of infection and hemorrhage.

Between the orbital septum and the levator aponeurosis in the upper lid is the pre-aponeurotic fat pad which is a forward extension of orbital fat. It is an important surgical landmark and its prolapse into weak areas of the septum is a major cause of baggy eyelids.

The levator palpebrae superioris muscle which elevates the lid takes origin from the lesser wing of the sphenoid bone just above the optic foramen and annulus of Zinn. It travels forward in close approximation to the underlying superior rectus muscle. As it crosses the equator of the globe the muscle fibers pass into a fibrous aponeurosis which fans out horizontally to occupy the entire orbital width. A thickened condensation of fibrous tissue, the superior suspensory ligament of Whitnall, extends across the orbit within this tendon, just at its junction with the muscular portion of the levator. Whitnall's ligament is attached to the orbital wall medially at the trochlea, and laterally to the capsule of the lacrimal gland and periosteum of the orbital wall. This ligament serves to support the levator and to change its vector force from horizontal in the orbit to vertical in the lid. As the aponeurosis passes forward into the upper lid it fans out to occupy the entire orbital width. It fuses with the distal fibers of the orbital septum about 4 to 6 mm above the tarsal plate, and sends fibrous slips that interdigitate between fibers of the orbicularis to insert into the intermuscular septae, forming a prominent lid crease. The aponeurosis attaches to the anterior aspect of the tarsal plate. Medial and lateral extensions of the aponeurosis forming the "horns" insert into the medial and lateral canthal tendons respectively. The levator muscle is innervated by the superior division of the third cranial nerve.

Müllers muscle is supplied by sympathetic fibers and lies just behind the levator aponeurosis. It originates from the distal fibers of the levator muscle and inserts onto the proximal border of the tarsal plate. In the lower lid analogous but less developed fibers take origin from the fascia of the inferior rectus muscle and pass to the lower border of the tarsus. Lockwood's ligament, or the inferior suspensory ligament, is a condensation of the capsules of the inferior oblique and inferior rectus muscles and spans the inferior orbit, helping to support the orbital contents. A fascial expansion from Lockwood's ligament and the inferior rectus sheath, the capsulopalpebral fascia, passes upward to insert into the inferior surface of the tarsus forming an analogue of the levator aponerurosis.

The tarsal plates are flat dense fibrous structures that give support to the eyelids. About 20 to 30 meibomian glands lie within the plate in each lid, and provide the important lipid component to the tear film.

Lining the posterior surface of both lids is the conjunctiva, a highly vascular mucous membrane that contains numerous mucous-secreating goblet cells, as well as small accessory lacrimal glands of Krause and Wolfring. From the eyelids the palpebral conjunctiva passes into the fornices and is continuous with the bulbar conjunctiva covering the globe.

The vascular supply of the eyelids is extensive. Arterial blood is derived mainly from the ophthalmic artery via the medial superior and inferior palpebral arteries that penetrate the orbital septum nasally. These run laterally as three arcades: the marginal arcades near the lid margins in the upper and lower lids, and the superior peripheral arcade that runs near the upper border of the tarsus in the upper lid. These arcades anastomose temporally with the lateral superior and lateral inferior palpebral arteries derived from the lacrimal artery. Further anastomotic branches join the external carotid system via the transverse facial and superficial temporal arteries laterally, and the dorsal nasal and angular arteries medially.

Venous drainage anterior to the tarsal plate is into the angular and superficial temporal veins. A deeper system, draining posterior to the tarsus, empties into tributaries of the ophthalmic veins.

Lymphatic vessels in the lateral two-thirds of the upper lid and the lateral one-third of the lower lid enter the preauricular lymph nodes. The medial one-third of the upper and medial two-thirds of the lower lids drain into the submaxillary nodes.

The sensory nerve supply to the lids is from the fifth cranial nerve. The supraorbital and supratrochlear branches of the ophthalmic division supply the upper lid with some branches of the infratrochlear and lacrimal nerve also contributing. The lower lid is supplied principally from infraorbital branches of the maxillary division of the trigeminal nerve, along with some contribution from the infratrochlear nerve nasally.

Congenital Anomalies

Epiblepharon. This is a rare congenital conditon that is often difficult to differentiate from entropion. It occurs in the lower eyelid and usually disappears spontaneously by the end of the first year of life. In epiblepharon, the lash-bearing margin of the lid is pushed against the globe by an accessory fold of skin, particularly in downgaze. The eyelid margin itself is normal in position, not turned in as in true entropion. Corneal damage is uncommon since the inturned lashes in infants are fine and soft. The condition therefore usually requires no treatment. If irritation is present, then surgical intervention is indicated. This consists of removing a small strip of skin and orbicularis muscle just below the lid margin. An alternative method is the placement of lid crease sutures.[42] In this procedure absorbable sutures are passed from the conjunctival surface below the tarsus to the skin surface in the position of the desired new lid crease. A scar band is formed which prevents overriding of skin and orbicularis muscle, thus correcting the epiblepharon.

Congenital Entropion. This most commonly involves the lower eyelid (Figure 1-2). The etiology is unknown. It has been stated that entropion is caused by a bundle of hypertrophied pretarsal orbicularis in these children. However, more recent evidence has failed to demonstrate this, and rather suggests that at least some of these cases result from congenital disinsertion of the lower eyelid aponeurosis.[47] If corneal irritation results, surgical correction becomes necessary. The procedure consists of removing a strip of skin and pretarsal orbicularis muscle from beneath

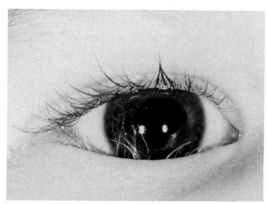

Figure 1-2. Congenital entropion of the lower eyelid.

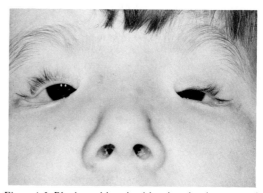

Figure 1-3. Blephorophimosis with epicanthus inversus and telecanthus.

the lid margin. If the eyelid aponeurosis is disinserted, it is repaired. The wound is closed with absorbable sutures through the skin margins and fixed to the epitarsus such that when tied the lashes are everted away from the globe.

Congenital entropion of the upper eyelid is quite uncommon, but more of a problem since damage to the cornea can be more severe. It is usually caused by a kinked tarsus. Treatment is surgical by fracturing the tarsal plate horizontally along its entire length. In closing this fracture, the posterior margin of the upper tarsal edge is sutured to the anterior margin of the lower tarsal edge so that the free margin of the lid is everted.

Coloboma. A coloboma is a full-thickness developmental defect that may involve the upper or lower lids, or both. The edges of the defect may be adherent to the bulbar conjunctiva and cornea, and dermoid lesions at the limbus may also be present. The cornea usually tolerates the resultant exposure reasonably well. Treatment is surgical and there is usually sufficient lid tissue present to achieve good cosmetic and functional results. The edges of the defect are carefully resected and an end-to-end anastomosis of the normal edges is performed as in repair of lid lacerations.[13] If the defect is large, a lateral canthotomy and cantholysis may be performed, and undermining of the lateral temporal tissues with temporal advancement may be necessary to achieve closure.

Blepharophimosis. This is a congenital, usually bilateral horizontal shortening of the palpebral fissures in the presence of normal eyelid structures. It is commonly associated with other defects such as ptosis, epicanthus inversus, telecanthus and ectropion of the lateral portion of the lower lid (Figure 1-3). Major reconstruction of the medial and lateral canthus are usually required for correction, and placement of a transnasal wire may be needed to shorten the intercanthal distance if significant telecanthus is present.

Distichiasis. Distichiasis is usually a congenital anomaly in which an accessory row of lashes turns backward toward the cornea (Figure 1-4). The

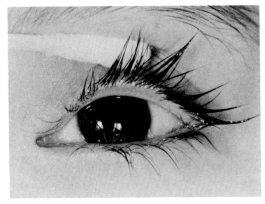

Figure 1-4. Congenital distichiasis.

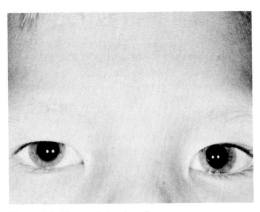

Figure 1-5. Congenital epicanthus.

condition may involve only a few lashes or the entire lid margin. If only a few additional lashes are present, they can be removed by electrolysis. More commonly there are too many lashes for effective removal by this method. In these cases the treatment is surgical. The eyelid is split into anterior and posterior lamellae and the offending lash follicles with the tarsus of the posterior lamella are excised by removing a 3 mm marginal strip. Excellent results can also be obtained by cryotherapy to the margin of the posterior lamella.[5]

Epicanthus. The epicanthus is a congenital fold of skin over the medial canthus which covers the caruncle (Figure 1-5). It may produce a pseudostrabismus. Most commonly this fold originates superiorly from the skin just below the brow, from the upper eyelid, or as an extension of the superior tarsal fold. The latter form is seen as the typical Mongolian fold. In Caucasians, epicanthus commonly disappears in early childhood as the bridge of the nose widens. When treatment is required, it is best delayed until 4 to 5 years of age. The basic defect consists of a vertical shortening of skin at the medial canthus. A realignment of skin can be achieved by any number of vertical skin lengthening procedures, such as the double Z-plasty or Y to V-plasty.

Ankyloblepharon. Ankyloblepharon is a congenital adherence of the lid margins that may vary from a single filamentous band to extensive adhesion of the entire lid margins. Treatment consists of simple separation of the lids with scissors or a scalpel. If the adhesion is extensive, sutures between the conjunctiva and skin may be necessary.

Congenital Ptosis. Congenital ptosis usually results from a developmental dystrophy or neurogenic weakness of the levator muscle. It is usually unilateral, but may be asymmetrically bilateral, and varies from slight to severe. It may be associated with other extraocular muscle abnormalities, the most common being involvement of the superior rectus muscle.

The condition is usually noted during the first few weeks or months of life. Some bilateral cases may not become apparent until later when the child is noted to be using the frontalis muscle to raise the lids above the visual axis.

Examination of a child with ptosis should include measurement of the position of the lids as well as the degree of levator function. The latter is evaluated by having the child look from the downgaze to the upgaze positions while immobilizing the brow. The presence or absence of a lid crease is also important since its presence indicates that some levator function exists (Figure 1-6). Synkinetic movements associated with opening of the mouth, clenching the jaws, and with chewing movements suggests presence of the Marcus-Gunn jaw-winking phenomenon. In this syndrome, misdirected nerve fibers from the trigeminal nerve seem to elevate the ptotic lid above its normal position when the muscles of mastication are activated.

Treatment of congenital ptosis in most cases is surgical. Its timing

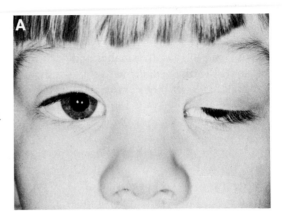

Figure 1-6. Congenital ptosis. Prior to surgery.

depends upon visual function. In general, if the visual axis are not obscured by the ptotic lid, it is best to delay repair until the child is 3 to 4 years old. Earlier intervention becomes necessary when occlusion amblyopia threatens visual acuity. The surgical procedure depends on the degree of levator function and the position of the lid. In ptosis cases with fair to good function, advancement of the levator aponeurosis will give good results. When ptosis is more severe and function is poor (3 to 4 mm) suspension of the tarsus to Whitnall's ligament will usually provide adequate height and contour. In cases of severe ptosis and less than 3 mm of function, suspension of the lid to the frontalis muscle, preferably with autogenous fascia lata, is the procedure of choice. In infants in whom the fascia lata is poorly developed, Supramid suture has given good temporary results, but this material may have to be replaced at a later date.

Eyelid Cysts

Milia. Milia are intracutaneous retention cysts caused by occlusion of pilosebaceous follicles. They commonly occur on the eyelids away from the lid margins. Milia appear as small, rounded, elevated, whitish lesions without associated inflammation. Although milia do not cause symptoms, they may be a cosmetic blemish that requires treatment. Superficial cysts may be removed with 5% salicylic acid and 10% sulfa ointment. They are also easily removed by making a small incision through the surface of the lesion with expression of the contained sebaceous material. The interior lining of the cyst cavity should be lightly cauterized with trichloroacetic acid.

Sebaceous Cysts. These cysts are related to milia, but are larger and result from the occlusion of the outlet from meibomian, Zeis or sebaceous glands. Such cysts may remain quiescent or grow to considerable size. Meibomian cysts are limited by the fibrous tarsal tissues and may undergo degenerative changes. They appear as elevated, yellowish lesions that may be associated with inflammatory reaction (Figure 1-7), and can be removed by surgical excision of the cyst with its enclosing walls. If infected, they may require drainage and hot compresses prior to total excision.

Zeis gland cysts are smaller and occur near the lid margins. They are rounded, whitish lesions with thin overlying skin that may rupture spontaneously or with hot compresses. Expression with gentle pressure will often evacuate the cysts. Larger cysts will require excision. They may also be treated by incision with cautery of the cyst walls.

Cysts of Glands of Moll and Sweat Glands.

Cysts of the sweat glands may result from sweat gland adenomas with dilation of the duct in the dermis, or from distension of the secretory tubules themselves. Moll gland cysts, also called sudoriferous cysts, occur on the lid margins. They enlarge slowly forming pinkish, transparent vesicle-like cysts that are more commonly seen on the lower lid near the punctum (Figure 1-8). These cysts may be uni- or multiocular depending upon whether the duct or tubule is involved in the cyst formation. Treatment consists of total excision, since failure to remove the walls will usually result in recurrence. Smaller cysts may be incised, drained, and the walls chemically cauterized. Since epitheliomas may originate in the cyst ducts, any tissue other than the thin-walled cyst should be submitted for histopathologic examination.

Epidermoid Cyst.

These most commonly result from epidermal rests sequestered into deeper tissues during embryogenesis. They may also arise from dermal appendages or from trauma with displacement of epidermis into deeper tissues. Epidermal cysts are slow-growing, elevated, rounded tumors of varying size with moveable skin overlying them. They are filled with keritinized material and there may be marked hyperplasia, necrosis and, occasionally, calcification. With rupture of the cyst a considerable foreign-body reaction results. Malignant degeneration is rare, but both squamous cell and basal cell carcinomas arising in epidermoid cysts have been described.[29,31,39]

Epidermoid cysts require excision with an attempt made not to rupture the cyst walls. If ruptured, the contents should be carefully washed away and the cyst walls completely excised.

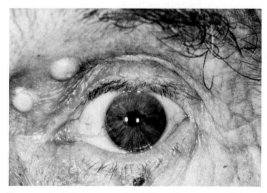

Figure 1-7. Sebaceous cysts of the left upper eyelid and medial canthus.

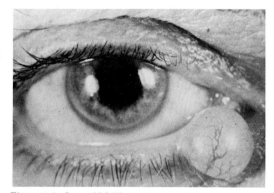

Figure 1-8. Cyst of Moll's gland—sudoriferous cyst.

Dermoid Cyst. Dermoid cysts are congenital rests of ectoderm consisting of a layer of epidermis with surrounding connective tissue which typically become incarcerated in bony suture lines. They may include skin appendages, and more rarely, smooth muscle, calcium and cartilage. The cyst is filled with keratinized debris and sebaceous material. There may be an associated inflammatory reaction if the contents leak out of the enclosing walls.

Dermoid cysts may occur in the eyelids where they most commonly involve the temporal portion (Plate IA). There may be deep orbital, sinus, or even intracranial extensions.

Because of the general increase in size and the danger of ruptures, we feel that dermoids should be removed. When surgery is considered, complete excision is usually possible, but may be difficult if the lesion is deep or involves bone. As with epidermoids, every attempt should be made to remove the entire cyst wall to prevent recurrence. Radiographic evaluation, particularly CT scanning and hypocycloidal tomography, and standardized echography may help to determine the size of the lesion and extent of bony involvement.

Epithelial Inclusion Cyst. These usually result from trauma or surgery at which time epithelial cells become sequestered beneath the surface. They may form a small cyst that remains stable, or which may enlarge and require excision. As with all epithelial cysts, the walls must be completely removed to prevent recurrence.

Inflammations and Granulomas

Chalazion. A chalazion is a chronic inflammatory granuloma within a meibomian gland. It appears to be caused by alterations in secretions with retention of secretory material due to plugging of ducts. The condition may be started and is aggravated by chronc blepharitis and low-grade bacterial infections involving the meibomian gland.

Clinically, the lesion presents as a firm nodule that increases in size over weeks or months. In chronic cases symptoms are minimal. There is much associated granulation tissue incited by retained material. The lesion most commonly is seen to bulge externally through the skin, and less commonly posteriorly through the conjunctiva. They may perforate these surfaces with the formation of marked granulation tissue.

The acute form of chalazion may also present as an inflamed, markedly tender nodule causing significant reaction in the adjacent lid (Plate IB). This results from infection, usually *Staphylococcus*, and may be associated with preauricular adenopathy. Such lesions frequently rupture spontaneously, and drain through the resulting fistula, usually on the conjunctival surface.

Once the inflammatory reaction has subsided, the final lesion is a small granuloma that requires no further treatment. However, during the acutely inflamed stage, medical treatment consists of hot packs four times daily, along with topical antibiotic ointment. Systemic antibiotics are not indicated unless adenopathy is severe and the infection marked enough to threaten an adjacent cellulitis.

When the chalazion does not respond to more conservative medical management after two weeks, or when the lesion is large and symptomatic, surgical drainage is indicated. Local anesthesia is injected subcutaneously around the lesion away from the lid margin and into the conjunctival fornix. Tetracaine is instilled into the eye and a chalazion clamp is applied to the lid. The lesion is incised usually vertically through the conjunctival surface, but when anterior just below the skin, an external approach using a horizontal incision may be necessary. The secretions and granulomatous tissue are curetted and the lining removed by sharp dissection. For conjunctival incisions the defect is left open to drain, and the patient is continued on hot packs and antibiotics for ten days.

Complications are uncommon, but include incomplete removal with persistent granulomatous tissue, perforation of the lid requiring suture repair, and excessive removal of tarsus with resulting lid margin deformity or damage to lashes.

Finally, it must be stressed that any atypical or recurring chalazion must be regarded as a possible neoplastic lesion until proven otherwise, and biopsy material must be submitted for histologic study. Adenocarcinoma of the meibomian glands, basal cell carcinoma, and squamous cell carcinoma, as well as metastatic carcinomas have all been mistaken for chalazia.

Foreign-Body Granuloma.

Foreign material implanted into the skin or conjunctiva may cause excessive inflammatory reaction and granuloma formation. This may result from abnormal scar deposition as with keloid formation, can be secondary to infection or hemorrhage, or to the presence of irritative materials such as dirt, wood or hairs following trauma, silica or talc, or metallic particles. Certain endogenous materials such as uric acid crystals in gout, or the ruptured contents of epidermoid or pilar cysts, can produce a foreign-body reaction.

Foreign-body granulomas contain macrophage infiltration around the foreign material, with lymphocytes and foreign-body type giant cells. Treatment consists of excision with meticulous removal of all inciting material.

Sarcoid Granuloma.

Sarcoidosis is a chronic multisystem disease of unknown etiology in which the skin may be involved in about one-third of cases. The nodular skin lesions can occur in the eyelid, conjunctiva and orbit, and there may or may not be associated uveitis. The lid lesions are soft, rounded, well-circumscribed nodules that may simulate a chalazion. They consist of epithelioid and giant cells of the Langhans type, with a light admixture if lymphocytes. Caseation necrosis is typically not seen.

Clinically, these lesions run a benign course with a tendency to spontaneous healing. If they become large, interfere with lid function, or cause significant cosmetic blemish, they may require excision. Systemic corticosteroids are used for the more severe pulmonary and intraocular complications of the disease.

Tuberculosis and Syphilis. Tuberculosis involving the eyelids most commonly results from reinfection and manifests itself as a form of lupus vulgaris. These lesions usually occur on the face and consist of epithelioid cells and giant cells typically of the Langhans type. An inflammatory infiltrate is present, more pronounced in the upper dermis, and leads to destruction of cutaneous structures with resultant scarring and fibrosis in areas of healing.

Clinically, lupus vulgaris appears as well-demarcated, reddish-brown patches associated with a small nodule. These increase in size and number, but with time undergo central ulceration and cicatrization. When both upper and lower lids are involved, lid deformity may result in ectropion and corneal exposure.

Syphilis involving the eyelid is rarely seen anymore. It may occur as a primary lesion where it presents as a nodule, usually at the lid margin, which soon ulcerates. The lesion consists of acanthosis of the epidermis with an underlying infiltrate of lymphocytes and plasma cells. Vascular endothelial proliferation and occlusion of capillaries and small vessels are seen. Secondary syphilis can involve the lids with a maculopapular rash.

There are no specific treatments for the above skin lesions in tuberculosis and syphilis, but once the diagnosis is made systemic therapy should be instituted. Evaluation and management are best undertaken by an internist or infectious disease specialist and individualized depending upon associated findings.

Bacterial Infections

Erysipelas. Erysipelas is an acute superficial cellulitis caused by group A *Streptococcus pyogenes*. The marked cellular infiltrate consists of neutrophils and a few lymphocytes. The process may extend down to the level of the orbital septum.

Clinically, the lesion appears as a well-demarcated, indurated reddish area with a distinct and often palpable advancing border. Facial involvement is common. Occasionally, bullae are present which may later suppurate. Preauricular and submandibular adenopathy is usually present. Complications are rare except in the most severe cases, and include necrosis and gangrene of the lids. Cultures of the skin or conjunctiva are usually unrewarding. Needle aspiration is contraindicated because of the danger of spread into deeper tissue planes.

Erysipelas is treated with penicillin G intravenously for two or three days, followed by oral penicillin for another week. If an abscess forms in the lid, this may need surgical drainage.

Impetigo. This is a superficial cutaneous infection caused by *Staphylococcus aureus* and group A *Streptococcus pyogenes*. It is most commonly seen in children under five or six years of age and is characterized by epithelial bullae containing numerous neutrophils with an inflammatory infiltrate within the dermis. As bullae rupture, a loose crust forms composed of fibrin and cellular debris. There is usually marked erythema of the lids with edema of the preseptal tissues (Figure 1-9). Regional adenopathy is present.

Treatment consists of warm soaks, removal of crusts, and application of topical antibiotics such as bacitracin. In infants, intravenous administration of penicillin G plus methacillin should be undertaken in the hospital.

Hordeolum.

A hordeolum or sty is a *Staphylococcus* infection of the lash follicle and associated gland of Zeis. Clinically, the lesion begins with a tenderness localized to the lid margin, but edema and induration may involve a larger area (Plate IC). After several days the lesion points with discharge of pus among the lashes. In some cases the process involutes without discharge. The condition is usually of short duration and resolves spontaneously, but rarely may lead to a spreading cellulitis when severe.

Treatment is medical, and surgical drainage is rarely necessary. Hot packs are applied four times daily to hasten pointing and drainage, and topical antibiotics are used to prevent the spread of infection. Following subsidence, efforts should be made to prevent recurrences with lid hygiene and, if necessary, the continued use of antibiotic ointment at bedtime. Treatment of predisposing factors, such as diabetes, blepharitis, acne vulgaris, etc., should also be undertaken.

Blepharitis.

Blepharitis is a subacute or chronic inflammation of the eyelid margins. It may be asymptomatic and neglected by the patient, but is not uncommonly associated with a secondary conjunctivitis or keratitis. Several types of the disorder have been distinguished.

In the squamous or seborrheic type no bacterial agent has been identified. Rather, seborrheic dermatitis is the basic skin lesion. It is associated with oily and flaking skin around the eyelids and eyebrows, with greasy scales forming at the base of the eyelashes. There is hyperemia of the lid margins (Plate ID). When chronic, lashes may be lost, there may be rounding of the posterior border of the lid, and associated chronic conjunctivitis. At this point the patient is usually quite symptomatic with complaints of tearing, photophobia and intolerance of air pollutants such as

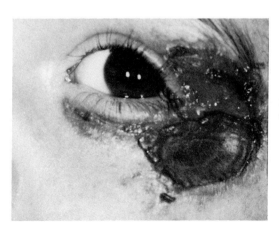

Figure 1-9. Impetigo involving the lateral canthus and both upper and lower eyelids.

smoke. *Pitysporum ovale* may be found among the marginal lid debris, but its role in the pathogenesis of the disease remains uncertain.

Treatment of seborrheic blepharitis must include simultaneous management of associated seborrhea of the skin and scalp. Inspisated purulent material is manually expressed from the meibomian gland and marginal scales are removed with frequent lid scrubs using a mild baby shampoo on cotton-tipped applicators. Topical selenium sulfide lotion rubbed into the lid margin may be helpful as are mild local steroid preparations for control of the more acute inflammatory process. Once the condition is under control lid scrubs and antibiotics continued once daily or several times weekly may minimize recurrences.

Staphylococcal blepharitis is a bacterial inflammation of the glands along the lid border. Crusts of desquamated epithelium accumulate along the eyelid margins and can be associated with ulceration, necrosis of ciliary follicles, scarring of the adjacent conjunctiva, and an inferior punctate keratitis. Scrapings of lid margin debris reveal *Staphylococcus* and numerous polymorphonuclear leukocytes. When severe and prolonged, the condition may lead to lid thickening and deformity of the lid margins with trichiasis.

Treatment consists of manual removal of crusts with debridement of ulcer craters. The lesions should be cultured to establish antibiotic sensitivities. At home the patient should continue frequent hot soaks followed by application of bacitracin or gentamicin ointment three or four times a day. Antibiotics must be continued at bedtime for at least a month after symptoms have disappeared. The use of steroids topically in conjunction with antibiotics will reduce inflammation and ultimate lid scarring, and will ameliorate symptoms. In persistent cases, systemic oxacillin or erythromycin may be effective in controlling the disease.

Viral Infections

Herpes Simplex. *Herpes simplex* dermatitis most commonly involves the face and genital region. When the eyelids and nose are affected a possible serious complication is the associated keratitis which, when recurrent, can cause significant corneal scarring. *Herpes simplex* is a DNA-virus that typically produces an intra-epidermal vesicle on the skin with marked destruction of epidermal cells. An inflammatory infiltrate usually accompanies these vesicles. Intranuclear viral inclusions may be seen with appropriate histologic scrapings from the base of these vesicles.

On the eyelids *herpes simplex* presents as a cluster of superficial, clear vesicles with a mild surrounding inflammatory base (Figure 1-10). These usually dry, slough, and heal in about seven to 10 days without residual scarring. Treatment is directed at preventing secondary infection with topical antibiotic ointments. Various solutions such as calamine lotion with 0.125% menthol and 0.25% phenol may hasten resolution. The use of antiviral agents, such as IDU, is not generally helpful for cutaneous lesions. Recurrence is common and such patients should always be examined carefully for ocular involvement.

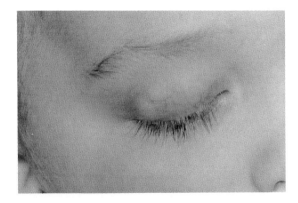

Plate I-A. Dermoid cyst in the temporal aspect of the right upper eyelid.

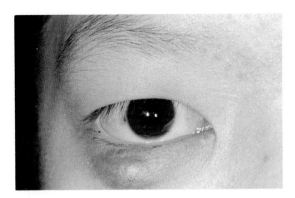

Plate I-B. Chalazion with marked inflammatory reaction.

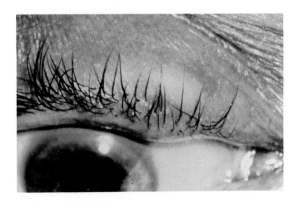

Plate I-C. External hordeolum.

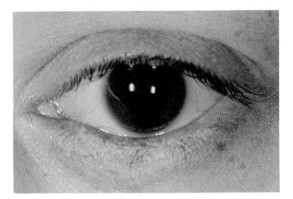

Plate I-D. Blepharitis of the lower eyelid.

Plate I-E. *Herpes zoster* in the distribution of the ophthalmic division of the left trigeminal nerve.

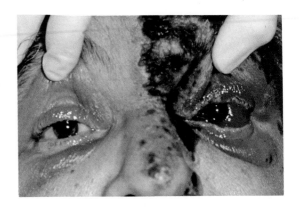

Plate I-F. Molluscum contagiosum.

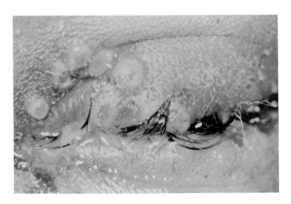

Plate I-G. Seborrheic keratosis.

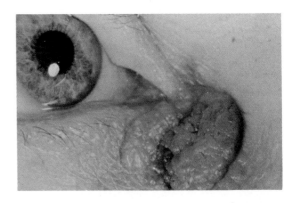

Plate I-H. Xanthalasma.

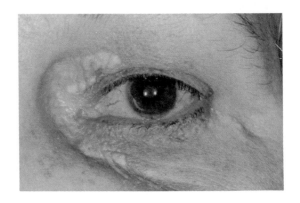

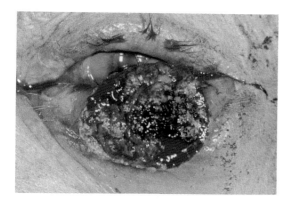

Plate II-A. Keratoacanthoma involving most of the lower eyelid.

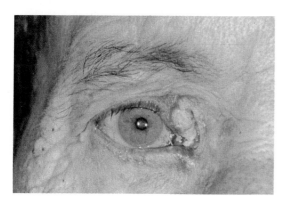

Plate II-B. Squamous cell carcinoma of the medial canthus.

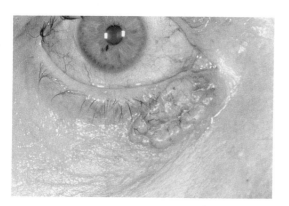

Plate II-C. Basal cell carcinoma.

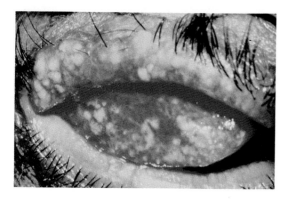

Plate II-D. Meibomian gland carcinoma involving the entire upper eyelid.

Plate II-E. Acquired melanosis.

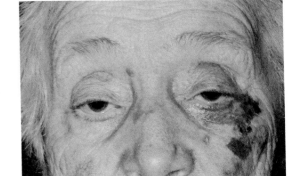

Plate II-F. Malignant melanoma.

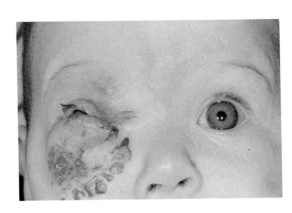

Plate II-G. Capillary hemangioma.

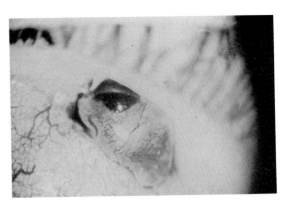

Plate II-H. Pyogenic granuloma.

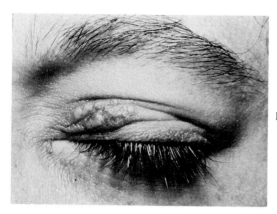

Figure 1-10. *Herpes simplex* involving the upper eyelids.

Herpes Zoster. *Herpes zoster* is caused by a DNA-virus and may involve the skin supplied by the ophthalmic division of the trigeminal nerve. The histologic appearance is similar to that of *herpes simplex*, but there is frequently more vasculitis and inflammatory infiltrate.[28]

Clinically, the dermatitis usually begins as a vesicular eruption in the distribution of the frontal branch of the ophthalmic nerve involving the forehead and eyelids, and typically not crossing the midline (Plate IE). Marked pain is common. Severe inflammatory reaction may be seen and the base of these lesions may appear hemorrhagic. With involvement of the nasociliary branch, iritis and keratitis may occur. The vasicular stage is followed by spontaneous drying and crusting.

Treatment consists of symptomatic relief of pain. Topical steroids will reduce the inflammatory reaction and subsequent scarring, and may lessen the severity of post-herpetic neuralgia, a not uncommon complication. As with *herpes simplex*, topical antibiotics are applied to prevent secondary infection. Very severe cases of post-herpetic neuralgia may require alcohol injections or even section of the nerve for relief.

Vaccinia. Vaccinia infection of the eyelids is uncommon. Infection occurs when a child scratches a vaccination site and then rubs the eye. Accidental contamination from other individuals is also a cause. The diagnosis is suggested by a pustular lesion near the lid margin accompanied by edema and erythema. The opposing lid margin may also be involved, and there is usually painful preauricular adenopathy. A history of recent vaccination and the presence of eosinophilic intracytoplasmic inclusion bodies on smears will help establish the diagnosis. Occasionally a secondary keratitis may be seen. The lid lesions usually heal with little scarring and conservative management with topical antibiotics is indicated to prevent secondary infection. In severe cases with corneal involvement vaccinia immunoglobulin has been reported to be helpful.

Verruca Vulgaris. Verrucae are small epidermal papillae of viral etiology. They are common on the hands, and are sometimes seen on the eyelids. Verrucae form circumscribed, firm, elevated papillomatous growths with a hyperkeratotic surface that tend to enlarge slowly (Figure

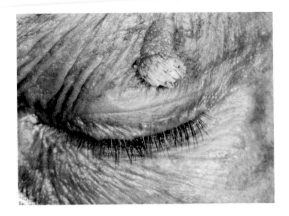

Figure 1-11. Verruca vulgaris.

1-11). When the lid margin is involved, they may cause a secondary conjunctivitis. Surgical excision or electrocautery will give satisfactory results. Cryotherapy and laser therapy may also control these lesions.

Molluscum Contagiosum. Molluscum contagiosum is a mildly contagious dermatologic disease caused by a filterable virus. The lesions consist of hyperplastic epithelial cells that grow downward into the underlying dermis as multiple lobules. Many cells contain large intracytoplasmic inclusion bodies that enlarge gradually displacing the nucleus to the periphery of the cell.

Clinically, molluscum appears as a variable number of small descrete, domed nodules with an umbilicated center (Plate IF). The lesions occur more commonly in children. They tend to occur along the lid margins and are usually asymptomatic. Occasionally they may cause a persistent conjunctivitis or keratitis that fails to respond to treatment until the molluscum is eradicated.

Treatment consists of unroofing the lesion with curettage of its contents and cauterization of the base. The lesion may also be excised or treated with cryotherapy. When associated conjunctivitis or keratitis persists, diligent search of the lid margins will frequently reveal additional small molluscum bodies.

Fungal Infections

Fungal infections involving the eye are rare. The clinical picture of chronic ulceration with histologic confirmation of the offending organism will establish the diagnosis. Treatment of fungal infections remains unsatisfactory, but Amphotericin B and Natamycin may have some therapeutic value. Actinomycosis does respond to penicillin, erythromycin and tetracycline, and Blastomycosis to stilbamidine.

Actinomycosis. Caused by *Actinomyces israelii*, involvement of the eyelids usully follows mild trauma to the lid with vegetable matter such as straw. The skin lesion is nodular and produces a greenish-yellow purulent discharge. It may result in formation of sinus tracts in the skin from deeper foci.

Sporotrichosis. This is caused by the fungus *Sporotrichum schenkii*. It forms multiple small subcutaneous abscesses that are usually painless. As the overlying skin breaks down, chronic ulcers may form. New nodules may form along draining lymphatics.

Blastomycosis. The causative agent is *Blastomyces dermatitidis*, and is seen most frequently in the southeastern United States. Acquired through traumatic contact with vegetable materials, it forms a chronic infection of the skin. The lesions appear as papillomatous growths that may break down and ulcerate. Lid involvement may also be seen in up to 25% of the patients with the systemic form of the disease.[18]

Coccidioidomycosis. The causative organism, *Coccidioidomyces immitis*, is common in the central valleys of California. This fungus produces a systemic illness that can involve the skin of the eyelids. Infection occurs by inhalation and exposure to contaminated dust. The skin manifestations appear as an erythema nodosum-like lesion that progresses to ulceration and purulent discharge. It is frequently accompanied by a phlectenular conjunctivitis, episcleritis, and superficial keratitis.[46] In some cases it may develop into a granulomatous mass.

Parasitic Infestations

Pediculosis. A common parasitic infestation of the eyelid is caused by the crab louse, *Phthirus pubis*. The nits appear as tiny, rounded, translucent masses firmly adherent to the base of the lashes, and may be mistaken for dandruff. Although removal of both nit and mature louse may be performed with forceps, treatment is best achieved with topical 1% gamma benzene hexachloride cream (Kwell). The cream is rubbed into the lashes with care taken not to get it into the eye, and organisms, including the nits, are manually removed. Treatment is repeated one week later to eradicate any adults resulting from nits missed on the first treatment. Daily application of yellow oxide of mercury with manual removal of lice and nits is also effective for lash infestation.

Scabies. Infestation with the mite *Sarcoptes scabei* may involve the eyelid skin along with infection in other parts of the body. It is transmitted by contact with other infected persons, and may also be obtained from cats, dogs, and other small mammals. The primary lesion is the mite's burrow, but papules and vessicles may also be present. An intense pruritis usually accompanies the infestation. Treatment is with 1% gamma benzene hexachloride cream (Kwell) repeated after one week, or with 10% Crotamiton cream (Eurax) applied to the affected areas and repeated 48 hours later. All infected areas of the body must be treated simultaneously, as well as potentially infected close contacts.

Benign Epidermal Tumors

Seborrheic Keratosis. This common lesion is entirely epidermal in origin and frequently presents variability in its appearance. All types have in common hyperkeratosis, acanthosis and papillomatosis, but each of these elements may predominate in specific lesions. Sharply demarcated keratin plugs are characteristic, and pigmentation is variable.

The lesions appear clinically as well-circumscribed slightly elevated, usually pigmented, warty tumors with a greasy-appearing surface (Plate IG). They are usually a few millimeters in size, and slowly enlarge. Because of their variable presentation, they may be confused with premalignant or even malignant tumors. In such cases, histopathologic examination is essential. The management of this lesion is mainly for cosmesis and diagnosis, and is easily achieved by surgical excision. The base of the tumor is sharply demarcated and lies entirely within the epidermis, facilitating its removal.

Xanthelasma. Xanthelasma is a common disorder most frequently seen around the eyelids in middle-aged female patients. It is the most common cutaneous lesion in patients with primary hypercholesteremia, but frequently occurs in individuals with normal serum cholesterol. Up to 30 to 40% of patients with xanthelasma will have an elevated serum cholesterol.[38] The extent of the disease varies from a few lesions of pinhead size to extensive involvement of both upper and lower lids. The lesions are usually bilateral, soft, yellowish, sharply demarcated, and slightly elevated (Plate IH). They are asymptomatic, but can cause a significant cosmetic blemish.

Treatment consists of uncovering any underlying serum lipid abnormality and instituting appropriate therapy. The skin lesions can be treated with tricholaracetic acid applied with great care. Surgical excision is more effective and is usually easily achieved in the upper lid because of loose eyelid skin. In the lower lid care must be taken in removing too much skin resulting in ectropion. When the lesion are large, partial excision may be necessary, or skin grafting required. Lesions not uncommonly recur.

Papilloma. Papillomas of the eyelids are very common epithelial tumors characterized by hyperkeratosis and papillomatosis. They are seen at the lid margin or on the skin of the lid, and may be multiple. When occurring on the margin they may cause a seconary conjunctivitis. Papillomas tend to be quite variable in appearance. They can be either sessile or stalked, associated with varying amounts of inflammation or pigment, and they are likely to have a vegetative surface with scales (Figure 1-12). They often cause a cosmetic defect and may become mechanically irritated. Also, there is a small incidence of malignant degeneration. Papilloma is the most

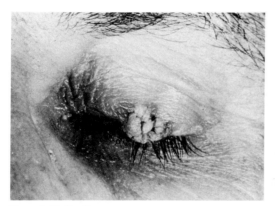

Figure 1-12. Papilloma.

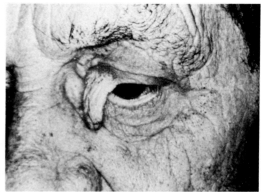

Figure 1-13. Cutaneous horn.

frequent misdiagnosis of basal cell carcinomas. For all these reasons, it is often advisable to remove such lesions. Surgical excision with histo-pathologic examination is the procedure of choice, although they can also be eradicated by cautery or cryotherapy.

Cutaneous Horn. Cornu cutaneum or cutaneous horn is a clinically descriptive term referring to an excessively hyperkeratotic papilloma (Figure 1-13). Other hyperkeratotic lesions, such as a filliform verruca, a seborrheic keratosis, a solar keratosis, keratoacanthoma, or even a squamous cell carcinoma, may at times present as a cutaneous horn. These lesions are uncommon, but can be striking in appearance. They tend to occur on the lid margins or at the canthi, and are more frequent in the elderly. There is a small tendency to malignant transformations, paralleling its occurrence in the underlying lesion.

Cutaneous horns can become quite large, producing not only a cosmetic defect, but occasionally a functional one as well. They are best removed by surgical excision.

Keratoacanthoma. Keratoacanthoma is a benign epidermal tumor that may appear on the eyelids. It predominates in Caucasians. It is usually a solitary lesion of irregular proliferations of epidermis with strands extending downward into the dermis. Cells are frequently atypical in appearance and contain many mitotic figures. An inflammatory infiltrate is usually present at the base, and a large central crater is filled with keratin. Initially the lesion appears as a maculopapular mass that becomes dome-shaped with a central crater (Plate IIA). It tends to grow rapidly over six to eight weeks, attaining a maximum size of 2 cm in diameter and 1 cm in height. Lesions may persist for several years, but typically regress slowly over four to six months, and may disappear with some residual scarring. Recurrences are rare.

Because of its appearance and rapid growth keratoacanthoma has frequently been misdiagnosed as a malignancy. However, because of its tendency to spontaneous involution, proper diagnosis and conservative management are important. Biopsy is frequently required.

The nature of treatment must be decided only after careful evaluation and biopsy examination to rule out a true squamous cell carcinoma which can easily be confused with keratoacanthoma. Resolution can often be hastened by removing the tumor flush with the skin followed by electrocautery or cryotherapy. Intralesional injection of steroids may also be helpful. Treatment of larger lesions may reduce the ultimate scarring that usually follows spontaneous involution.

Inverted Follicular Keratosis.

This is a variant of pseudoepitheliomatous hyperplasia, or may arise as an irritated seborrheic keratosis. The lesion is characteristically a papillomatous mass of proliferating epidermal cells which appears to be inverted on itself with small concentrically arranged whorl-like squamous eddies centrally. The mass presents as a solitary nodule on normal skin. Malignant transformation is said not to occur.[50]

Treatment should be conservative. If removal is done for cosmesis, simple surgical excision is performed with histologic confirmation.

Pseudoepitheliomatous Hyperplasia.

This lesion tends to occur in areas of chronic inflammation such as in granulomas and ulcers, in stasis dermatitis, lupus vulgaris, and in basal cell carcinomas. Histologically the tumor shows irregular epidermal proliferation with invasion of the dermis, small horn pearl formation, and mitotic figures with inflammation. It may resemble a low-grade squamous cell carcinoma.

Treatment involves excision including, when possible, the inciting lesion. Biopsy material should be submitted for histologic confirmation.

Calcifying Epithelioma.

Calcifying epithelioma of Malherbe is a benign hamartomatous tumor of uncertain histogenesis, but may originate from primitive undifferentiated epithelial cells, and differentiate toward hair follicle cells. The lesion is located in the lower dermis and may extend into the subcutaneous fat. It is often encapsulated and calcification, though frequent, is not a consistent finding. Typically the lesion manifests as a painless, freely moveable hard nodule covered by normal skin. It occurs more commonly in younger individuals of both sexes, and is frequently located in the upper lid or brow region.[36] Hemorrhage into the lesion may occasionally occur. Treatment consists of surgical excision.

Trichoepithelioma.

Trichoepithelioma is a rare benign epidermal tumor that represents a hamartoma of immature hair matrix cells. The lesion has a typical histologic appearance of numerous horn cysts composed of a fully keratinized center surrounded by basal cell epithelioma-like cells. These horn cysts represent abortive attempts at hair-shaft formation, and there is some variability in the degree of differentiation seen. Occasionally, there may be rupture of a cyst with foreign-body giant cell reaction and calcium deposition.

Trichoepitheliomas are congenital, although they generally appear clinically in adolescence and gradually increase in size and number. They are usually multiple, rounded, slightly elevated, firm, skin-colored nodules from 2 to 8 mm in diameter occurring most commonly on the face, and may be found on the eyelids. Treatment involves complete excision.

Benign Sweat Gland Tumors. These are relatively rare, slow-growing tumors that are usually misdiagnosed as other lesions. They have been classified in a number of different entities based on histopathology, including syringoma, cylindroma, clear cell hidradenoma and apocrine cystadenoma. They are usually said to be most common in young adults, but one recent study showed a predominance in the fifth and sixth decades of life.[35]

Clinically they appear as well-circumscribed, small, slightly elevated, superficial tumors 2 to 3 mm in diameter that tend to become cystic. The lesions are asymptomatic, are generally multiple, and involve the lower lid more frequently than the upper lid. These tumors can be confused with other lesions, including highly malignant sweat gland carcinomas,[23] and therefore treatment should be complete surgical excision for histologic diagnosis. Multiple lesions may be treated with electrocautery.

Benign Sebaceous Gland Tumors. This group includes senile sebaceous hyperplasia and true sebaceous adenoma. The former occurs on the face in older patients. It may be multiple, and appears as small, soft, yellowish, slightly umbilicated lesions, usually 2 to 3 mm in diameter. Sebaceous hyperplasia may be seen as an isolated entity or in association with tuberous sclerosis where they are seen chiefly over the malar eminences. No treatment is required.

Sebaceous adenoma is exceedingly rare on the eyelid. When present, it is usually solitary and appears as a smooth, firm, rounded, elevated, sometimes pedunculated mass. It must be distinguished from adenocarcinoma of the sebaceous gland. Excisional biopsy with tissue confirmation is the treatment of choice.

Benign Meibomian Gland Tumors. Included here is hyperplasia of the meibomian glands in which there is overgrowth and multiplication of normal glandular elements, and adenoma of the meibomian glands where there is loss of the normal glandular arrangement. The latter appears clinically as a slow-growing, firm nodule arising from within the tarsus. It is generally asymptomatic. Because of the possibility of malignancy, these lesions should be completely excised.

Pre-malignant Epidermal Tumors

Senile Keratosis. Senile keratosis may occur on exposed skin surfaces in older individuals with a history of many years of exposure to sunlight. They are more common in patients with a fair complexion. The keratoses appear as multiple lesions measuring less than 10 mm in diameter, with a hard, slightly elevated surface of dry scales firmly adherent to a mildly erythematous base. The nodules vary in color from reddish, to brown, to greyish-black, and usually occur on atrophic skin. The incidence of squamous cell carcinoma arising from these tumors is given as 20 to 25%,[33] but such lesions do not, as a rule, metastasize.[30] Senile keratoses must be followed closely for such transformation. If doubt exists, the lesion should be excised for tissue examination by a pathologist.

Xeroderma Pigmentosum. This is a rare pre-malignant recessively inherited disease in which sunlight precipitates an abnormal reaction in the epidermis and upper dermis. The basic pathology is defective repair of DNA. Ocular involvement may be seen in 70% of such patients.[34] Early lid lesions consist of erythema with scaling and small areas of hyperpigmentation resembling freckles. These lesions are hyperkeratotic with a perivascular inflammatory infiltrate. The skin then becomes atrophic, with telangiectases and more irregular pigmentation. Eventually, the entire lower lid may be lost. Ultimately, various malignant tumors arise, usually basal cell carcinoma or squamous cell carcinoma, but also malignant melanoma and, rarely, fibrosarcoma.[22,24]

Involvement of the eye results from atrophy of the lid skin leading to entropion or ectropion, symblepharon formation, and eventual loss of the entire lid with severe corneal exposure. There is no specific treatment for this disease and therapy is directed at removing malignant lesions and dealing with the ocular complications before useful vision is lost.[43]

Malignant Epidermal Tumors

Intraepithelial Epithelioma. Also known as Bowen's disease of skin, intraepithelial epithelioma represents an intraepithelial squamous cell carcinoma-in-situ. As such, it behaves biologically like a pre-malignant lesion, although morphologically it has features more typical of squamous cell carcinoma. Characteristically, the basal layer remains intact. However, in a small percentage of cases the basal layer may be violated in some areas, thus giving rise to a true invasive squamous cell carcinoma.[28]

Clinically, the lesion appears as a slightly elevated, reddish to brownish, sharply demarcated area that may show areas of crusting and ulceration. The lesion enlarges slowly at its periphery. It is most common in older individuals where it is usually seen at the limbal conjunctiva. It occurs much less commonly on the eyelids. Some 2 to 3% of such lesions will become invasive.[45] Although this tumor is somewhat radiosensitive and also responds to cryotherapy, proper management involves complete surgical excision with histologic examination for evidence of invasiveness.

Squamous Cell Carcinoma. Squamous cell carcinoma tends to occur most commonly on exposed areas of skin damaged by sunlight, or arise in other pre-existing lesions such as senile keratoses, chronic ulcers, burn scars or areas of chronic lid inflammations. These tumors may be rather indolent, but in general grow rapidly. The incidence of metastases is 0.5 to 5.0%.[1,30]

Clinically, these tumors begin as elevated keratinized areas. The center often ulcerates and is covered by a crust that overlies granular tissue that bleeds easily. The lesion may resemble a basal cell carcinoma or occasionally form a fungating, verrucous mass without ulceration (Plate IIB).

Because of its local invasiveness and potential for metastasis, early identification and treatment is important. One must be aware of the various pre-existing lesions that may give rise to squamous cell carcinomas, and any suspicious lesions must be biopsied. Although the tumor responds to radiation and cryotherapy, because of the unacceptable recurrence rates with these methods, Mohs' microsurgical excision with histologic control of all margins must be considered the treatment of choice whenever possible.[3]

Basal Cell Carcinoma.

Basal cell carcinomas occur most commonly on the face, particularly the periorbital area. They represent the most frequently encountered malignancy on the eyelids. Such tumors are seen principally in middle-aged to elderly individuals in whom chronic exposure to sunlight, chemical or mechanical injury, or chronic irritations have been predisposing factors. Fair-skinned individuals are particularly prone to this disease. Basal cell carcinomas occur most frequently on the lower lid, followed in decreasing order by the medial canthus, upper lid, and lateral canthus.[29]

The lesions appear clinically in various forms. In the nodular variety the tumor begins as a small, elevated, waxy nodule with telangiectatic vessels on its surface, which slowly enlarges and eventually undergoes central ulceration. The ulcer crater typically is surrounded by a rolled, "pearly" border (Plate IIC). There may be a variable amount of pigmentation, and the lesion may even show cystic changes. As growth continues, the lesion may take on an atypical appearance and can easily be confused with a benign tumor such as a papilloma. The morpheaform or sclerosing variety manifests as a firm, slightly elevated, yellowish plaque with ill-defined borders. The limits of this tumor frequently extend far beyond the clinically apparent edges of the lesion, and it may be deeply infiltrative into the lid or orbit. Basal cell carcinomas grow slowly by peripheral extension. Distant metastases are exceptionally rare. The patient is usually asymptomatic and thus many years may elapse before the lesion comes to medical attention. As ulceration ensues, chronic irritation and frequently bleeding herald medical consultation.

If left untreated the course is progressive enlargement and local invasion of orbit, bones, paranasal sinuses, sclera, and even brain. Mortality rates were as high as 11% among advanced cases in the past.[7] Any lesion suspected of being a basal cell carcinoma must be biopsied. Various uncontrolled modes of treatment have their proponents, notably radiation and cryotherapy.[19] In neither, however, is there any control of residual tumor, and recurrence rates of 5% to 20% are common. Recurrent tumors are frequently more invasive and more difficult to eradicate. It is in this group that the highest mortality rates are seen. More recently hematoporphyrin derivative phototherapy has shown good initial results in treating tumors of the skin, but it suffers from the same lack of histologic control as cryotherapy and radiation.

The most effective treatment is Mohs' microsurgical excision with histologic control of all margins,[32] followed by immediate reconstruction of the defect or granulation in selected cases.[3] This procedure provides maximum preservation of normal eyelid tissue, and has been shown to have the lowest recurrence rates currently available. Standard frozen-section monitoring at surgery is the next best alternative to the Mohs' technique.

Sebaceous and Meibomian Gland Carcinoma.

Adenocarcinoma of the meibomian gland is an uncommon lesion, representing about 2% of malignant eyelid tumors in the United States. A recent study revealed the incidence to be far greater among Chinese; it was 33% of malignant lid tumors.[37] It tends to occur in older individuals during the fifth and sixth decades, and is more common in females. The tumor involves the upper lid in two-thirds of cases.

Clinically, this tumor appears as a small, firm nodule without ulceration, and often resembles a more benign lesion, such as a chalazion unresponsive to usual treatment.[8,48] A more diffuse growth pattern with conjunctival changes may simulate a chronic blepharoconjunctivitis or trachoma (Plate IID). Eventually, the lid margin becomes distorted with loss of lashes, and a large papillomatous or fungating mass results with invasion of the orbit and paranasal sinuses. Metastatic spread to regional lymph nodes is common and occurs early in the course of the disease. Overall mortality rates are high even when treated early.

It is clear that early recognition and treatment is essential in the management of this disease. Any patient with a chalazion-like lesion recurrent after repeated curettage, or unresponsive to conventional medical therapy, requires biopsy, as does recurrent or persistent unilateral blepharoconjunctivitis. Wet biopsy tissue must be submitted for fat stains which are crucial to the diagnosis. Once the diagnosis is established, treatment consists of wide surgical excision, preferably by Mohs' microsurgical excision. For larger lesions involving the orbit, primary exenteration appears to result in lower mortality rates.[37]

Radiation therapy may be of some value in inoperable cases. Metastases to regional lymph nodes or to distant sites are not uncommon.

Sweat Gland Carcinoma.

Although very rare, adenocarcinomas of the sweat glands and Moll's glands have been reported to occur on or around the eyelids.[27,35] Such tumors do not show a characteristic clinical appearance and may present as a recurrent chalazion-like lesion. These are aggressive tumors, locally recurrent, and with a high rate of metastasis. Treatment consists of total excision with histologic control. A metastatic evaluation of regional lymph nodes is important, as is periodic follow-up examination. Recurrences may require extenteration.

Pigmented Eyelid Lesions

These lesions may be formed either by nevus cells or by melanocytes.

Those composed of nevus cells are the pigmented nevi, and may occur in the epideris or within the dermis. Those formed from melanocytes may originate in the epidermis, or from dermal melanoblasts giving rise to Blue nevi and oculodermal melanocytosis. Both nevus cells and melanocytic lesions may undergo malignant transformation.

Oculodermal Melanocytosis and Blue Nevi.

Oculodermal melanocytosis is a rare lesion involving the eye and skin of the eyelid and face in the distribution of the trigeminal nerve. Eighty-five percent of reported cases are among Japanese, and the incidence among Blacks appears to be greater than that for Caucasians. In about one-half of affected cases pigmentation first becomes manifest during the first few months of life; in the other half, it is not evident until later, usually during puberty.

The skin nevus is typically flat, blue to brown in color, with irregular and indistinct borders. It most frequently involves the zygomatic region, eyelids, and temple. The lesion typically enlarges and darkens during puberty and under hormonal influences such as menstruation and pregnancy. The eye is involved in 60% of cases. When it is, the sclera is always pigmented, and the iris, choroid and ciliary body may also be involved.

The nevus arises from intradermal melanoblasts. Malignant transformation to melanoma has been reported in 4.5% of cases overall, but among Caucasians the incidence appears to be much greater.[14] There is no specific treatment of oculodermal melanocytosis as the depth and diffuse nature of the nevus makes cosmetic surgery difficult or impossible. Management of malignancy must be tailored to the individual case.

The blue nevus is a rare lesion on the eyelid. It is related to oculodermal melanocytosis in that it forms from deep intradermal melanoblasts, but in the blue nevus these are grouped into nests that disrupt local dermal architecture. Clinically, lesions are sharply outlined, firm, rounded nodules, bluish in color. Malignant transformation occurs rarely, if at all. Surgical excision is usually easily accomplished for cosmetic purposes.

Melanocytic Nevi.

Nevi are common lesions occurring on the eyelids and conjunctiva. They vary considerably in their clinical appearance. Although usually present from birth, they may not become pigmented until later in childhood or even into adulthood. They are almost always benign, although some have malignant potential. The major clinical varieties are the junctional nevus, the compound nevus, and the intradermal nevus.

The junctional nevus is the type represented by most flat or slightly elevated nevi (Figure 1-14). It is smooth, circumscribed, hairless, and pigmented various shades of brown. The single nevus cells or cell nests occur within the lower epidermis, not penetrating into the dermis below. Because of their junctional activity, there is a low potential for malignant degeneration.

The compound nevus shows features of both a junctional and intradermal nevus. Nevus cells are seen within the epidermis and in the upper dermis. As with purely junctional nevi, these lesions have a low malignant potential.

Intradermal nevi show little or no junctional activity, the cords and nests

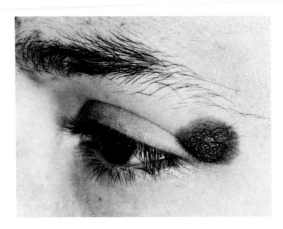

Figure 1-14. Junctional nevus.

of nevus cells lying largely or wholly within the upper dermis. These nevi form the common mole, may have a papillomatous growth form, and frequently contain hair. They do not undergo malignant transformation.[2]

Nevi occurring on the eyelids primarily cause a cosmetic defect. If necessary, they can be removed by shave biopsy. Larger lesions may require more major resection followed by plastic reconstruction. Certainly, any nevus that is enlarging should be biopsied for histologic examination.

Acquired Melanosis. Acquired melanosis of the skin is important because of the significant incidence of malignant transformation within these lesions, and because of the difficulty in distinguishing benign from malignant tumors.

The most common acquired pigmented lesion is the ephelis or freckle. This represents a hyperpigmentation of the basal layer of skin, and is of cosmetic significance only. Easily confused with freckle is lentigo benigna which is a smooth, dark-brown pigmented lesion measuring a few millimeters in diameter. These occur in older patients, are frequently multiple on exposed areas of skin, and may coalesce to form irregularly-shaped patches. They differ from freckles in that the number of melanocytes is increased with elongation of the rete ridges.

Pre-cancerous melanosis, including lentigo maligna, is a distinct lesion resulting from a neoplastic proliferation of dendritic melanocytes in the lower epidermis. It begins as an irregular or diffuse pigmented, flat lesion that varies from dark brown to black in color (Plate IIE). It tends to grow peripherally in some areas while regressing in others. The lesion usually arises in older patients on exposed areas of skin; commonly on the face where the eyelids may be involved. There is a high tendency for transformation into invasive malignant melanoma, occurring on average after approximately 10 years.[28] Such transformation begins with irregular induration, followed by nodule formation, and may be accompanied by areas of ulceration. Management of patients with pre-cancerous melanosis consists of following them closely for any evidence of transformation. Any suspicious areas should be treated by surgical excision with frozen-section control of all margins.

Malignant Melanoma. Malignant melanoma is a rare tumor that may arise from normal-appearing skin, but usually arises from a pre-existing pigmented lesion such as a junctional nevus or area of pre-malignant melanocytosis. These are highly aggressive cancers with a significant mortality rate. They are frequently misdiagnosed.

Clinically, malignant melanoma appears as a gradually enlarging pigmented mass that may have some surrounding inflammatory reaction (Plate IIF). The surface may show some crusting and bleeding, or frank ulceration. Pigmentation is variable, and occasionally may be absent. Metastasis usually occurs early via lymphatics to regional lymph nodes, and later by hematogenous spread to the liver, lungs and skin. Prognosis is greatly favored by absence of metastases. The depth of penetration of the lesion into the underlying dermis has also been shown to be a very important prognostic criterion.[40] In general, these lesions tend to be recognized too late, and treated too conservatively. Because of the diffuse nature of these tumors, local excision alone tends to be inadequate, and recurrence rates are exceedingly high. Mohs' microsurgical excision or wide excision with frozen-section control is necessary. The use of electrocautery or cryotherapy alone, without histologic control, is contraindicated. Cryotherapy to the excisional bed or to superficial melanomas has proved to be a beneficial adjunct to surgery, particularly for conjunctival lesions.[9,25] For more extensive lesions exenteration may be indicated.

Vascular Tumors

Capillary Hemangioma. This is the most common vascular tumor on the eyelid. It typically arises shortly after birth and rapidly increases in size during the first six to 12 months of life. These lesions are usually sharply circumscribed, bright red, elevated, often lobulated areas (Plate IIG). They are composed of endothelial cell proliferations in which capillary lumina develop as the lesion matures. A capsule is not present, and the tumor extends into the subcutaneous tissues and beyond the limits of the visible lesion. In the typical course of growth, fibrosis progressively replaces the capillaries leading to a gradual shrinkage of the tumor. Most capillary hemangiomas have regressed by the age of 6 to 7 years.

Because of this spontaneous regression, treatment is usually not indicated. However, in some cases, large lesions of the eyelid may obscure the visual axis with resultant amblyopia, making treatment unavoidable. Although surgical excision is easy and preferable for small hemangiomas, by the time they are large enough to cause amblyopia surgery is difficult and will cause excessive scarring. Reduction in the size of such lesions, sufficient to clear the visual axis, may be achieved by various modalities, notably x-ray therapy or locally injected corticosteroids. Some workers advocate a short course of systemic steroids which will effectively shrink the tumor mass in most cases. The use of sclerosing agents injected into the tumor has also been successful.

Cavernous Hemangioma. The cavernous hemangioma may occur isolated in the lid, but frequently also involves the orbit. The lesion consists of large, irregular cavernous spaces filled with blood and lined with endothelium. Most, if not all, of these tumors contain some admixture of capillary and cavernous components. A fibrous capsule-like covering is frequently present. The lesion appears as a raised, soft and compressible mass with normal overlying skin (Figure 1-15). Cavernous hemangiomas of the lid are more commonly seen in children where the mass can be noted to enlarge and darken with crying or other valsalva maneuver.

Treatment by surgical excision is easily accomplished when the child is of pre-school age. Occasionally, however, because of the size and interference with vision, surgery must be performed at an even earlier age. Care should be taken to remove the entire tumor intact as bleeding can be extensive.

Nevus Flammeus. Also known as port wine stain, this form of capillary hemangioma is most commonly found on the occiput not associated with other malformations. It occurs on the face in the distribution of the trigeminal nerve, frequently associated with malformation of larger blood vessels as in Sturge-Weber or Klippel-Trenaunay syndromes (Figure 1-16). The typical deep red, flat lesion is composed of capillary ectasias in the dermis and subcutaneous layers. It is primarily of cosmetic concern, but its presence should alert a search for other manifestations of associated diseases. In particular, the patient with Sturge-Weber syndrome must be aware of the possibility of central nervous system complications and of secondary glaucoma.

Treatment for the cosmetic blemish is with cover creams. Recent use of the argon laser for removal of these lesions has been encouraging.

Lymphangioma. This tumor more commonly occurs in the conjunctiva, but may involve the face, eyelids and orbit. It presents as a bluish or purplish, soft, compressible mass that may be superficial or deeply seated. It grows slowly and at times may enlarge precipitously from hemor-

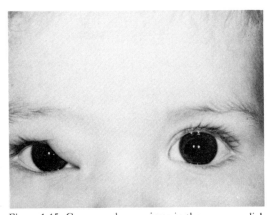

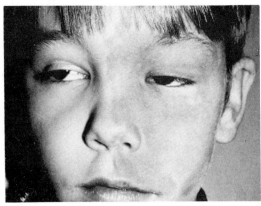

Figure 1-15. Cavernous hemangioma in the superomedial anterior orbit.

Figure 1-16. Nevus flameus in a patient with Sturge-Weber syndrome.

rhage within. Lymphangiomas are composed of dilated lymphatic channels lined with endothelium, and containing lymph and lymphocytes. Because of their tendency to invade adjacent tissues, early recognition and complete surgical excision is recommended when possible.

Hemangioendothelioma. These are tumors of endothelial cells without capillary formation. The benign hemangioendothelioma is a congenital lesion that tends to grow rapidly and may involve the orbit as well as the lid. If recognized early it should be excised completely, but the tumor tends to be sensitive to x-rays. A malignant variety of this lesion is very rare, but has been reported in the lid and orbit. It presents as a dusky red plaque or nodule infiltrating the skin and which may show ulceration. Treatment is total excision, but recurrences are common, and the outcome is frequently fatal due to metastatic spread.

Hemangiopericytoma. The hemangiopericytoma is a rare tumor of pericytic proliferation which may occur in the eyelid or orbit. It appears as a reddish, sometimes tender mass that enlarges slowly. Although most of these lesions are benign, a malignant form exists. As with other such lesions, early diagnosis is important, and complete surgical excision is the preferred treatment.

Pyogenic Granuloma. Pyogenic granuloma is now believed to be an acquired proliferation of endothelium and capillary channels embedded in a loose, edematous stroma, histologically similar to a capillary hemangioma. The lesions are rare on the eyelids, but when present show a predilection for the lower lid. They are several millimeters to several centimeters in size, slightly pedunculated, smooth nodules, often covered by a dark crust (Plate IIH). The tumor bleeds easily with slight trauma. In early lesions there is no inflammation, but because of erosion of the epithelium, older lesions frequently become infected and ulcerated, taking on the appearance of an infectious granuloma with secondary inflammatory changes.

Treatment is best carried out by excision of the lesion with chemical or thermal cautery of the base. Epithelialization with minimal scarring results.

Neurogenic Tumors

Neurofibroma. A neurofibroma is a benign tumor of peripheral nerve sheaths, and may involve the eyelid and orbit. Although it can occur in isolation, neurofibroma is usually seen in part of von Recklinghausen's disease, a dominantly inherited syndrome affecting peripheral and cranial nerves (Figure 1-17). Neurofibromas consist of a diffuse Schwann cell proliferation with some involvement of mesodermal endoneural cells. They usually first appear in childhood or adolescence, and enlarge slowly in size and number. These tumors are generally flesh-colored, soft, globular

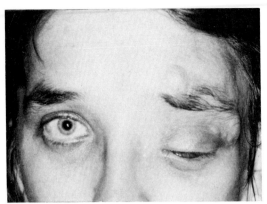
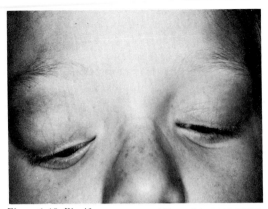

Figure 1-17. Neurofibromatosis involving the left orbit and eyelids.

Figure 1-18. Plexiform neuroma of the right upper eyelid.

masses that may form localized nodules on the skin. They can also cause a diffuse thickening of skin into large, pendulous and flabby masses. When cellular proliferation is restricted within the nerve sheath, a plexiform neuroma of distinct clinical appearance, the so-called "bag of worms," results, and is not uncommonly seen in the eyelids (Figure 1-18). Upper lid involvement is frequently associated with marked mechanical ptosis. Degeneration to a malignant Schwannoma may occur in cutaneous neurofibromas, but is extremely rare, reported in only two of 678 patients.[12]

The neurofibroma does not respond to x-radiation. Treatment is surgical excision and reconstruction when necessary. Because of the diffuse nature of the tumor complete removal is usually not possible and recurrence is common. Tumor growth frequently stabilizes after maturity, and it is best to delay surgery until then. However, severe ptosis threatening amblyopia in a child, or severe cosmetic psychological considerations may justify early intervention.

Neurilemmoma. Neurilemmomas, also known as Schwannomas, occur as benign tumors of peripheral and cranial nerves. They may be found on the lids or in the orbit. These tumors are well-circumscribed, encapsulated proliferations of Schwann cells containing few or no nerve fibers. Clinically, they appear as asymptomatic subcutaneous masses that may be soft due to partial cystic degeneration. The lesions may attain a size of several centimeters. Treatment is by surgical excision which is easily accomplished due to its well-circumscribed capsule. Malignant degeneration is rare.

Other Tumors of Mesenchymal Origin

Rhabdomyosarcoma. Rhabdomyosarcoma is a malignant tumor arising from undifferentiated striated muscle precursor cells. It may occur in the lid and orbit where it is the most common primary orbital malignancy in childhood. Seventy-five percent of reported cases occur in children under 10 years of age, with an average age at diagnosis of 7 to 8 years.[6,20,26,41] The incidence is slightly higher in males. Patients usually appear with a rapid progression over weeks to months of a lid mass, or with lid edema, ptosis and proptosis. Metastases to lungs and bone are common, and the mortality rate with any form of treatment is extremely high. Exenteration has been the standard treatment. More recently, radiotherapy of 5,500 rads in fractionated doses to the lesion and ipsilateral lymph nodes, along with adjuvant chemotherapy has proven to be at least as effective as radical surgery.[10,15]

Fibroma and Fibrosarcoma. Fibromas are rare lesions, but they have been reported to occur in the eyelid. Histologically there are two types; those composed predominantly of fibroblasts and referred to as fibromas, and those containing an admixture of fibroblasts and histiocytes, called histiocytomas (Figure 1-19). The two types grade into one another. Fibromas are encapsulated tumors appearing clinically as reddish or yellowish-brown nodules. They may be firm or soft depending upon the amount of collagen present. Treatment is surgical excision.

The fibrosarcoma is also quite rare and usually demonstrates low-grade malignancy. It presents as a reddish to bluish nodule, frequently with satellite lesions. It is resistant to x-rays, and management consists of wide excision.

Keloid. Keloids are hypertrophic scars resulting from trauma or surgery. They are common particularly in highly pigmented persons. In the earliest stages keloids resemble normal wound healing with fibroplasia and fibrosis. This is followed by sclerosis and hyalinization of the collagen bundles which gradually replace the normal papillary dermis. Keloids are red, raised and firm scars with a smooth and shiny surface that extends beyond the limits of the original injury. Patients who have demonstrated keloid formation in the past should avoid further surgery unless necessary. Once a keloid has formed treatment consists of steroid injections or excision with minimal disturbance of adjacent normal tissue. A subcuticular stainless steel wire suture, along with ACTH administration, may significantly reduce the foreign-body inflammatory reaction which further incites keloid formation.[11] X-ray therapy to the scar line immediately after surgery may also minimize the reactive fibrosis. Fortunately, the eyelids are less prone to keloid formation than the thicker skin elsewhere.

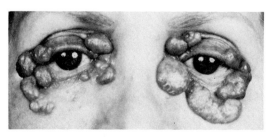

Figure 1-19. Fibrous histiocytoma involving all four eyelids.

Lymphomatous Tumors

Lymphomas. These represent a group of neoplasms frequently arising from multiple foci. Lymphomas are composed chiefly of immature and mature elements of the lymphoid-reticular system. The exact cell type is variable, and these tumors may exhibit anything from a non-specific well-differentiated inflammatory infiltrate of histiocytes and mature lymphocytes, to a tumor composed of immature stem cells with numerous mitotic figures. Lymphomas may occur in the eyelid, on the conjunctiva, or in the orbit, and are frequently bilateral (Figure 1-20). The cutaneous lesions may present as plaques or nodules, often rubbery in consistency. When the anterior orbit is involved, such as the lacrimal gland, the mass may protrude into the upper lid where it is easily palpable. If a biopsy reveals the presence of lymphoma, a thorough search for systemic disease must be made. If discovered, the patient should be referred to an oncologist for management. A local lid or orbital lesion is best treated with radiation.

Reticulum Cell Sarcoma. This undifferentiated lymphoid tumor usually presents initially as a solitary lesion, frequently in the skin. It is composed principally of immature reticulum cells with some admixture of mature histiocytes. If leukemia develops, it is a monocytic leukemia. Histologically, reticulum cell lymphoma may be difficult to differentiate from histiocytosis as seen in Hand-Schuller-Christian or Letterer-Siwe disease. These tumors are radiosensitive, and chemotherapy is indicated for the systemic disease.

Mycosis Fungoides. Mycosis fungoides is a rare clinical entity that may be associated with any of several lymphomatous diseases, and may involve the eyelids. Clinically, this lesion affects the skin predominantly and begins as a sharply outlined, erythematous eruption with scaly patches resembling eczema or psoriasis. This is followed by the development of well-demarcated, slightly indurated plaques that often show some central clearing resulting in ring-like patches. These are followed by rounded or lobulated, raised tumors, usually brownish-red in color. They frequently undergo ulceration. The lesions consist of a multiplicity of cell types located in the upper dermis. These include immature and atypical histiocytes and reticulum cells with various inflammatory cells including

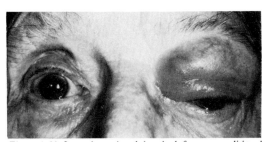

Figure 1-20. Lymphoma involving the left upper eyelid and anterior orbit.

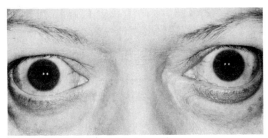

Figure 1-21. Thyroid ophthalmopathy.

lymphocytes, eosinophils and plasma cells. As with other lymphomas, surgery is indicated for biopsy and tissue diagnosis, but treatment consists of local radiation for control of lid or orbital masses, and chemotherapy for the systemic disease.

Metabolic and Autoimmune Disorders

Thyroid Ophthalmopathy. Thyroid disease is very common and usually involves the eyelids to some extent. It is seen most frequently in middle-aged females. Progression of the ophthalmic complications of this disease often follows achievement of the euthyroid state. The most common eye findings are lid edema and lid retraction, especially temporally (Figure 1-21). The latter may or may not be associated with significant proptosis. Structural changes occur in the levator muscle and its aponeuosis with fatty infiltration and fibrosis. The sympathetic muscles in the upper and lower eyelids receive overstimulation in early thyroid ophthalmopathy, and undergo fibrosis, contracture, and fatty infiltration in later stages. The lid retraction may be severe enough to cause symptomatic corneal exposure. Treatment in early stages consists of artificial tears and bland ointments at bedtime. Surgical recession of the levator aponeurosis and extirpation of sympathetic muscles in upper eyelids is very effective in correcting lid retraction when symptoms or cosmetic deformity become significant. Lower lid recession is achieved by disinsertion of the lower eyelid retractors.

Collagen-Vascular Diseases. This is a complex group of diseases with multi-systemic effects. Many are characterized by cutaneous lesions that often are found on the eyelids. Systemic lupus erythematosis is a diffuse systemic disease mainly affecting young females. The typical facial rash may be associated with erythema and edema of the lids. In the chronic discoid form of the disease plaques resembling severe blepharitis may involve the lower lids with loss of lashes and, when severe, eventual ectropion.

Polyarteritis nodosa is another systemic collagen disease often associated with lid edema, usually as a result of renal complications, but may also follow exudative lesions of the lid connective tissues.

In dermatomyositis the lids may be involved in the widespread dermatitis, with pitting edema and occasionally ptosis.

Scleroderma is a chronic disorder that results in brawny edema and hypertrophy of connective tissues, followed by atrophy. When the lids are affected, significant distortion of structure may result.

Erythema multiforme is a disease affecting the mucous membranes but may involve the lid margins by extension from the conjunctiva. Complications include trichiasis, symblepharon formation with entropion, and severe dry eyes.

Treatment of these disorders should be aimed at the systemic manifestations and will often include systemic steroids, and may require cytotoxic agents. Local application of steroids may reduce some of the inflammatory reaction. More specific management of trichiasis or cicatricial lid changes should be dealt with on an individual basis.

Psoriasis. Psoriasis is a chronic disorder of skin that may affect the lids in up to 10% of cases. The etiology is unknown and may be inherited in a dominant pattern. The typical lesion is a sharply demarcated plaque with reddish borders and covered with fine silvery scales. The disease may vary from mild and relatively asymptomatic to severe with associated psoriatic arthritis. When the lid margins are involved, trichiasis and ectropion may result. Some control may be obtained by local cleansing of the lesions and the application of steroid creams.

Ocular Pemphigoid. Cicatricial pemphigoid is a disease of unknown etiology, but appears to have an immunologic basis. It affects mucous membranes, including the conjunctiva. It is a chronic, progressive illness characterized by subconjunctival inflammation and fibrosis in about 80% of patients.

The earliest stage may present as a chronic conjunctivitis that progresses to conjunctival shrinkage, blunting of the fornices, symblepharon formation, trichiasis, distichiasis, and severe sicca syndrome. Resulting corneal involvement leads to vascularization and opacification with severe loss of vision in some cases. Surgical intervention for the cicatricial lid changes often results in exacerbation of the inflammatory reaction. Medical treatment is with artificial tears and ointments, and with steroids, both topical and systemic. More recently the use of cytotoxic agents in conjunction with steroids has given encouraging results in managing these patients and allowing surgical procedures without worsening of the inflammatory response.[16]

Seborrhea. Seborrheic dermatitis is a poorly-defined chronic inflammatory disease that mainly affects hair-bearing areas. Its occurrence on the eyelids is usually in association with seborrhea elsewhere on the body. The etiology is unknown. Histologic findings are non-specific and include parakeratosis, acanthosis, and epidermal intracellular edema, with a chronic infiltrate in the dermis. Clinically, seborrheic dermatitis occurs in areas with a large number of sebaceous glands and in patients with excessive sebum production. Lesions consist of brownish-red areas of pale erythema with sharp borders and overlying yellowish greasy scales. They are often pruritic. The associated blepharitis characteristically shows erythema and swelling of the lid margins and morning crusting. The disease may alternate from periods of relative inactivity to severely inflamed states. The condition is aggravated by heat and excessive perspiration.

Treatment is by cleaning with mild shampoo to remove scales, and control of dandruff with selenium sulfide suspension (Selsun). A mild topical steroid cream such as 0.01% fluocinolone may be used to control inflammation. If secondary infection is present topical antibiotics should be added. If severe, systemic Tetracycline is the drug of choice. Systemic steroids are reserved for severe, spreading disease not controlled by local measures.

Motility Disturbances

Myasthenia Gravis. This is a disease of the neuromuscular junction that manifests as weakness of striated muscle. About one-half of affected patients present initially with ocular symptoms, most commonly ptosis, but also various degrees of ocular motility disturbances. The ptosis is usually bilateral, but may be unilateral, and is typically asymmetric. Muscular weakness is more extreme later in the day and is related to fatigue. The diagnosis can be made from the clinical history and a Tensilon test. In the latter intravenously administered Tensilon should result in a dramatic improvement in the ptosis or strabismus. The test should be performed by persons experienced in its use and prepared to deal with its potential complications.

Treatment of Myasthenia Gravis is with systemic anticholinesterase agents such as Mestinon. If there is no improvement in the ptosis on maximum medical therapy, or the patient becomes refractory to these drugs, levator aponeurotic surgery will correct or improve the ptosis in most cases. However, because of the variable nature of the ptosis, extreme conservation in surgical correction is warranted, and only after at least two years of stability.

Myokymia. This is an involuntary fasciculation of striated muscle seen commonly in the eyelid. Episodes may be initiated by fatigue or stress. The treatment is medical and carbamazepine (Tegretol) may offer relief of symptoms in some cases.

Essential Blepharospasm. A disease of unknown etiology, essential blepharospasm is a paroxysmal contraction of facial muscles supplied by the 7th cranial nerve. It usually is seen in persons over 45 years of age. The disease begins with occasional involuntary blinking which becomes more frequent with longer episodes of eye closing over several months to years. Symptoms are quite variable, ranging from a mild annoyance to severe visual disability (Figure 1-22). Many patients are unable to read, drive a car, or even to watch television. With constant orbicularis contraction, the frontalis muscle is used in an attempt to break the spasm. Brow droop and stretching of upper eyelid skin become common associated findings.

A variety of drugs have been advocated for control of these spasms, including Choline, Clonopin, Elavil, Valium, and Orphenadrine. Although a few patients report some improvement in symptoms, these drugs are largely disappointing in their effect. Surgical correction for severe cases includes selective 7th nerve sectioning. This procedure often gives some relief, but in 50 to 75% of cases the spasms recur over a three to five year period. A serious potential complication is facial palsy. More recently, an

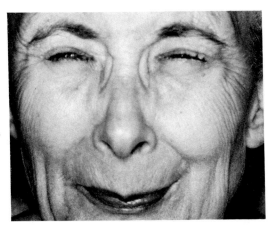

Figure 1-22. Essential blepharospasm.

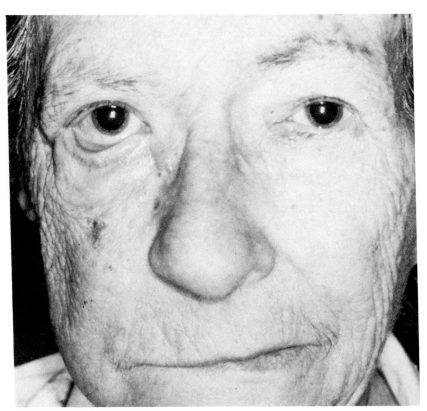

Figure 1-23. Bell's palsy.

extended version of an older surgical procedure has been introduced in which the orbicularis, procerus and corrugator muscles are extirpated, with simultaneous correction of the brow ptosis and redundant upper lid skin.[21] The results have been very encouraging and offer significant relief of symptoms in most patients. A new procedure involves local injection of botulinum toxin into the area of orbicularis muscle. Preliminary results have been good, but spasms recur and the procedure must be repeated every three to six months.

Bell's Palsy. This common facial paralysis is seen most frequently in older patients. When complete it results in epiphora, paralytic ectropion, and lagophthalmos (Figure 1-23). Exposure keratitis may result in corneal damage. Although most patients with Bell's palsy eventually recover spontaneously, significant symptoms or exposure may require early intervention. This is usually accomplished by a lateral tarsorrhaphy to correct the lagophthalmos and provide protection to the cornea. The tarsorrhaphy can be reversed at a later date if needed.

Malposition of Lids and Lashes

Acquired Ptosis. Acquired ptosis has been classified into a number of types, the most common ones being senile, traumatic, myogenic and neurogenic ptosis.

Senile ptosis is the most frequently encountered type in the older age group. It results from a thinning of the levator aponeurosis with local dehiscences or even frank disinsertion from the tarsus (Figure 1-24). It is characterized by a ptotic lid with good levator function, and a high or absent lid crease. The lid position typically is ptotic in both up and down gaze positions. Careful examination and transillumination may reveal the edge of the disinserted aponeurosis. Occasionally the patient will give a history of old trauma or surgery on the involved side.

Traumatic ptosis may follow injury to the levator muscle or its aponeurosis or to its nerve supply. It may not be recognized early after injury because of concomitant edema or hematoma. Any laceration involving the upper eyelid should be explored if lid function appears compromised.

Myogenic or neuromyopathic ptosis includes several entities, but in all the basic pathology involves dysfunction of the levator muscle. This may result from myasthenia gravis, progressive external ophthalmoplegia, or primary muscular dystrophy. There also appears to be a myopathy of unknown etiology that affects the levator muscle without involvement of other extraocular muscles, and is characterized by fatty infiltration of both the muscle and its aponeurosis.

In neurogenic ptosis the lesion may be located anywhere between the cerebral cortex and the nerve to the levator muscle. Other neurologic findings and extraocular muscles dysfunctions are frequently present, and will aid in localization of the lesion. In Horner's syndrome, neurogenic ptosis results from sympathetic denervation to Muller's muscle. The syndrome consists of ptosis, miosis, ipsilateral anhidrosis, and apparent endophthalmos. Preganglionic and postganglionic lesions should be differentiated as the former may represent significant pathology.

Most cases of acquired ptosis are treated surgically. There are two general classes of operative procedure for the correction of a ptotic eyelid;

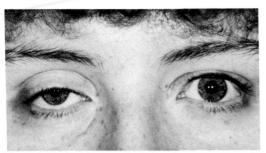

Figure 1-24. Acquired ptosis due to levator aponeurosis disinsertion.

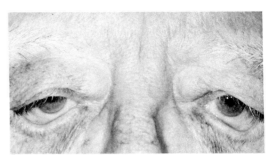

Figure 1-25. Senile ectropion of both lower eyelids.

levator shortening and frontalis suspension. Of these, aponeurotic surgery is the procedure of choice, and provides excellent results in most patients. Modifications of this procedure may be used even with poor levator function. The operation consists of a lid incision through the area of the upper lid crease, with resection or advancement of the levator aponeurosis and reattachment to the tarsal plate. The operation is performed under local anesthesia with adjustment of lid height and contour after examination of the patient in the upright position.

When levator function is very poor or non-existent eyelid suspension to the frontalis muscle, preferably with autogenous facia late, may be used.

The treatment of myogenic and neurogenic ptosis depends upon its specific cause. Aponeurotic surgery will usually provide adequate results in myogenic ptosis and in some cases of neurogenic ptosis. The use of cholinesterase inhibiting drugs has relieved symptoms in Myasthenia Gravis, but some patients will require levator shortening to correct residual ptosis. Ptosis from nerve palsy following trauma may improve spontaneously, and should be observed for at least six months before attempting surgical correction.

Ectropion. Ectropion is a condition in which the eyelid margin is turned outward away from the globe. It results in epiphora, hypertrophy of conjunctiva, and, when marked, exposure of the cornea.

Involutional or senile ectropion results from a laxity of the pretarsal orbicularis and is often associated with laxity of the medial and lateral canthal tendons as well (Figure 1-25). Repair is best achieved with a lid shortening procedure such as the lateral tarsal strip operation or its equivalent.[4] Medial canthal tendon plication may be required in some cases.

Paralytic ectropion may follow facial nerve palsy and results from loss of orbicularis muscle support to the lid margin. If caused by a Bell's palsy, recovery may occur spontaneously. If due to a cerebrovascular accident, trauma, or prior surgery, surgical correction will usually be needed. A lid shortening procedure will give adequate results.

In cicatricial ectropion the lid is mechanically pulled outward because of shortening of the outer lamella of the eyelid following traumatic, surgical, thermal, chemical or infectious injury (Figure 1-26). Correction should be delayed until all scarring has stabilized. Surgery may be difficult and must include removal of all scarred tissues. Skin lengthening procedures are required, and for minimal cicatricial changes a skin flap may suffice. For more extensive changes, myocutaneous flaps or skin grafts will usually be needed.

Entropion. In entropion the eyelid margin is turned inward against the globe, frequently resulting in corneal damage from mechanical irritation by the lashes. Acute spastic entropion is caused by ocular inflammation or injury and frequently follows surgery such as cataract extraction (Figure 1-27). It is usually transient in nature and affects mainly the lower lid. Treatment is elimination of the causative agent. If surgery becomes necessary, the fornix suture technique of Quickert[42] will correct the defect in most cases.

Involutional or senile entropion is the most common form seen in older patients. It is seen in the lower eyelid and results from a relaxation of the lower border of tarsus and a stretching or disinsection of the lower eyelid retractors. Correction consists of reinsertion of the retractors either alone or in conjunction with a lid shortening procedure. Cautery of the skin and orbicularis muscles along the length of the lid at the lower tarsal region may correct the condition in its early stages by causing a thermal shrinkage of the lax portion of the lid.

Cicatricial entropion is caused by conjunctival scarring and contraction resulting from trauma, thermal or chemical injury, or from infection such as trachoma. Treatment is surgical and consists of a marginal tarsoconjunctival rotation operation which may be used in either the upper or lower lid.

Trichiasis. Trichiasis is an abnormality of the eyelid margin in which some of the lashes are misdirected towards the globe. This results in corneal damage and symptoms of foreign body sensation. This may result from conjunctival shrinkage disorders or from chronic inflammation or distortion of the lid margin from infection or trauma. In mild cases where only a few lashes are involved, repeated epilation or electrocautery or block excision of a portion of the eyelid may relieve symptoms. When extensive, especially if there is associated keratitis, tarsal rotation procedures may be

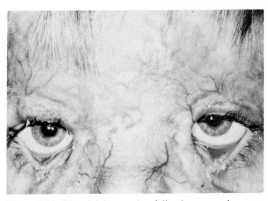

Figure 1-26. Cicatricial ectropion following severe burns to the eyelids.

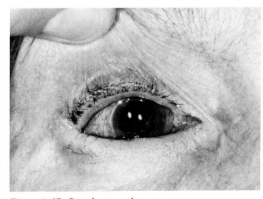

Figure 1-27. Spastic entropion.

indicated. The best results are achieved easily with cryotherapy to the mid margin containing the offending lashes. A double freeze-thaw-refreeze cycle to minus 20 degrees centigrade is used with thermocouple control of temperature at the level of the lash follicles. However, even cryotherapy is not without complications particularly in the conjunctival shrinkage disorders.

Aging Processes

Dermatochalasis. In dermatochalasis senile atrophy of the skin of the eyelids produces a loose, thin, redundant fold (Figure 1-28). It usually involves the upper lids and may be so severe as to overhang the lid margin to partially obscure the visual axis. The laxity is generally restricted to the skin and subcutaneous tissue, but some cases are associated with degeneration and relaxation of the underlying orbicularis muscle as well. The latter situation in the lower lid results in sagging and may produce malpositions of the lid margin or lacrimal punctum. If the orbital septum becomes weakened also, there may be protrusion of orbital fat, accentuating the baggy appearance of the lids (see below).

Correction of this condition is surgical. In the upper lid a carefully planned excision of both skin and orbicularis muscle usually gives gratifying results. For the lower lid, a far more conservative approach is recommended, since excess skin removal can result in the common complication of inferior scleral show, or more rarely, even frank ectropion. Good cosmetic results can be achieved with a lateral shortening of a skin-muscle flap and suspension of the orbicularis muscle to the deep tissue of the lateral incision. Usually very little, if any, vertical shortening of skin is required, especially if fat is removed.

Protrusion of Orbital Fat. This refers to the bulging of orbital fat into the eyelids due to laxity of the orbital septum, excessive fat, or both

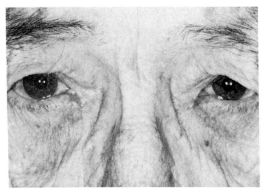

Figure 1-28. Dermatochalasis.

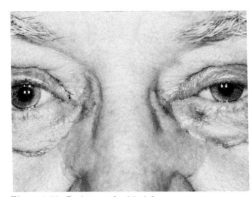

Figure 1-29. Prolapse of orbital fat.

(Figure 1-29). It is frequently symmetrical. It may be seen in isolation in the younger patient, but is more commonly associated with dermatochalasis in older individuals.

Treatment is by opening the septum and the individual fat pockets, typically three in the lower lid and two in the upper lid. The fat is removed by clamping with a hemostat, excising the fat, and cauterizing. Care must be taken not to pull orbital fat excessively and to achieve meticulous hemostasis to avoid the major complication of orbital hemorrhage. The orbital septum is not closed and redundant skin may be removed prior to skin suturing. If only excess fat is present without significant der-matochalasis, a transconjunctival approach may be utilized to avoid exter-nal scars. This is especially useful in the younger patient.

Trauma

Lacerations. Most lacerations of the eyelids require surgical repair for adequate cosmetic and functional results (Figure 1-30). Unless there is several corneal exposure, such repair can usually be delayed until optimal facilities and personnel are available, and until a thorough evaluation of the eye for concomitant injuries has been made.

Any laceration that has become infected requires medical treatment with appropriate antibiotics prior to any surgical repair. Small or even large skin-muscle lacerations not involving deeper structures are best sutured when initially seen. Avulsions of large areas of eyelid may be repaired by undermining adjacent areas and sliding flaps into the defect. Care must be taken to evaluate the underlying levator aponeurosis, and, if transected, this must be reattached.

Through-and-through lacerations involving the lid margin must have exacting closure to avoid lid margin notching.[13] It may be necessary to excise additional tissue along the margins of the defect to provide healthy surfaces for suturing. The medial and lateral canthal tendons should be carefully examined for disinsertion in cases of severe trauma.

When lacerations involve the medial one-third of the lid, the integrity of the canalicular system must be established. If transected, an attempt at primary anastomosis should be made with the use of the operating micro-scope. Silicone stents placed through the system are essential to prevent stenosis and closure at the repair site.

When significant lid tissue is lost, major reconstruction will be required by any of a number of oculoplastic techniques. Tissue may be borrowed from adjacent lids, from the opposite lid, or from the cheek or temple with the use of sliding flaps.

Burns. Eyelid burns are relatively common injuries. Exposure to sun or ultraviolet lamps may cause a first-degree burn with erythema and edema, and there may also be an associated keratitis. This usually heals without sequellae, and symptomatic relief may be achieved with cold compresses.

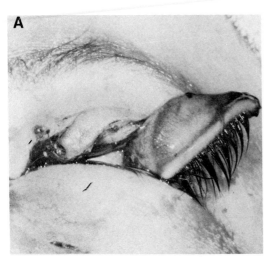 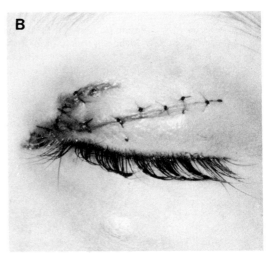

Figure 1-30A and B. Lacerations of upper and lower eyelids. A. Prior to repair; B. After plastic repair.

More severe burns causing partial or full-thickness skin loss will invariably result in scarring, with cosmetic disfiguring and usually ectropion. If extensive destruction of tissue has resulted, and the cornea is threatened by exposure, immediate steps must be taken to protect the eye by tarsorrhaphy of the remaining lids, placement of grafts over the tarsoconjunctival layer, or placement of a plastic film or moisture chamber over the damaged lids. Extensive debridement of eyelid tissues should be avoided. Prevention of secondary infection is important, and the use of prophylactic antibiotics follows the same principles as for burns elsewhere on the body. The role of topical steroids is controversial; they will reduce the ultimate scarring of the lids and shrinkage of the conjunctiva, and will help control the intraocular inflammation that frequently accompanies such injuries. However, steroids may make the control of infection more difficult, especially if the cornea is damaged.

With extensive loss of eyelid skin, grafting is necessary. If required, this is best done early in the course of the injury, using split-thickness grafts. Later, after contracture is complete, full-thickness grafts give better results.

Summary

Visual recognition and awareness of disease processes are essential ingredients for the management of eyelid disorders. Congenital and involutional disorders should be recognized and treated appropriately. Neoplasms should be diagnosed histopathologically and treated with appropriate degrees of surgery. Systemic diseases may be recognized when presenting with adnexal manifestations.

References

1. Ackerman LV, deRegato JA: *Cancer,* 2nd Ed. St. Louis: Mosby, 1954.
2. Allen AC, Spitz S: Malignant melanoma. *Cancer* 6:1, 1953.
3. Anderson RL, Ceilley RI: A multispecialty approach to the excision and reconstruction of eyelid tumors. *Ophth* 85:1150, 1978.
4. Anderson RL, Gordy DD: The tarsal strip procedure. *Arch Ophth* 97:2192, 1979.
5. Anderson RL and Harvey JT: Lid splitting and posterior lamella cryosurgery for congenital and acquired distichiasis. *Arch Ophth* 99:631, 1981.
6. Ashton N and Moyon G: Embryonal sarcoma and embryonal rhabdomyosarcoma of the orbit. *J Clin Pathol* 18:599, 1965.
7. Birge HL: Basal cell carcinoma mixed basal cell carcinoma and squamous cell epithelioma. *Arch Ophth* 19:700, 1938.
8. Boniuk M and Zimmerman LE: Sebaceous carcinoma of the eyelids, eyebrows, caruncle, and orbit. *Tr Am Acad Ophth Otolaryngol* 72:619, 1968.
9. Brownstein S, Jakobiec FA, Wilkinson RD, et al: Cryotherapy for precancerous melanosis (atypical melanocytic hyperplasia) of the conjunctiva. *Arch Ophth* 99:1224, 1981.
10. Chess J, Ni C, Xin RQ, et al: Rhabdomyosarcoma. *In* Ni C and Albert DM (Eds): Tumors of the eyelid and orbit: A Chinese-American collaborative study. *Int Ophth Clin* 22(1):163, 1982.
11. Conway H: *Tumors of the skin.* Springfield: C.C. Thomas, 1956.
12. D'Agostino AN, Soul EA, Miller RH: Sarcoma of the peripheral nerves and somatic soft tissues associated with multiple neurofibromatosis (von Recklinghausen's disease). *Cancer* 16:1015, 1963.
13. Divine RD and Anderson RL: Techniques in eyelid wound closure. *Ophth Surg* 13:283, 1982.
14. Dutton JJ, Anderson RL, Schelper R, et al: Oculodermal melanocytosis and orbital malignant melanoma. In press.
15. Ellsworth RM: Rhabdomyosarcoma of the orbit. Symposium on surgery of the orbit and adnexa. *Tr Acad New Orleans Acad Ophth.* St. Louis: Mosby and Co, 1974.
16. Foster CS, Wilson CA and Eakins MB: Immunosuppression therapy for progressive ocular cicatricial pemphigoid. *Ophth* 89:340, 1982.
17. Fox SA: Affections of the lids. *Int Ophth Clin* 4(1):1, 1964.
18. Francois J and Rysselaere M: *Oculomycoses.* Springfield: CC Thomas, 1972.
19. Fraunfelder FT, Zacarian SA, Limmer BL and Wingfield D: Cryosurgery for malignancies of the eyelid. *Ophth* 87:461, 1980.
20. Frayer WC and Enterline HT: Embryonal rhabdomyosarcoma of the orbit in children and young adults. *Arch Ophth* 62:203, 1959.
21. Gillum WN and Anderson RL: Blepharospasm surgery: An anatomic approach. *Arch Ophth* 99:1056, 1981.
22. Hadida E, Marill FG and Savage J: Xeroderma pigmentosum. *Ann Derm Syph* 90:467, 1963.
23. Haneveld GT and Hamburg A: Sweat gland tumor of the eyelid with conjunctival involvement. *Ophthalmologica* 179:73, 1979.
24. Hollander L and Krugh FJ: Cancer of the eyelids. *Am J Ophth* 29:244, 1944.
25. Jakobiec FA, Brownstein S, Wilkinson RD, et al: Combined surgery and cryotherapy for diffuse malignant melanoma of the conjunctiva. *Arch Ophth* 98:1390, 1980.
26. Jones IS, Reese AB and Kraut J: Orbital rhabdomyosarcoma: An analysis of 62 cases. *Am J Ophth* 61:721, 1966.
27. Khalil M, Brownstein S, Cordeer F and Nicolle D: Endocrine sweat gland carcinoma of the eyelid with orbital involvement. *Arch Ophth* 98:2210, 1980.
28. Lever WF: *Histopathology of the Skin,* 4th Ed. Philadelphia: Lippincott, 1967.
29. Love WR and Montgomery H: Epithelial cysts of the skin. *Arch Derm Syph* 47:185, 1943.
30. Lund HZ: How often does squamous cell carcinoma of the skin metastasize? *Arch Derm* 92:635, 1965.
31. McDonald LW: Carcinomatous change in cysts of the skin. *Arch Derm* 87:208, 1963.
32. Mohs FE: Chemosurgery for skin cancer. *Arch Derm* 112:211, 1976.

33. Montgomery H and Dorfel J: Verruca senilis and keratoma senile. *Arch Derm Syph* 166:286, 1932.

34. Newsome D, Kraemer K and Robbins J: Repair of DNA in xeroderma pigmantosum conjunctivitis. *Arch Ophth* 93:660, 1975.

35. Ni C, Dryja TP and Albert DM: Sweat gland tumors in the eyelids: A clinicopathological analysis of 5 cases. *In* Ni C and Albert DM (Eds): Tumors of the eyelid and orbit: A Chinese-American collaborative study. *Int Ophth Clin* 22(1):1, 1982.

36. Ni C, Kimball GP, Craft JL, et al: Calcifying epithelioma: A clinicopathological analysis of 67 cases with ultrastructural study of two cases. *In* Ni C and Albert DM (Eds): Tumors of the eyelid and orbit: A Chinese-American collaborative study. *Int Ophth Clin* 22(1):1, 1982.

37. Ni C, Searl SS, Kuo PK, et al: Sebaceous cell carcinoma of the ocular adenxa. *In* Ni C and Albert DM (Eds): Tumors of the eyelid and orbit: A Chinese-American collaborative study. *Int Ophth Clin* 22(1):23, 1982.

38. Pedace FJ and Winkelmann RK: Xanthalasma palpebrarum. *JAMA* 193:893, 1965.

39. Peden JC: Carcinoma developing in sebaceous cysts. *Ann Surg* 128;1136, 1948.

40. Peterson RF, Hazard JB, Dykes ER, et al: Superficial malignant melanoma. *Surg Gynecol Obstet* 119:37, 1964.

41. Porterfield JT and Zimmerman LE: Rhabdomyosarcoma of the orbit: A clinicopathologic study of 55 cases. *Virchows Arch Pathol Anat* 335:329, 1962.

42. Quickert MH and Rathbun E: Suture repair of entropion. *Arch Ophth* 85:304, 1971.

43. Reese A and Wilber J: The eye manifestations of xeroderma pigmentosum. *Am J Ophth* 26:901, 1947.

44. Ronchese F: Melanomata pathologically malignant, clinically non-malignant, in a case of xeroderma pigmentosum. *Arch Derm Syph* 68:335, 1953.

45. Stout AF: Malignant manifestations of Bowen's disease. *NYS J Med* 39:801, 1939.

46. Trowbridge DH: Ocular manifestations of coccidioimycosis. *Tr Pac Coast Oto-Ophth Soc* 33:229, 1952.

47. Tse DT: Aponeurosis disinsertion in congenital entropion. *Arch Ophth* 101:436, 1983.

48. Wagoner MD, Beyer CK, Gander TR and Albert DM: Common presentation of sebaceous gland carcinoma of the eyelids. *Ann Ophth* 14:159, 1982.

49. Zacarian SA: Cancer of the eyelids—a cryosurgical approach. *Ann Ophth* 4:473, 1972.

50. Zimmerman LE: Surgical pathology of the eye and ocular adnexa. *In* Ackerman LV (Ed), *Surgical Pathology,* 2nd Ed. St. Louis: Mosby, 1959.

Chapter 2

The Patient
with Proptosis

Thomas C. Spoor, MD, MS

THE PATIENT WITH PROPTOSIS

Introduction

The eye is surrounded by the orbit, containing fat, vessels, nerves and extraocular muscles (Figure 2-1). The orbit is separated by periorbita and bone from the adjacent brain and sinuses (Figure 2-2). Intracranial or sinus diseases invading the orbit may present, therefore, as proptosis or visual dysfunction. Conversely, primary ocular or orbital disease may spread to contiguous intracranial structures or the paranasal sinuses. Cognizance of these relationships allows you to better evaluate the patient with proptosis or periorbital trauma. This chapter will stress orbital disorders in adults commonly presenting to the practicing ophthalmologist: idiopathic orbital inflammation, infection, lacrimal tumors, metastatic tumors, and dysthyroid orbitopathy are commonly encountered and should be recognized by all ophthalmologists. Disorders in children—inflammation, infection and tumor (specifically rhabdomyosarcoma)—should be differentiated by the primary ophthalmologist prior to referral or treatment.

Any presumed infectious or inflammatory mass not responding to treatment, an unusual lid mass, or unexplained ptosis in a child under sixteen years of age should be considered a rhabdomyosarcoma until proven otherwise. This is a histologic diagnosis; early biopsy is the key to making it correctly. The ophthalmologist should suspect rhabdomyosarcoma whenever dealing with an unexplained orbital or adnexal problem in a child. Its potential lethality if undiagnosed, and curability when diagnosed and treated early, make rhabdomyosarcoma *the* diagnosis of exclusion in spite of its relative rarity.[1] Early referral for appropriate treatment with a combination of supravoltage irradiation and chemotherapy may be gratifying for both physician and patient.

Ultrasonography is a valuable adjunct to orbital diagnosis in the hands of some clinicians;[2] but for the practicing ophthalmologist, an orbital CT scan affords peace of mind and valuable information when evaluating the patient with proptosis. An orbital study with 2 mm sections should be specified and appropriate reconstructions (coronal, oblique or sagittal) obtained. Computed tomography has facilitated the evaluation and management of orbital disorders and a basic knowledge of CT anatomy should be part of every ophthalmologist's armamentarium (see Chapter 10).

The initial evaluation of a patient presenting with an orbital problem should differentiate true proptosis from pseudoproptosis. Common causes of pseudoproptosis include unilateral axial myopia (1 mm length/3 diopters myopia), or contralateral ptosis or enophthalmus causing the normal side to appear proptotic.

Once an orbital problem has been identified, a complete history and ophthalmological exam are necessary. Ask specifically about thyroid dys-

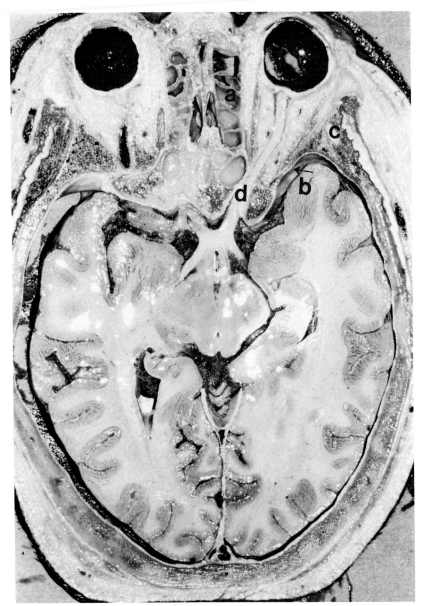

Figure 2-1. Section through mid-axial plane of right orbit demonstrating relationship between the orbit and a) ethmoid sinus, b) temporal lobe in middle cranial fossa, and (➤) sphenoid ridge, c) temporalis fossa and lateral orbital wall, d) optic canal.

function or remote malignancy, both common causes of proptosis. The degree of proptosis should be documented by exophthalmometry and the amount of hyper or hypoophthalmia determined. Visual acuity and color vision are documented and formal perimetry obtained if either are abnormal. Pupils should be inspected for significant anisocoria. The presence of an afferent defect or light/near dissociation should be noted. Anisocoria due to sympathetic or parasympathetic dysfunction should be recognized and differentiated. Extraocular motility, especially versions and ductions,

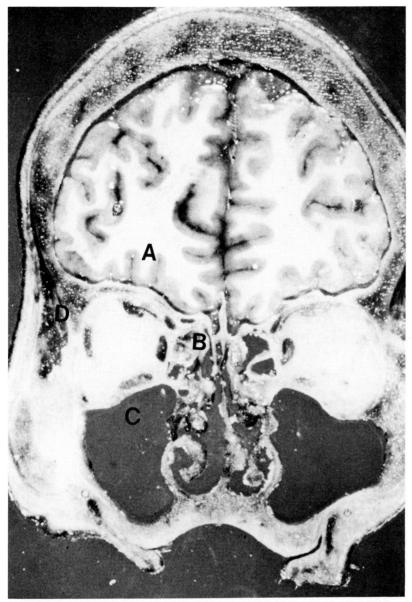

Figure 2-2. Coronal section through mid-orbit demonstrating relationships between orbit and a) anterior cranial fossa, b) ethmoid sinus, c) maxillary sinus, d) lateral orbital wall and temporalis fossa.

should be evaluated in all cardinal fields of gaze and lids observed for ptosis, retraction and lag. Corneal reflexes and infraorbital sensation should be evaluated. Orbital resistance to retropulsation can be determined by comparing the ease of pressing each globe into the orbit. Intraocular pressure should be measured in both primary and upgaze. Slit lamp exam and funduscopy complete the examination.

Anatomic Relationships. The orbit is bound superiorly by the

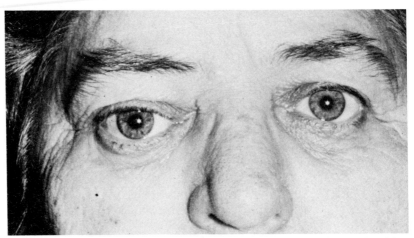

Figure 2-3. Patient with mucocele of right frontal sinus. Note proptosis and depression of right eye.

frontal sinus and anterior cranial fossa. Neoplasms of the frontal sinus can involve the orbit. Frontal sinus mucoceles (Figure 2-3) classically present as slowly progressive proptosis and hypoophthalmia.

The anterior cranial fossa and frontal lobes overlie the orbital roof (Figure 2-2). Trauma to the superior orbit may penetrate the anterior cranial fossa and warrant neurosurgical evaluation and intervention. Occult intracranial injury should always be considered when evaluating ocular and orbital trauma (Figure 2-4A & B).

The lacrimal gland lies in the superior temporal quadrant of the orbit. It may be involved by infection, inflammation, benign or malignant neoplasms. These patients may present with proptosis or a palpable orbital mass. Visual dysfunction and pain may or may not be present depending upon the underlying process.

Deep to the orbit lies the sphenoid sinus and middle cranial fossa. Infections and neoplasms in the sphenoid sinus may present as orbital pain accompanied by visual or oculomotor dysfunction due to parasellar cranial nerve involvement.[3]

Aneurysms, dural and carotid cavernous fistulas and sphenoid ridge meningiomas are middle cranial fossa problems that may initially present as orbital dysfunction: proptosis, visual loss or oculomotor palsies (Figure 2-1). The diagnosis of aneurysms or carotid cavernous fistula can usually be easily made after appropriate clinical and CT examination. Dural cavernous fistulas and sphenoid ridge meningiomas may be more difficult to diagnose.

Dural cavernous fistulas are a small arteriovenous fistula involving a small dural arteriole and the cavernous sinus. Antecedent trauma may or may not have occurred, but these fistulas often appear spontaneously.[4] Patients with dural-cavernous fistulas are often asymptomatic, presenting with a red-eye unresponsive to medical treatment.[5] Supraorbital pain and diplopia secondary to a mild sixth nerve paresis may occur. Signs are usually mild and include dilated conjunctival vessels, (arterialized veins) mild

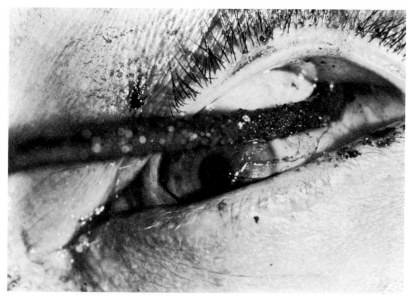

Figure 2-4A. Penetrating injury to left orbit by metal rod (courtesy of J.S. Kennerdell, M.D.).

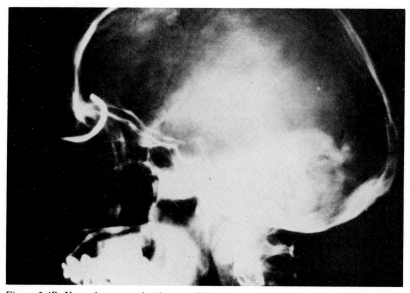

Figure 2-4B. X-ray demonstrating intracranial involvement.

proptosis and sixth nerve paresis (Figure 2-5). Objective bruits may be auscultated or subjective bruits elicited by careful history. Definitive diagnosis is made by complete selective cerebral angiography. A presumptive diagnosis can be made by demonstrating an enlarged superior ophthalmic vein by computed tomography or ultrasonography, in the appropriate clinical setting. Many dural-cavernous fistulas close spontaneously, and unless visual dysfunction progresses, conservative management is advocated.[4]

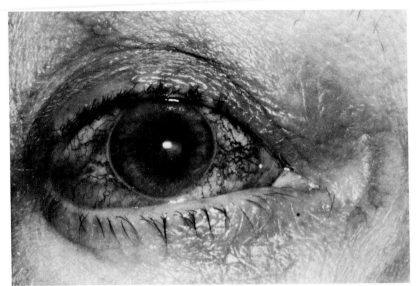

Figure 2-5. Patient with a dural-cavernous fistula OD demonstrating mild proptosis and arterialization of conjunctival vessels.

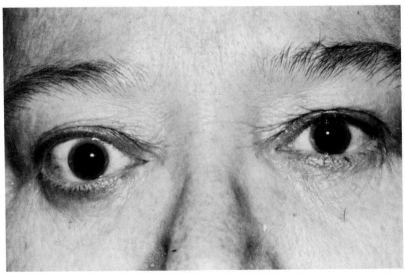

Figure 2-6. Patient with right sphenoid ridge meningioma with mild proptosis and no visual dysfunction.

Patients with sphenoid ridge meningiomas may present to the ophthalmologist with proptosis, visual dysfunction due to optic nerve compression or motility dysfunction (Figure 2-6). Computed tomography may demonstrate a markedly enlarged sphenoid ridge (Figure 2-7) with or without orbital involvement. Treatment is in the realm of the neurosurgeon; and the results may be less than excellent.[6] The surgeon should strive to obtain adequate decompression with sparing of the oculomotor and optic nerves, maintaining integrity of extraocular motility and visual function. The thin lamina papyracae forms the medial wall of the orbit separating it from the ethmoid sinus (Figure 2-1). Neoplasms and infections in the sinus can easily penetrate this thin barrier and involve the orbit (Figure 2-8). Analogously, orbital contents may become entrapped in a medial wall fractured by blunt trauma. The maxillary sinus lies inferior to the orbit (Figure 2-2). As with the ethmoid sinus, infection and neoplasms here may involve the orbit and orbital contents may become entrapped if the bony floor is fractured after blunt trauma (Figure 2-9A & B).

All ophthalmologists should be conversant with the diagnosis and treatment of common orbital disorders. These include dysthyroid orbitopathy, metastatic tumors, idiopathic orbital inflammation (pseudotumor), orbital infections, lacrimal fossa lesions and trauma. These entities are common enough to present regularly to the practicing ophthalmologist. Dysthyroid orbitopathy is sufficiently common that I have devoted an entire chapter to it (see Chapter 3).

Metastatic Tumors. The tumors most commonly metastasizing to the orbit are breast carcinoma in the female and lung carcinoma in the male.[7]

Breast carcinoma is particularly insidious. The patient in Figure 2-10A presented with orbital metastasis 21 years after a "successful" mastectomy. Computed tomography demonstrated the orbital mass (Figure 2-10B). Biopsy confirmed the clinical suspicion of adenocarcinoma of the breast. When evaluating a patient with proptosis, it is very important to specifically inquire about past malignant disease and any previous surgery. The accurate diagnosis of orbital metastatic disease is based upon suspicion and a complete medical history. Breast and prostatic carcinomas and cutaneous malignant melanomas may present with orbital manifestations (decreased vision, diplopia, ptosis and proptosis and pain) years after the primary tumor was diagnosed. This information must be specifically requested. In my experience, breast is the most common tumor metastatic to the orbit followed by lung, prostate and cutaneous melanoma. Other primary tumor sites in patients with carcinoma metastatic to the orbit include kidney, testicle, thyroid, pancreas and gastrointestinal tract.[7]

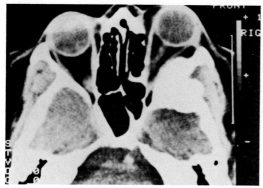

Figure 2-7. CT scan from patient in Figure 2-6, demonstrating marked hypertrophy of sphenoid ridge.

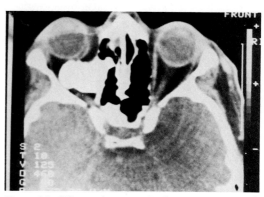

Figure 2-8. CT scan demonstrating large osteoma extending into orbit from adjacent ethmoid sinus.

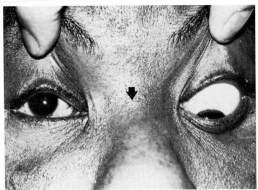

Figure 2-9A. Limited depression of right eye after incarceration of right inferior rectus in orbital floor fracture.

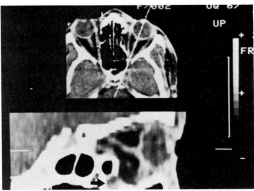

Figure 2-9B. CT scan (oblique reconstruction) documenting entrapment of inferior rectus in posterior fracture site on orbital floor (⬆).

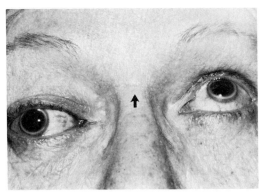

Figure 2-10A. Orbital metastasis presenting as an "elevator palsy," 21 years after mastectomy for carcinoma of breast.

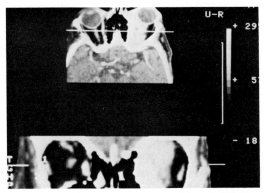

Figure 2-10B. CT scan from patient in Figure 2-10A demonstrating diffuse infiltration of orbit by metastatic tumor.

Idiopathic Orbital Inflammation (Pseudotumor). Idiopathic orbital inflammation is common; presenting symptoms and signs depend in part upon which orbital structures are inflamed. The etiology is unknown, however most cases are exquisitely responsive, at least initially, to systemic corticosteroids. Computed tomography has enabled us to specifically identify the inflamed orbital structures and correlate their involvement with the presenting orbital dysfunction.

Myositis. Patients with acute orbital myositis present with pain and diplopia. Their orbits are swollen, tender to touch, and attempted ductions are limited and painful (Figure 2-11). The presenting extraocular motility dysfunction depends upon which muscles are inflamed and to what extent. The patient in Figure 2-11 had isolated involvement of the right medial rectus with painful restricted adduction, but normal abduction, whereas other patients may have extensive right medial rectus involvement on computed tomography (Figure 2-12) and limitation of both abduction and adduction. With medial rectus myositis, the adjacent ethmoid sinus may or

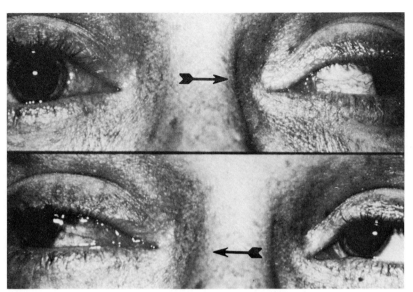

Figure 2-11. Patient with myositis of right medial rectus and defective ocular adduction, but full abduction.

may not be involved. When involved (Figure 2-13), the sinusitis resolves as quickly as the myositis after treatment with systemic corticosteroids.

The girl in Figure 2-14 presented with ptosis and evidence for inflammation in the superior orbit. Her CT scan demonstrated enlargement of her levator as well as the palpable preseptal mass (Figure 2-15). The response to systemic corticosteroids should be dramatic and complete. Twenty-four hours after receiving 60 mg prednisone this girl had a marked subjective and objective response (Figure 2-16); seventy-two hours later her appearance was nearly normal.

Patients with inflammation in the vicinity of the trochlea may present with a pseudo-Brown's syndrome (Figure 2-17). Those with multiple muscle involvement may present with excessive orbital swelling, pain and

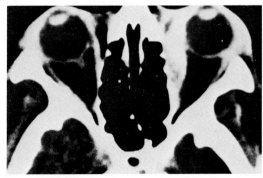

Figure 2-12. CT scan demonstrating markedly enlarged medial rectus.

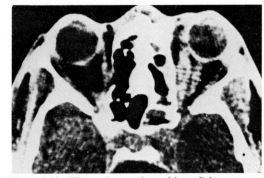

Figure 2-13. CT scan from patient with medial rectus myositis and adjacent sinusitis.

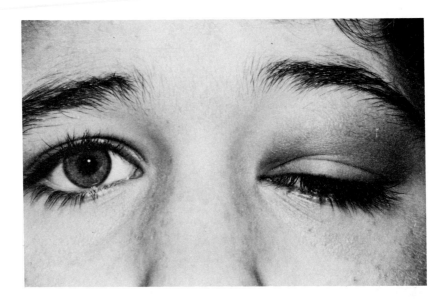

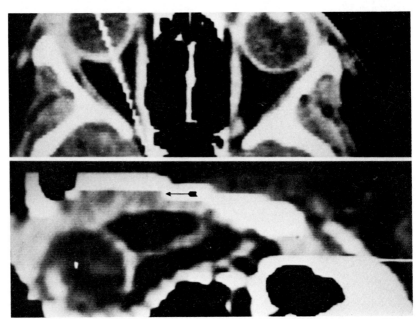

Figure 2-15. CT scan demonstrating enlargement of the levator and preseptal mass on oblique reconstruction.

chemosis (Figure 2-18). There may be no recognizable pattern to the motility dysfunction.

An atypical CT appearance or incomplete response to corticosteroids should prompt further evaluation and biopsy if necesssary to rule out a neoplasm masquerading as orbital inflammation. The patient in Figure 2-19 presented with clinical idiopathic orbital inflammation and responded dramatically to systemic corticosteroids. CT scan was atypical (Figure 2-20) demonstrating a ring enhancing mass adjacent and above the medial rectus.

The patient remained asymptomatic after her course of prednisone had been completed. Since her initial scan was atypical, it was repeated and revealed a residual mass remaining superior and adjacent to the medial rectus (Figure 2-21) which proved to be metastatic cutaneous melanoma.

Treatment of orbital myositis is with systemic corticosteroids. Initially, I use 60-100 mg of prednisone, depending upon the size and age of the patient. Signs and symptoms should dramatically resolve within 24-48 hours. The prednisone is rapidly tapered and discontinued over three to

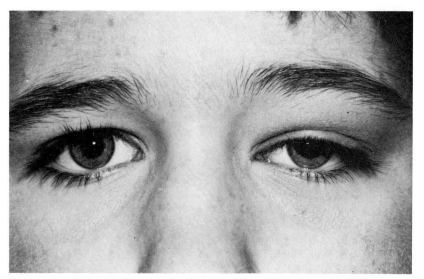

Figure 2-16. Partial resolution of ptosis and preseptal mass 24 hours after initiation of systemic prednisone.

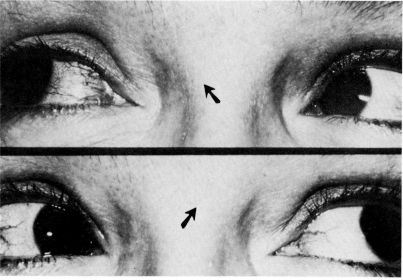

Figure 2-17. Pseudo-Brown's syndrome secondary to orbital inflammation. Note failure of right eye to fully elevate in adduction.

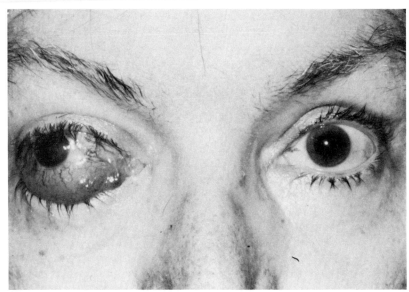

Figure 2-18. Multiple muscle involvement with orbital myositis. Note excessive orbital swelling and conjunctival chemosis. Motility was restricted in all fields of gaze. (Photo courtesy Dr. James Rush.)

four weeks. If symptoms recur, the dose of prednisone at which they recurred is doubled and maintained for one week, then tapered again. For example, the girl in Figure 2-14 dramatically improved at an initial dose of 60 mg prednisone per day. She remained asymptomatic until her daily prednisone dose was 10 mg per day. At this time her pain and lid swelling recurred. Prednisone was increased to 20 mg daily and after a week very slowly tapered to 2½ mg per week at which level she remained asymptomatic. Patients refractory to or intolerant of corticosteroids may benefit from low dose orbital irradiation (2000 rads).[14]

The course of acute orbital myositis is variable. Most patients resolve of orbital inflammation. A painful steroid responsive optic neuropathy should prompt a search for a compressive mass lesion or occult fungal infection.[23] The following case is illustrative:

A 48-year-old lady was referred with a painful optic neuropathy OS. Visual acuity was 20/20 OD, counting fingers OS with a dense central scotoma. Skull x-rays and CT scans were essentially normal. A diagnosis of inflammatory retrobulbar neuritis was made and she was begun on prednisone 80 mg/day. Within 48 hours her pain was gone and her acuity returned to 20/20. As steroids were tapered, acuity decreased to counting fingers and pain recurred. Reinstitution of systemic steroids again alleviated the pain and acuity returned to 20/40. One week later, she returned with a painful, frozen orbit and amaurotic eye. Three weeks later she died of an intracranial aspergillosis infection.[23]

Patients with perineuritis may have a swollen disc as well as the other signs of periscleral inflammation described previously. Perineuritis as a

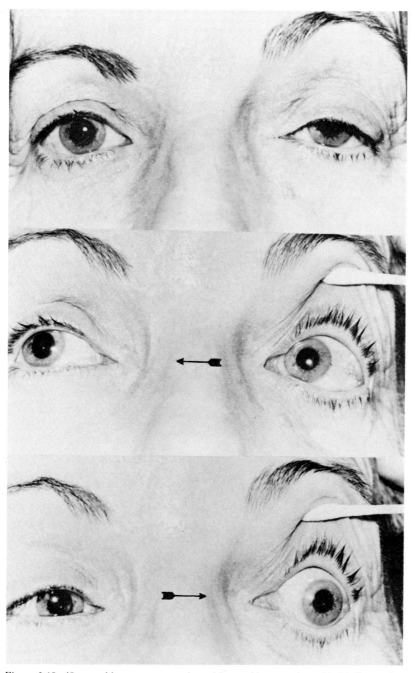

Figure 2-19. 48-year-old woman presenting with steroid responsive orbital inflammation. Note ptosis and restricted adduction and abduction of left eye (pupils dilated Latrogenically).

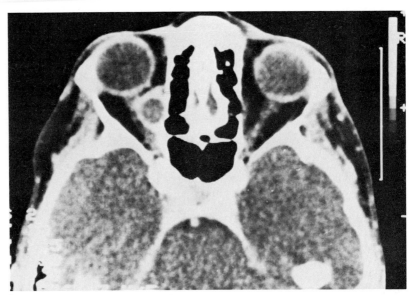

Figure 2-20. CT scan from patient in Figure 2-19 demonstrating ring enhancing mass adjacent to medial rectus.

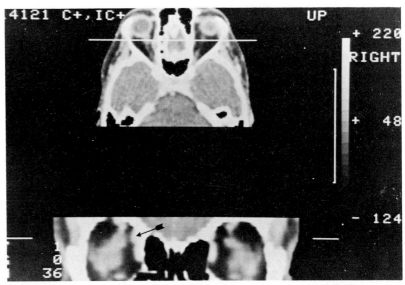

Figure 2-21. CT scan from patient in Figure 2-19 six weeks after complete resolution of her clinical symptoms. Residual mass is present adjacent to and above left medial rectus (◆).

manifestation of secondary syphilis is increasingly prevalent in our promiscuous society but, fortunately, is treatable. Appropriate serologic testing should be obtained in *any* patient with unexplained perineuritis.[24,25]

Perineuritis results from a loose inflammatory infiltration of the optic nerve sheath. Patients present with minimal symptoms of visual dysfunction and signs of disc swelling—often bilateral. Those with associated encephalitis or meningitis will have neurologic signs, swollen discs and good visual function. Subsequently the diagnosis of papilledema secondary to elevated intracranial pressure is made. After the lumbar puncture reveals normal CSF pressure the diagnosis of perineuritis can be made.[24]

Perineuritis may also be associated with more remote orbital inflammation such as in an orbital vasculitis. Definitive causes of perineuritis include syphilis, sarcoidosis. These treatable etiologies should be sought.

Orbital Infections

Orbital infections may threaten both vision and life. Subsequently, they should be treated promptly, appropriately and aggressively. Pre-septal cellulitis and dacryocystitis are relatively benign soft tissue infections, not confined by the orbital septum. Post-septal infections are confined to a closed space behind the orbital septum and as expanding masses can cause irreversible loss of vision and motility defects. Post-septal infections include diffuse orbital cellulitis, localized abscesses and sub-periosteal abscesses.

Pre-Septal Cellulitis. Pre-septal cellulitis is an infection localized to the eyelid, anterior to the orbital septum (Figure 2-25). It may result from lid trauma or an adjacent sinusitis. These patients are usually mildly febrile (100° F) and may have a minimal WBC count elevation (10-15,000). Visual acuity, pupils and extra-ocular motility are normal. The entire infectious process is localized anterior to the orbital septum. Treatment consists of systemic antibiotics, or incision and drainage if the abscess is fluctuant. An underlying sinusitis should be appropriately treated by an otorhino-laryngologist.

Dacryocystitis. Dacryocystitis is an infection of an obstructed lacrimal sac, most commonly presenting in infants and the elderly. Tenderness, erythema and fluctuance over the medial canthal area are common (Figure 2-26). Expression of pus by pressure over the lacrimal sac is diagnostic.

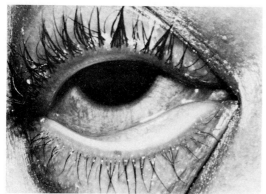

Figure 2-22. Patient with periscleritis. Eye is inflamed and tender to touch with minimal anterior segment inflammation.

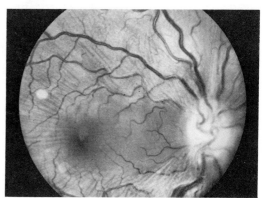

Figure 2-23. Neuroretinal edema and folds secondary to periscleritis.

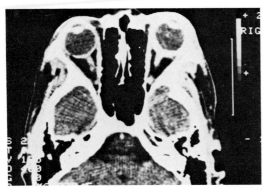

Figure 2-24. CT scan with contrast from patient with peri-scleritis. Note thickening of the sclero-uveal rim increasing after intravenous contrast.

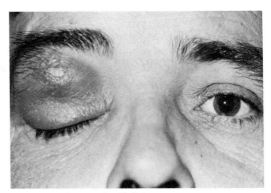

Figure 2-25. Preseptal cellulitis.

Temporary treatment is with systemic antibiotics (Keflex 500 mg q6h) and incision and drainage. Definitive treatment after the acute infection is quiescent entails nasolacrimal probing in the infant and dacryocystorhinostomy in the adult.

Post-Septal (Orbital) Cellulitis. Orbital cellulitis is an acute bacterial infection of the orbital contents. Expansion may cause blindness; posterior extension may cause death secondary to cavernous sinus thrombosis. It is a serious infection, especially in debilitated patients.[26] In the pre-antibiotic era 25% of patients died and 25% lost vision from complications of orbital cellulitis.[27] Even today, misdiagnosed or mistreated patients may rapidly lose vision in the affected eye.[28] The following case is illustrative:

> A ten-year-old boy presented to the emergency room complaining of headache and a red eye. X-rays revealed a pansinusitis. An ophthalmology consultant documented 5 mm of proptosis, 20/20 visual acuity, normal pupillary reactions and full extraocular motility. Systemic antibiotics were started and pus drained from the maxillary sinus via a Caldwell-Luc incision. Postoperatively the boy remained febrile and visual acuity deteriorated to 20/400. An afferent pupil was present and extraocular motility restricted. Computed tomography demonstrated a large, medial sub-periosteal abscess, which was then drained. Visual acuity has remained 20/400.

This case illustrates the need for compulsive evaluation and treatment of the patient with an orbital abscess. Vision can be rapidly lost, even while being treated with appropriate intravenous antibiotics.[28]

In the absence of injury, lid, tooth, or facial infections, orbital cellulitis is usually secondary to an adjacent sinusitis. Orbital complications of acute sinusitis have been classified as inflammatory edema, orbital cellulitis, cavernous sinus thrombosis, orbital abscess and sub-periosteal abscess (SPA).[29,30] The former three may respond to medical therapy—high dosage of appropriate intravenous antibiotics. Orbital and sub-periosteal abscesses may require prompt surgical drainage to obviate mechanical compression of the optic nerve and visual loss due to elevated orbital pressure.[27] Early drainage also allows appropriate cultures to be obtained and antibiotic therapy modified as needed.

It may be difficult to differentiate a diffuse orbital cellulitis from an abscess on clinical grounds. Both patients may be febrile with elevated WBC counts and manifest lid edema, proptosis, chemosis, impaired ocular motility and decreased vision and an afferent pupil. Lateral displacement of the globe and impaired adduction are suggestive of a medial sub-periosteal abscess (Figure 2-27). The site of the abscess can also be accurately localized by computed tomography and aid surgical exploration (Figure 2-28).

Initial management should include broad spectrum intravenous anti-biotics and computed tomography with coronal reconstructions. Specific antibiotic recommendations are not offered since selection changes so rapidly and resistant strains emerge and may vary from institution to institution. I recommend initial broad spectrum coverage of gram positive and gram negative bacteria with a cephalosporin or staphicidal penicillin (nafcillin or methacillin) and an aminoglycoside. Ampicillin or chloramphenicol should be added to cover Hemophilus in a child less than five years old. Antibiotics can be modified as culture results are obtained or as the clinical response dictates.

If a sub-periosteal abscess is detected on computed tomography, it should be promptly drained. This is a relatively easy and safe extra-orbital procedure that allows you to both decompress the orbit, relieving pressure on the optic nerve, and obtain appropriate culture material. These abscesses are poorly penetrated by intravenous antibiotics and may continue to expand causing visual loss in spite of apparently appropriate antibiotics.[28] Intraorbital abscesses are not as technically easy to drain, carry a higher surgical morbidity and may resolve with appropriate antibiotic treatment. These may be treated more conservatively and followed to resolution if they respond to systemic antibiotics. Abscesses not responding to 24-48 hours of medical therapy require surgical drainage.

Lacrimal Fossa Masses. Superior-temporal orbital masses require prompt evaluation and treatment. Etiologies may be infectious, inflam-

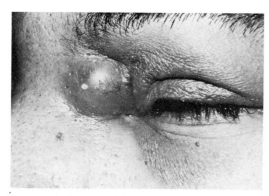

Figure 2-26. Dacryocystitis.

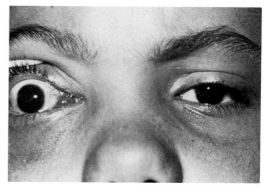

Figure 2-27. Orbital cellulitis. (Courtesy of Dr. Thomas Slamovitz, MD)

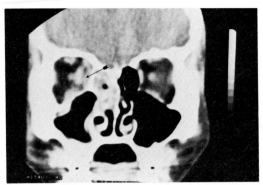

Figure 2-28. CT scan from patient in Figure 2-27—coronal reconstruction demonstrates abscess in right orbit (▲) from adjacent ethmoid sinusitis.

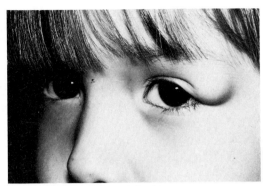

Figure 2-29. Dermoid cyst left orbit.

matory, or neoplastic. Benign neoplasms, such as benign mixed tumors or dermoids, have an excellent prognosis after appropriate surgical removal. Malignant neoplasms include lymphomas and epithelial carcinomas. These must be differentiated histopathologically since their treatment and prognosis are markedly different.

Lacrimal fossa masses may be differentiated by history (duration, pain), examination, and computed tomography. Details of the differential diagnosis of lacrimal masses have been elegantly described by Wright, et al.[31,32] A scheme for the clinical and CT diagnosis of lacrimal fossa masses has been recently described by Jakobiec, et al.[32] I will review the differential diagnoses of masses in the superior temporal orbit.

Dermoid Cyst. Dermoid cysts often occur in the region of the lacrimal gland. Typically, dermoids are diagnosed in childhood, presenting as a painless subcutaneous mass with a regular configuration (Figure 2-29). They are firm, immobile to palpation, and not attached to overlying skin. They rarely present with alarming symptoms of pain, rapid growth or visual loss or demonstrate erythema or swelling of the overlying skin.[34] Less commonly, these cysts may present in later life.

Computed tomography demonstrates an extraconal mass with well defined margins and a low-absorption center (Figure 2-30). Fluid may be present in the cyst secondary to sebaceous material and lipid. Plain x-rays may reveal a sharply defined cyst-like bony defect sometimes with sclerotic margins. A presumptive diagnosis can usually be made prior to surgery based upon the clinical presentation and computed tomographic findings. Computed tomography should be obtained prior to surgery for these lesions may extend deeply into the orbit and require lateral orbitotomy for removal.

Complete surgical removal is the appropriate treatment. The surgical approach is dictated by the location, size and degree of orbital involvement by the tumor.

Benign Mixed Tumors. Benign mixed tumors (BMT) may be diag-

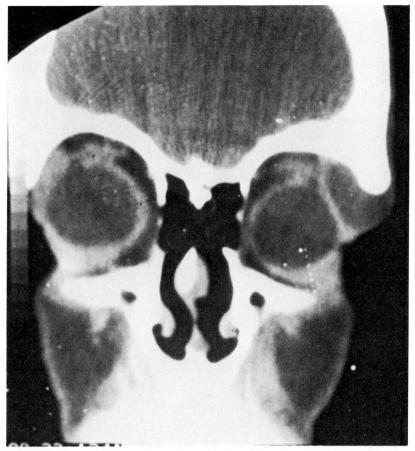

Figure 2-30. Coronal CT scan from patient with dermoid cyst demonstrating well-encapsulated hypodense orbital mass.

nosed by history, exam, and computed tomographic findings.[31-33] These patients present with painless proptosis of long duration without inflammatory signs or symptoms (Figure 3-31). Visual acuity may be minimally decreased due to choroidal stria, or stretching and displacement of the optic nerve due to a large mass effect, but such decreased acuity is unusual. A mass may be palpable in the superior temporal quadrant.

Plain x-rays may reveal compressive changes (fossa formation) in the lacrimal region without erosion of the bone. Computed tomography (Figure 2-32) demonstrates rounded or globular soft tissue outlines with smoothly encapsulated margins. Contiguous bone may be molded demonstrating compressive fossa formation.[33]

The combination of the characteristic clinical presentations and computed tomographic findings necessitates the preoperative diagnosis of benign mixed tumor and the need for an extended supero-lateral orbitotomy.[31,32] To obviate recurrence or malignant degeneration of a BMT, the tumor must be removed *in toto* and the capsule not violated. This necessitates meticulous microsurgical orbital techniques.[35]

A painful, rapidly developing mass in the superior temporal quadrant

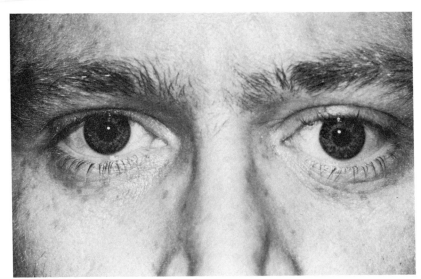

Figure 2-31. Subtle proptosis of left eye in patient with a large benign mixed tumor of lacrimal gland.

requires prompt attention. Differential diagnostic possibilities include dacryoadenitis (inflammation), lymphoma, or epithelial carcinoma of the lacrimal gland. Since treatment and prognosis are markedly different for each of these entities, they must be differentiated.

Dacryoadenitis. Acute dacryoadenitis may be infectious or secondary to idiopathic orbital inflammation (pseudotumor). Patients present with a short history (days) of swelling and pain in the superior temporal orbit. The lids may be swollen, the conjunctiva chemotic. Patients with infectious dacryoadenitis may be febrile with an elevated WBC, have a purulent discharge and preauricular or cervical lymphadenopathy. Symptoms and signs should resolve promptly with appropriate systemic antibiotics.

Inflammatory dacryoadenitis (pseudotumor) is common. These patients also present with pain, swelling and chemosis. However, they are generally afebrile, have a normal WBC count, no lymphadenopathy, and x-rays are normal. Computed tomography documents the size and extent of the mass. Response to systemic corticosteroids should be rapid and dramatic with a prompt resolution of signs and symptoms. If acute dacryoadenitis does not resolve with appropriate treatment, the lacrimal gland should be biopsied to determine the etiology for chronic dacryoadenitis and to rule out a lymphoma or an epithelial carcinoma.

Lymphomas. Lymphomatous lesions of the lacrimal gland range in severity from reactive lymphoid hyperplasia to malignant lymphomas with systemic manifestations. These rarely present with inflammatory signs and symptoms. Most commonly patients present with progressive swelling of the eyelid and a palpable non-tender mass in the vicinity of the lacrimal gland (Figure 2-33). Computed tomography will demonstrate the size and extent of the mass which may be quite remarkable (Figure 2-34).

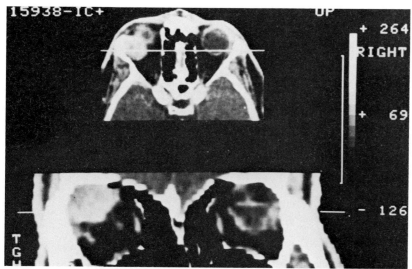

Figure 2-32. Axial (above) and coronal (below) CT scans of benign mixed tumor of left lacrimal gland. Note well-encapsulated mass molding adjacent bone.

Lacrimal glands involved with inflammatory or lymphoid conditions usually demonstrate diffuse, compressed and molded enlargement on computed tomography without associated bone defects.[34] Compressive thinning of adjacent bone by a lymphoma has recently been described[36] but bony changes are very unusual[33] and usually mitigate against the diagnosis of lymphoma.

These lesions should be biopsied through the eyelid either trans-marginally as described by Nesi and Smith[37] or transseptally. The specimen obtained should be large enough to allow the pathologist to perform appropriate studies. Prior consultation with the pathologist ensures that he will perform appropriate studies, including cultures, touch prep, or electron microscopy, as indicated to make an accurate diagnosis. Lymphomatous lesions are best treated with orbital irradiation, appropriate dosage depending upon whether they are benign or malignant. Lymphomas may

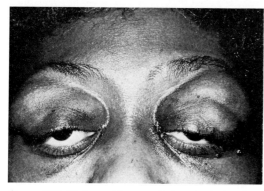

Figure 2-33. Patient with systemic lymphoma involving both lacrimal glands.

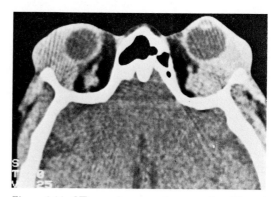

Figure 2-34. CT scan demonstrating extensive, bilateral lymphoma involving both lacrimal glands.

respond initially to systemic steroids. Incomplete response warrants a biopsy.

Epithelial Carcinoma. Patients with epithelial carcinomas of the lacrimal gland characteristically have a short, rapidly progressive, painful course (Figure 2-35). These symptoms are shared with other rapidly expanding lacrimal masses. X-rays and computed tomography may demonstrate bony erosion not found with inflammatory or lymphomatous lesions. Although these lesions are globular in outline, their margins may be irregular denoting infiltration and absence of encapsulation (Figure 2-36).

Biopsy is necessary for a definitive diagnosis and differentiation between chronic inflammation, lymphomas and epithelial malignancies. Biopsy should be through the eyelid either transseptally or transmarginally to preserve the periosteal barrier if the lesion proves to be an epithelial carcinoma.

If an epithelial carcinoma, i.e., adenocystic carcinoma, is diagnosed on permanent section, surgical treatment should be radical—combining orbital exenteration with radical orbitectomy if the tumor is confined within periosteum and there is no evidence for orbital apex involvement. This is best accomplished through the combined efforts of a neurosurgeon and oculoplastic surgeon.

This surgery is somewhat deforming (Figure 2-37) but the prognosis without radical surgery is dismal and the terminal manifestations of this tumor equally deforming and grotesque (Figure 2-38).

Those patients with extension of tumor beyond the periosteum and erosion of bone and who are not operable for "cure" may benefit from less radical surgery, i.e., exenteration plus irradiation. Irradiation is not curative, but may be palliative and prolong survival. The patient described in Figure 2-38 had extensive bony involvement at the time of surgery and exenteration was not performed. The tumor relentlessly involved his eye, orbit, maxillary sinus and temporal fossa grossly disfiguring his face (Figure 2-38). The terminal event was uncontrollable hemorrhage from an internal maxillary artery eroded by tumor.

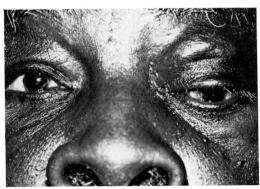

Figure 2-35. Patient with adenocystic carcinoma of left lacrimal gland.

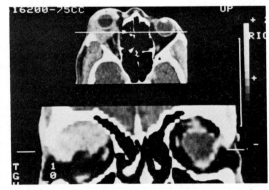

Figure 2-36. CT scan, axial (above) and coronal (below) from patient with adenocystic carcinoma of lacrimal gland (Figure 2-35). Note irregular margins and erosion of bone.

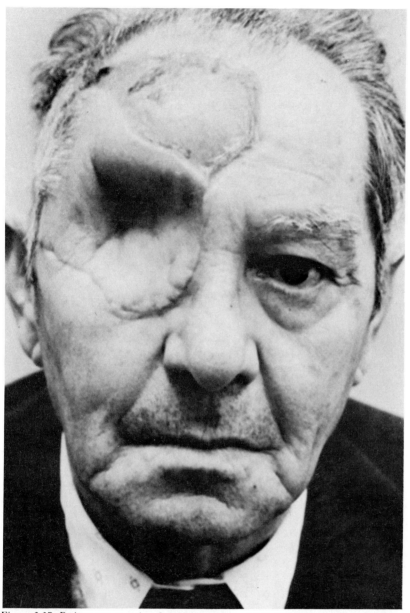

Figure 2-37. Patient two months after orbitectomy and full-thickness skin graft (courtesy Eugene Quindlen, M.D.).

There is no good treatment for adenocystic carcinoma of the lacrimal gland. Prognosis is dismal with conventional exenteration and radiation therapy. Chemotherapy is ineffective. Tumor spreads through the haversian system in bone and perineurally. The rationale for radical orbitectomy is to excise subclinical microscopic disease in hopes of completely extirpating the tumor. Time will tell whether this radical therapy enhances long-term survival. Recurrent or residual tumor may be treated with high dose

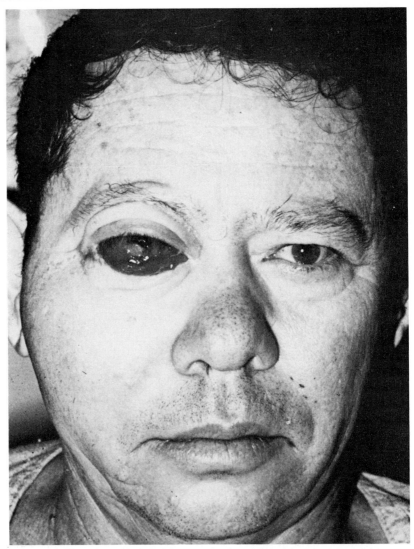

Figure 2-38. Extensive orbital, facial and ocular involvement by adenocystic carcinoma of lacrimal gland.

radiation therapy. This is palliative, not curative, but does seem to prolong survival.

Summary

Common orbital disorders can be diagnosed by a complete history, careful examination and computed tomography. Diagnosis is aided by understanding the anatomic and functional relationships between the orbit and contiguous brain and sinuses. This knowledge coupled with an understanding of common orbital disorders, should enable the clinician to better manage the patient with proptosis.

References

1. Nicholson DH, Green WR: *Rhabdomyosarcoma in pediatric ocular tumors*. New York: Masson, 1981, pp 247-254.
2. Byrne SF, Glaser JS: Orbital tissue differentiation with standardized echography. *Ophthalmology* 90:1071-1090, 1983.
3. Lew D, Southwisk S, Montgomery WW, Weber AL, Baker AJ: Sphenoid sinusitis. *New Engl J Med* 309:1149-1154, 1983.
4. Grove AS: The dural shunt syndrome. *Ophthalmology,* 91:31-44, 1984.
5. Phelps CD, Thompson HS, Ossoinig KS: The diagnosis and prognosis of atypical carotid cavernous fistula (The Red Eye Syndrome). *Am J Ophthalmol* 93:523-536, 1982.
6. Bommal J, Thibaut A, Brotemi J, Born J: Invading meningiomas of the sphenoid ridge. *J Neurosurgery,* 53:587-599, 1980.
7. Ferry A, Font R: Carcinoma metastatic to the eye and orbit: A clinicopathologic study of 227 cases. *Arch Ophthalmology,* 92:276, 1974.
8. Slavin RL, Glaser JS: Idiopathic orbital myositis. *Arch Ophthalmol,* 100:1261-1265, 1982.
9. Spoor TC, Hartel WC: Orbital myositis. *J Clin Neuro-Ophthalmol* 3:67-74, 1983.
10. Bullen CL, Younge BR: Chronic orbital myositis. *Arch Ophthalmol,* 100:1749-1751, 1982.
11. Weinstein GS, Dresner SC, Slamovits TL, Kennerdell JS: Acute and subacute orbital myositis. *Am J Ophthalmol,* 96:209-217, 1983.
12. Ludwig I, Tomsak RL: Acute recurrent orbital myositis. *J Clin Neuro-Ophthalmol* 3:41-47, 1983.
13. Eshaghian J, Anderson RL: Sinus involvement in inflammatory orbital pseudotumor. *Arch Ophthalmol,* 99:627-630, 1981.
14. Sergott RC, Glaser JS, Charynlu K: Radiotherapy for idiopathic orbital pseudotumor. *Arch Ophthalmol* 99:853-856, 1981.
15. Jakobiec FA: Orbital inflammations. *In:* Jones IS, Jakobiec FA: *Diseases of the Orbit.* Hagerstown: Harper & Row, 1979, p. 216.
16. Rush JA, Kennerdell JS, Donim JF: Acute periscleritis—a variant of idiopathic orbital inflammation. *Orbit* 1:221-230, 1982.
17. Bertelson TI: Acute sclerotenonitis and ocular myositis complicated by papillitis, retinal detachment. *ACTA Ophthalmol (Kbh)* 39:136-152, 1960.
18. Benson WE, Shields JA, Tasman W, Crandall AJ: Posterior scleritis: a cause of diagnostic confusion. *Arch Ophthalmol* 97:1482-1486, 1979.
19. Smith JL, Taxdal DSR: Painful ophthalmoplegia: the Tolosa-Hunt syndrome. *Am J Ophthal* 61:1466-1472, 1966.
20. Domin JF, Borti A: Orbital myositis: its relationship to the Tolosa-Hunt syndrome. *In:* Smith JL (ed): *Neuro-ophthalmology Update.* USA: Masson 1977, pp 99-103.
21. Mottow LS, Jakobiec FA: Idiopathic orbital pseudotumor in childhood. I. Clinical characteristics. *Arch Ophthalmol* 96:1410, 1978.
22. Mottow-Lippa L, Jakobiec FA, Smith M: Idiopathic inflammatory orbital pseudotumor in childhood. II: Results of diagnostic tests and biopsies. *Ophthalmology* 88:565-575, 1981.
23. Spoor TC, et al: Aspergillosis—Presenting as a steroid responsive optic neuropathy. *J Clin Neuro-ophthalmol* 2:103-107, 1982.
24. Miller NR: *Clinical Neuro-ophthalmology,* 4th Ed. Baltimore: Williams & Wilkins, 1982, p 253.
25. Rush JA, Ryan EJ: Syphilitic Optic Perineuritis. *Am J Ophthalmol* 92:404-406, 1981.
26. Krohel G, Krauss HR, Christensen RE, Minkler D: Orbital Abscess. *Arch Ophthalmol* 98:274-276, 1980.
27. Jakobiec FA: Orbital Inflammations. *In:* Jones IS, Jakobiec FS (eds): *Diseases of the Orbit.* Hagerstown: Harper & Row, 1979, p 238.
28. Harris GJ: Subperiosteal abscess of the orbit. *Arch Ophthal,* 101:751-757, 1983.
29. Chandler JR, Langerbrunner DJ, Stevens ER: The pathogenesis of orbital complications in acute sinusitis. *Laryngoscope* 80:1428, 1970.
30. Schramm VL, Myers EN, Kennerdell JS: Orbital complications of acute sinusitis: evaluation, management and outcome. *Ophthalmology* 86:221-229, 1978.

31. Wright JE, Stewart WB, Krohel GB: Clinical presentation and management of lacrimal gland tumours. *Brit J Ophthalmol* 63:600-606, 1979.
32. Stewart WB, Krohel GB, Wright JE: Lacrimal gland and fossa lesions: an approach to diagnosis and management. *Ophthalmol* 86:886-895, 1979.
33. Jakobiec FA, Yeo JH, Trokel SL, Abbott GF: Combined clinical and computed tomographic diagnosis of primary lacrimal fossa lesions. *Amer J Ophthalmol* 94:785-807, 1982.
34. Howard GM: Cystic tumors. *In:* Jones IS, Jakobiec FS (eds): *Diseases of the Orbit.* Hagerstown: Harper & Row, 1979.
35. Kennerdell JS, Maroon JC: Microsurgical approach to intraorbital tumors. *Arch Ophthalmol,* 94:1333-1336, 1976.
36. Harris GJ, Dixon T, Haughten V: Expansion of the lacrimal gland fossa by a lymphoid tumor. *Am J Ophthalmol,* 96:546-547, 1983.
37. Smith B, Nesi F: Orbital Tumors. *In:* Smith, B, Nesi, F: *Ophthalmic Plastic Surgery.* St. Louis: C.V. Mosby, 1981.

Chapter 3

Dysthyroid Orbitopathy

Walter C. Hartel, MD
John S. Kennerdell, MD

DYSTHYROID ORBITOPATHY

Introduction

Since the initial classic description of thyroid ophthalmopathy by Graves' and Basedow in the 19th century,[1] ocular findings in association with systemic thyroid disease have been catalogued and classified. Despite the long-standing recognition of this disorder our understanding of its pathogenesis remains limited and treatment is merely palliative. Clinical difficulties encountered in management range from simple recognition with mild involvement to severe compressive optic neuropathy. This chapter, in addition to highlighting clinical findings and treatment modalities, will outline a treatment oriented classification of dysthyroid ophthalmopathy.

Pathogenesis

The etiologic mechanism producing dysthyroid orbitopathy is unknown. Pathologically, there is infiltration of extraocular muscles, orbital fat, and skin by lymphocytes, plasma cells, macrophages and mast cells. In addition, both extraocular muscles and orbital fat contain increased amounts of mucopolysaccharides, predominantly hyaluronic acid. The round cell infiltration and attendant edema can cause gross extraocular muscle enlargement up to five times normal thickness.[2,3]

Numerous attempts to isolate a specific humoral factor responsible for the development of dysthyroid ophthalmopathy have met with minimal success. Levels of long-acting thyroid stimulator (LATS), antibodies to thyroglobulin, and thyroid stimulating immunoglobulins (TSI) have not been shown to correlate with the clinical activity of ocular disease.[4] Investigations of the cellular immune system in Graves' patients have been directed at evaluating T-lymphocyte populations. The relationship of various lymphocyte subpopulations to steroid responsiveness in patients with dysthyroid orbitopathy may suggest multiple mechanisms for ultimate tissue alteration.[5] No precise inflammatory mechanism has been demonstrated. Likewise, no causative relationship between systemic thyroid disease and dysthyroid ophthalmopathy has been proven, though their clinical coincidence suggests such a link.

Clinical Diagnosis of Systemic Thyroid Disease

Systemic symptoms of hyperthyroidism include weakness, weight loss, nervousness, and palpitations. Physical examination frequently reveals tachycardia, atrial arrhythmias, thyromegaly and tremor. The hypothyroid patient may complain of cold intolerance, lethargy, poor appetite and constipation. Clinical signs include bradycardia, adynamic ileus, and auditory deficiency. When thyroid disease is suspected on a systemic or ocular basis, analysis of circulating thyroid hormones is carried out initially by ordering testing of T3 RIA, T4 RIA, T3 Resin Uptake, and TSH levels.

The development of radioimmunoassay techniques has increased the accuracy of hormone quantification and eliminated the errors with past techniques produced by exogenous iodine intake.[6] The concentrations of both primary circulating thyroid hormones, T3 (triiodothyronine) and T4 (thyroxin), can be measured to nanogram sensitivity. Both values are needed to identify those patients excreting excess T3 while maintaining normal T4 concentrations (T3 thyrotoxicosis).[7]

The T3 resin uptake value indicates unbound thyroxin binding globulin sites and is used, in conjunction with the serum T4 concentration, to indicate the level of bioavailable or "free" T4. This may be expressed as a "free thyroxin index" (FTI) which is the total T4 value multiplied by the T3 RU fraction. Alternatively, but less reliably, the free T4 may be determined by direct serum analysis.

Serum levels of thyroid stimulating hormone (TSH) may also be determined by radioimmunoassay. High circulating TSH levels indicate primary hypothyroidism or Hashimoto's thyroiditis.[8]

Should the above preliminary thyroid screening studies indicate a euthyroid state in the presence of dysthyroid ocular signs, the pituitary-thyroid axis must be evaluated. Up to two-thirds of patients with euthyroid Graves' disease will have a pituitary-thyroid axis that functions without regulatory feedback control of TSH secretion by circulating T3 and T4.[4] In the past, this deregulation was revealed by the Werner suppression test,[9] where oral intake of T3 over a seven-day period failed to significantly suppress subsequent radioactive iodine uptake. The thyrotropin releasing hormone (TRH) stimulation test yields the same information and is easier to perform.[10] Serum T3 levels are drawn at intervals following intravenous injection of TRH. Failure of the expected TSH rise 30 minutes after injection indicates abnormal hypothalamic-pituitary regulation of TSH secretion.

A small percentage of patients with dysthyroid ophthalmopathy will have normal systemic thyroid studies, including TRH testing.[11] The existence of this patient subpopulation underscores the need to treat dysthyroid ocular disease as an entity separate from systemic thyroid disease. Several observers have commented on the prevalence of dysthyroid ocular findings in Graves' patients who are hypothyroid following treatment with radioactive iodine.[12,13] In our clinical experience, control of the systemic thyroid state, including normalization of hormone levels, has no effect on the progression or stability of the dysthyroid ophthalmopathy.

Clinical Diagnosis of
Dysthyroid Ophthalmopathy

Dysthyroid ophthalmopathy may be found in almost any age group though it is uncommon in pediatric patients.[14,15] Individuals who present with mild ophthalmopathy usually pose more of a diagnostic rather than therapeutic problem. Periorbital swelling, conjunctival hyperemia, and lid abnormalities prompt patient presentation with a change in cosmetic appearance. Early lid retraction, often intermittent, must be differentiated from other causes of lid elevation, including dorsal midbrain syndromes and aberrant regeneration following third nerve paresis.[4] Dynamic evidence of lid dysfunction includes lid lag on downgaze (von Graefe's sign) and infrequent or incomplete blinking (Stellwag's sign). Poor tear film dispersion often leads to mild exposure keratopathy.

Dysthyroid orbitopathy characteristically is a disease of exacerbation followed by remission, with an initial congestive phase manifest by chemosis and orbital inflammation. During such congestive periods, extraocular movement may be affected resulting in diplopia primarily on an inflammatory basis. Most often, however, long-standing motility disorders are the result of an infiltrative process resulting in extraocular muscle dysfunction and enlargement.

A restrictive disorder is documented by forced duction testing. Following topical anesthesia with 10% cocaine or 4% lidocaine, the globe is grasped with toothed forceps near the insertion of the restricted muscle. As the patient attempts to look in a direction opposite this muscle, an attempt is made to rotate the globe into the field of gaze, often unsuccessfully. Free movement suggests a neuropathic process rather than a restrictive myopathy.

Extraocular muscle enlargement may be verified by ultrasonography[16-18] (Figure 3-1) and computed tomography[4,19-23] (Figures 3-2A, B). To successfully document dysthyroid disease, the ophthalmologist must maintain good communication with a neuroradiologist and obtain multiple thin section orbital images. In order of frequency, the muscles most often affected are the inferior rectus, medial rectus, superior rectus/levator complex and lateral rectus.[24]

The differential diagnosis of restrictive myopathy from extraocular muscle enlargement includes orbital myositis, contiguous sinus inflammation, and carotid cavernous fistula. Patients with orbital myositis experience much more pain and discomfort than those with thyroid ophthalmopathy. Individuals with sinusitis and contiguous orbital inflammation exhibit systemic signs of infection, pain with pressure over the involved sinus, and evidence of sinus inflammation on plain films and computed tomography. Additional findings with dural or carotid cavernous fistula include an audible bruit on clinical examination and dilatation of the superior ophthalmic vein demonstrable with ultrasound and computed tomography. On CT

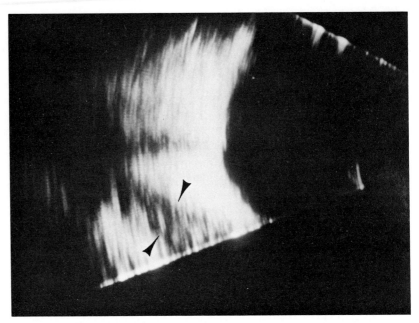

Figure 3-1. B-scan ultrasonography demonstrating an enlarged inferior rectus muscle (Arrows).

imaging, dysthyroid muscle enlargement usually spares the muscle tendons[25] as opposed to the diffuse enlargement of muscle and tendons seen in the other disorders.

Dysthyroid orbitopathy is the leading cause of unilateral and bilateral exophthalmos in adults.[26] Proptosis is a direct result of extraocular muscle enlargement and the swelling of orbital fat. Hertel exophthalmometry[27] remains the most reliable method of measuring the amount of forward displacement of the globes. Serial readings should be taken with the same base setting.

Increasing intraorbital pressure causes an increased resistance to manual retrodisplacement of the globe. When markedly enlarged extraocular mus-

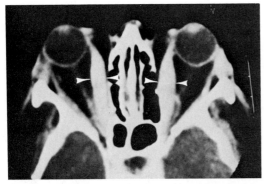

Figure 3-2A. Computerized tomography, axial projection, demonstrating bilaterally enlarged medial rectus muscles (Arrows).

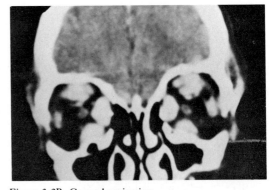

Figure 3-2B. Coronal projection.

cles play a major role in the exophthalmos and intraorbital pressure rise, a 3 mm or greater difference in intraocular pressure measurements may be seen comparing primary and upgaze.[28]

Proptosis and lid retraction can lead to severe corneal exposure and ulceration (Figure 3-3A, B). The keratitis is usually present over the inferior cornea, though central erosion may be present in advanced cases.

Compressive optic neuropathy, resulting most often from direct apical optic nerve pressure by muscle enlargement, constitutes the most severe form of dysthyroid disease threatening vision. The initial ocular exam of any patient with probable dysthyroid ophthalmopathy should include assessment of color vision, the relative pupillary responses, and visual field testing. While the most frequent abnormalities are central scotomata and inferior arcuate defects,[29,30] peripheral depression may also result in a location dependent upon the actual point of apical compression. On funduscopy the disc may be normal, edematous, or in neglected cases, atrophic.

The diagnosis is confirmed by demonstrating progressive visual field loss and extraocular muscle enlargement with ultrasound or computed tomography. In the absence of demonstrable apical muscle enlargement on computed tomography, other glaucomatous, inflammatory, or compressive etiologies for the optic nerve dysfunction should be sought.

Therapeutic Classification and Treatment

Werner first proposed the classification of the Eye Changes of Graves' Disease which comprehensively outlined the major findings in dysthyroid ophthalmopathy to the American Thyroid Association in 1969[31,32] (Figure 3-4). While this classification does provide a method for categorizing ocular involvement of increasing severity, it does not give the clinician a methodical approach to patient management. A similar but condensed classification (Figure 3-5) identifies five categories of clinical presentation to guide therapeutic intervention. The severity of disease within each category

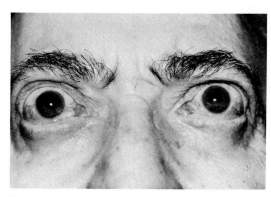

Figure 3-3A. Left inferior corneal exposure resulting from severe exophthalmos and lid retraction.

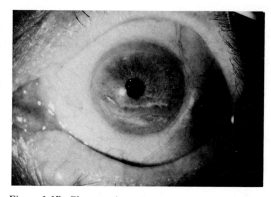

Figure 3-3B. Close-up, left eye.

ABRIDGED CLASSIFICATION OF EYE
CHANGES OF GRAVES' DISEASE

CLASS*	DEFINITION
0	No physical signs or symptoms
1	Only signs, no symptoms (signs limited to upper eyelid, retraction, stare & eyelid lag)
2	Soft tissue involvement (symptoms & signs)
3	Proptosis
4	Extraocular muscle involvement
5	Corneal involvement
6	Sight loss (optic nerve involvement)

*Each class usually, but not necessarily, includes the involvement indicated in the preceding classes.

Figure 3-4. Reprinted from Werner SC: Modification of the classification of the eye changes of Graves' disease. Am. J. Opthalmol. 83:725, 1977.

THERAPEUTIC CLASSIFICATION OF
DYSTHYROID OPHTHALMOPATHY

CATEGORY	TREATMENT
I. CONGESTION	LUBRICANTS STEROIDS
II. LID RETRACTION	LUBRICANTS LID SURGERY
III. MYOPATHY	PRISMS MUSCLE SURGERY
IV. EXOPHTHALMOS	STEROIDS ORBITAL DECOMPRESSION
V. OPTIC NEUROPATHY	STEROIDS RADIATION THERAPY ORBITAL DECOMPRESSION ANTIMETABOLITES

Figure 3-5.

varies and patients often present with several categories of involvement. Most individuals with soft signs of thyroid ophthalmopathy can simply be followed clinically at periodic intervals for the development of further disease. More severe ophthalmopathy is best managed using a treatment approach based upon the primary category of presentation.

Congestion. Patients with mild orbital congestion and symptoms suggestive of mild exposure keratopathy may benefit from ocular lubricants, even in the absence of corneal staining. For those that present with corneal erosion and proptosis without active infection during a congestive phase of ophthalmopathy, short-term treatment with prednisone at a daily dose of 80-100 mg decreases the inflammatory orbitopathy facilitating topical treatment. Topical corticosteroids should never be used in this disorder because they are ineffective and inhibit corneal healing leading to the possibility of corneal ulceration. Acute extraocular muscle dysfunction from severe orbital congestion also responds in the early phase to systemic corticosteroids.

Lid Retraction. Artificial tears delivered periodically while awake and ointment at bedtime relieve the symptoms of mild corneal exposure. Persistent keratopathy due to lid retraction is best handled surgically. Topical sympathetic inhibitors such as guanethidine,[33,34] bethanidine,[35] and thymoxamine[36] may temporarily lower the upper lid but provide equivocal long-term efficacy.

Lid surgery is directed at correcting retraction that has been clinically stable for at least 12 months, except in those cases where corneal healing is refractory to conservative management.[37-39] Restoring normal lid position provides corneal protection as well as cosmetic improvement (Figures 3-6A, B). Mueller's muscle resection, usually performed from a conjunctival approach, can lower the upper lid position by 1-2 mm. With 2 mm or more of retraction, levator recession[40,41] or myotomy[42,43] must be added. A marginal suture left in place through the upper lid and taped to the cheek will minimize postoperative contracture and lid elevation.

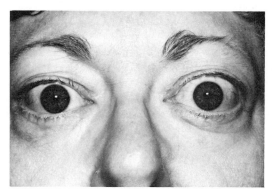

Figure 3-6A. Bilateral upper eyelid retraction.

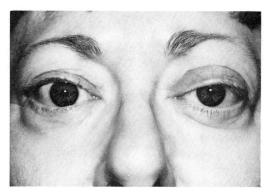

Figure 3-6B. Same patient following bilateral Mueller's muscle resection and left levator myotomy.

Advanced retraction of either upper or lower lids necessitates graft placement between the levator aponeurosis and tarsus or, in the case of the lower lid, between lower lid retractors and tarsus.[44] When eye bank sclera is used, a 50% postoperative shrinkage of the graft material is expected. Currently under clinical investigation, free upper to lower tarsal transplantation for lower lid retraction seems to be superior to exogenous grafting in our hands at this time. Sometimes, though less optimal, tarsorrhaphy may be required to adequately protect the cornea.

Myopathy. Dysthyroid myopathy frequently results in a stable horizontal or vertical motility disturbance following resolution of the congestive period of dysthyroid ocular disease. Restrictive myopathy causing diplopia in the primary and reading positions should be treated surgically only when the measured deviation has been constant for six months and there are no signs of active orbital congestion. Use of spectacle prisms may provide symptomatic relief for those patients with small angle deviations and the recent onset of a motility defect. As with most restrictive motility disorders, recession of the fibrotic muscle is the procedure of choice.[37,45-47] If intraoperative forced duction testing following recession reveals a significant residual restriction, a marginal myotomy can be done as part of the primary surgery. This approach results in satisfactory postoperative alignment with restoration of binocularity in up to two-thirds of select patients following one operation.[48] Alternatively, adjustable suture techniques hold promise for patients with lesser degrees of muscle fibrosis.[24,49]

Proptosis. Exophthalmos from acute orbital congestion may be temporarily decreased with high dose systemic corticosteroids. Individuals with exophthalmos of 25 mm or more and corneal exposure not controlled with more conservative means are candidates for orbital decompression. Decompressive surgery is also recommended for severe disfiguring proptosis leading to psychologic decompensation.[50]

A two-wall decompression involves partial removal of the medial orbital wall and floor. This may be accomplished either by a transantral (Ogura)[51,52] or anterior approach[53-56] and provides 3-7 mm of decompression. The three-wall decompression combines the anterior approaches above with a modified Kronlein lateral orbitotomy for decompression of the lateral wall.[57,58] This procedure provides 6-10 mm of globe retrodisplacement and allows for apical decompression under excellent surgical exposure. Patients with over 30 mm of proptosis may require partial resection of the orbital roof as well by a team comprised of both the orbital surgeon and neurosurgeon.[59,60] Adequate access for the four-wall decompression may be obtained through the combined lateral/anterior approaches providing up to 17 mm of decompression[50] (Figures 3-7A, B).

Optic Neuropathy. Treatment of dysthyroid optic neuropathy is directed at reduction of apical optic nerve compression by the enlarged extraocular muscles.[61] Fifty percent or more of patients with dysthyroid optic neuropathy will respond over the short term to high dose systemic corticosteroids at a daily dose of 80-100 mg.[29,62] At least partial recovery of

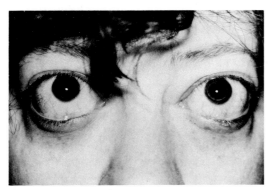

Figure 3-7A. Advanced thyroid exophthalmos.

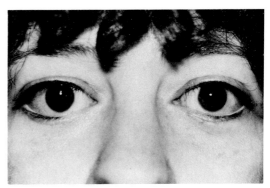

Figure 3-7B. Same patient following bilateral four-wall orbital decompression.

vision and field usually occurs within one week for steroid responders. Spontaneous remissions do occur, and a small number of individuals will maintain acuity and a full visual field while the steroid dose is tapered over a period of months.

Radiation therapy,[63,64] consisting of 1500 to 2000 rads of external beam irradiation delivered to the orbital apex, can be used effectively in patients with systemic contraindications for corticosteroids or those patients on high dose prednisone who rebound on a tapering dose schedule.[65] The full effect of radiation treatment may not be evidenced for several weeks after initiation of therapy, making this modality unsuitable for rapidly progressive compression.

Due to extraocular muscle enlargement located primarily in the posterior orbit, compressive optic neuropathy can occur without marked proptosis. Most of these patients may be adequately decompressed with a two-wall procedure. With greater exophthalmos a three- or four-wall decompression is indicated. Whichever procedure is employed, care must be taken to ensure decompression posteriorly to alleviate compression at the orbital apex.

Most patients respond favorably to decompressive surgery. Antimetabolites such as cyclophosphamide have been tried with some success in exceptional patients with concomitant systemic neoplasms or progressive disease after decompression.[66] Further investigation into the use of these drugs is warranted.

Summary

Dysthyroid ophthalmopathy is a disorder of unproven etiology characterized pathologically by round cell infiltration of orbital muscles and fat. Though the association of ocular findings with systemic thyroid disease is well established, the stability or progression of ophthalmopathy is independent of systemic disease control. Clinical findings include orbital and ocular congestion, lid retraction, extraocular muscle restriction/dysfunction, exophthalmos and compressive optic neuropathy.

A treatment oriented classification of dysthyroid orbital manifestations guides therapeutic intervention. Patients with mild orbital and ocular congestion require no specific intervention and are best simply followed. Severe congestive orbitopathy responds to short-term systemic corticosteroids. Lid retraction is amenable to a variety of surgical techniques, each designed to restore normal lid position, provide corneal protection, and improve the appearance of the patient. Dysthyroid myopathy and secondary diplopia are managed with spectacle prisms for small deviations and muscle surgery for more advanced motility deficits. The goal is binocular vision in the primary and reading positions. Orbital decompression is indicated for patients with proptosis of 25 mm or more than is markedly disfiguring or causes severe exposure keratopathy. The choice of surgical procedure is based upon the amount of globe retrodisplacement needed. Apical optic nerve compression is treated acutely with systemic steroids. External beam irradiation to the posterior orbit may satisfactorily decrease muscle enlargement to halt progressive optic neuropathy in some cases. Rapidly progressive loss of acuity and field refractory to systemic steroids is an indication for decompressive surgery. Care must be taken during surgery to adequately decompress the posterior orbit at the position of apical compression.

The ophthalmologist must take full responsibility for management of the ocular abnormalities in thyroid disease. Appropriate intervention is determined by the primary category of ophthalmopathy present.

References
1. Duke-Elder. Vol. XIII. p 935-938, St. Louis: Mosby 1974.
2. Kroll AJ, Kuwabara T: Dysthyroid ocular myopathy. Anatomy, histology and electron microscopy. *Arch Ophthalmol* 76:244, 1966.
3. Riley FC: Orbital pathology in Graves' disease. *Mayo Clin Proc* 47:975, 1972.
4. Sergott RC, Glaser JL: Graves' ophthalmopathy: a clinical and immunologic review. *Surv Ophthalmol* 26:1, 1981.
5. Sergott RC, Felberg NT, Savino PJ, Blizzard JJ, Schatz NJ: Graves' ophthalmopathy—immunologic parameters related to corticosteroid therapy. *Invest Ophthalmol Vis Sci* 20:173, 1981.
6. Fisher DA: Advances in the diagnosis of thyroid disease. I. *J Pediat* 82:1, 1973.
7. Marsden P, McKerron CG: Serum triiodothyronine concentration in the diagnosis of hyperthyroidism. *Clin Endocrinol* 4:183, 1975.
8. Fisher DA: Advances in the diagnosis of thyroid disease. II. *J Pediat* 82:187, 1973.
9. Werner SC, Spooner M: A new and simple test for hyperthyroidism employing L-triiodothyronine and the twenty-four hour I^{31} uptake method. *Bull NY Acad Med* 31:137, 1955.
10. Ormunton NJ, Alexander L, Evered DC, Clark F, Bird T, Appleton D, Hall R: Thyrotrophin response to thyrotrophin-releasing hormone in ophthalmic Graves' disease: correlation with other aspects of thyroid function, thyroid suppressibility and activity of eye signs. *Clin Endocrinol* 2:369, 1973.
11. Solomon DH, Chopra IJ, Chopra UC, Smith FJ: Identification of subgroups of euthyroid Graves' ophthalmopathy. *N Engl J Med* 296:181, 1977.
12. Almqvist S, Algvere P: Hypothyroidism in progressive ophthalmopathy of Graves' disease. *Acta Ophthalmol* 50:761, 1972.
13. Barbosa J, Wong E, Doe RP: Ophthalmopathy of Graves' disease: outcome after treatment with radioactive iodine, surgery or antithyroid drugs. *Arch Int Med* 130:111, 1972.
14. Young LA: Dysthyroid ophthalmopathy in children. *J Pediatr Ophthalmol Strab* 16:105, 1979.

15. Uretsky SH, Kennerdell JS, Gutai JP: Graves' ophthalmopathy in childhood and adolescence. *Arch Ophthalmol* 98:1963, 1980.
16. Werner SC, Coleman DJ, Franzen LA: Ultrasonographic evidence of consistent orbital involvement in Graves' disease. *N Engl J Med* 290:1447, 1974.
17. Mickler DS, Ogden C: Ultrasound in early thyroid ophthalmopathy. *Arch Ophthalmol* 98:277, 1980.
18. Coleman DJ, Jack RL, Franzen LA, Werner SC: High resolution B-scan ultrasonography of the orbit: eye changes of Graves' disease. *Arch Ophthalmol* 88:465, 1972.
19. Hilal SK, Trokel SL, Coleman DJ: High resolution computerized tomography and B-scan ultrasonography of the orbits. *Tr Am Acad Ophthalmol Otolaryngol* 81:607, 1976.
20. Hilal SK, Trokel SL: Computerized tomography of the orbits using thin sections. *Semin Roentgenol* 12:137, 1977.
21. Kennerdell JS, Maroon JC: CT scan appearance of dysthyroid orbital disease. *Ann Ophthalmol* 10:153, 1978.
22. Grove AS: Orbital disease: examination and diagnostic evaluation. *Ophthalmology* 86:854, 1979.
23. Trokel SL, Hilal SK: Recognition and differential diagnosis of enlarged extraocular muscles in computed tomography. *Am J Ophthalmol* 87:503, 1979.
24. Scott WE, Thalacker JA: Diagnosis and treatment of thyroid myopathy. *Ophthalmology* 88:493, 1981.
25. Trokel SL, Jakobiec FA: Correlation of CT scanning and pathologic features of ophthalmic Graves' disease. *Ophthalmology* 88:553, 1981.
26. Grove AS: Evaluation of exophthalmos. *N Engl J Med* 292:1005, 1975.
27. Tengroth B, Bogren H, Zackrisson U: Human exophthalmometry. *Acta Ophthalmol* 42:864, 1964.
28. Zappia RJ, Winkelman JZ, Gay AJ: Intraocular pressure changes in normal subjects and the adhesive muscle syndrome. *Am J Ophthalmol* 71:880, 1971.
29. Trobe JD, Glaser JS, Laflamme P: Dysthyroid optic neuropathy. *Arch Ophthalmol* 96:1199, 1978.
30. Trobe JL: Optic nerve involvement in dysthyroidism. *Ophthalmology* 88:488, 1981.
31. Werner SC: Classification of the eye changes of Graves' disease. *Am J Ophthalmol* 68:646, 1969.
32. Werner SC: Modification of the classification of the eye changes of Graves' disease. *Am J Ophthalmol* 83:725, 1977.
33. Gay AJ, Wolkstein MA: Topical guanethidine therapy for endocrine lid retraction. *Arch Ophthalmol* 76:364, 1966.
34. Millar GT: Guanethidine drops in thyroid eye disease. *Trans Ophthalmol Soc UK* 38:677, 1968.
35. Skinner SW, Miller JE: Permanent improvement of thyroid related upper eyelid retraction from bethanidine. *Am J Ophthalmol* 67:764, 1969.
36. Dixon RS, Anderson RL, Hatt MU: The use of thymoxamine in eyelid retraction. *Arch Ophthalmol* 97:2147, 1979.
37. Schimek RA: Surgical management of ocular complications of Graves' disease. *Arch Ophthalmol* 87:655, 1972.
38. Putterman AM, Urist M: Surgical treatment of upper eyelid retraction. *Arch Ophthalmol* 87:401, 1972.
39. Dixon R: The surgical management of thyroid-related upper eyelid retraction. *Ophthalmology* 89:52, 1982.
40. Putterman AM: Surgical treatment of thyroid-related upper eyelid retraction: graded Mueller's muscle excision and levator recession. *Ophthalmology* 88:507, 1981.
41. Harvey JT, Anderson RL: The aponeurotic approach to eyelid retraction. *Ophthalmology* 88:513, 1981.
42. Grove AS: Levator lengthening by marginal myotomy. *Arch Ophthalmol* 98:1433, 1980.
43. Grove AS: Upper eyelid retraction and Graves' disease. *Ophthalmology* 88:499, 1981.
44. Dryden RM, Soll DB: The use of scleral transplantation in cicatricial entropion and eyelid retraction. *Tr Am Acad Ophthalmol Otolaryngol* 83:669, 1977.
45. Dyer JA: Ocular muscle surgery in Graves' disease. *Tr Am Ophth Soc* 76:125, 1978.

46. Ellis FD: Strabismus surgery for endocrine ophthalmopathy. *Ophthalmology* 86:2059, 1978.
47. Sugar HS: Management of eye movement restriction (particularly vertical) in dysthyroid myopathy. *Ann Ophthalmol* 11:1305, 1979.
48. Evans D, Kennerdell JS: Extraocular muscle surgery for dysthyroid myopathy. *Am J Ophthalmol* 95:767, 1983.
49. Jampolsky A: Current techniques of adjustable strabismus surgery. *Am J Ophthalmol* 88:406, 1979.
50. Kennerdell JS, Maroon JC: An orbital decompression for severe dysthyroid exophthalmos. *Ophthalmology* 89:467, 1982.
51. Ogura JH, Thawley SE: Orbital decompression for exophthalmos. *Otolaryngol Clin North Am* 13:29, 1980.
52. Small RG, Meiring NL: A combined orbital and antral approach to surgical decompression of the orbit. *Ophthalmology* 88:542, 1981.
53. McCord CD, Moses JL: Exposure of the inferior orbit with fornix incision and lateral canthotomy. *Ophthal Surg* 10:53, 1979.
54. Leone CR, Bajandas FJ: Inferior orbital decompression for dysthyroid optic neuropathy. *Ophthalmology* 88:525, 1981.
55. Anderson RL, Linberg JV: Transorbital approach to decompression in Graves' disease. *Arch Ophthalmol* 99:120, 1981.
56. Linberg JV, Anderson RL: Transorbital decompression: indications and results. *Arch Ophthalmol* 99:113, 1981.
57. Trokel SL, Cooper WC: Orbital decompression, effect on motility and globe position. *Ophthalmology* 86:2064, 1979.
58. McCord CD: Orbital decompression for Grave's disease: exposure through lateral canthal and inferior fornix incision. *Ophthalmol* 88:533, 1981.
59. MacCarty CS, Kenefick TP, McConahey WM, Kearns TP: Ophthalmopathy of Graves' disease treated by removal of roof, lateral walls, and lateral sphenoid ridge: Review of 46 cases. *Mayo Clin Proc* 45:488, 1970.
60. Riley FC: Surgical management of ophthalmopathy in Graves' disease: transfrontal orbital decompression. *Mayo Clin Proc* 47:986, 1972.
61. Kennerdell JS, Rosenbaum AE, El-Hoshy MH: Apical optic nerve compression of dysthyroid optic neuropathy on computed tomography. *Arch Ophthalmol* 99:807, 1981.
62. Panzo GJ, Tomsak RL: A retrospective review of 26 cases of dysthyroid optic neuropathy. *Am J Ophthalmol* 96:190, 1983.
63. Donaldson SS, Bagshaw MA, Kriss JP: Supervoltage orbital radiotherapy for Graves' ophthalmopathy. *J Clin Endocrinol Metab* 37:276, 1973.
64. Ravin JG, Sisson JC, Knapp WT: Orbital radiation for the ocular changes of Graves' disease. *Am J Ophthalmol* 79:285, 1975.
65. Brennan MW, Leone CR, Janaki L: Radiation therapy for Graves' disease. *Am J Ophthalmol* 96:195, 1983.
66. Bigos ST, Nisula BC, Daniels GH, Eastman RC, Johnston HH, Kohler PO: Cyclophosphamide in the management of advanced Graves' ophthalmopathy: a preliminary report. *Ann Int Med* 90:921, 1979.

Chapter 4

Strabismus: Nonsurgical Treatment

Edward R. O'Malley, MD
Eugene M. Helveston, MD

STRABISMUS: NONSURGICAL TREATMENT

The goals of strabismus treatment are equal vision, ocular alignment and improved binocularity. For each case of strabismus there are sensory and motor obstacles which must be overcome.

The sensory defects include uncorrected refractive errors, suppression amblyopia, anomalous retinal correspondence and eccentric fixation. Motor obstacles to binocularity include orbital and extramuscular anatomic alterations, changes in the extraocular muscles which affect their ability to contract and relax, cranial nerve palsies, and overacting and underacting muscles.

Burian divided sensory-motor problems into the categories of "dynamic" and "static."[1] Dynamic processes such as the role of accommodative convergence or the presence of anomalous retinal correspondence are due to potentially reversible abnormalities in the relationship between the eye and the central nervous system. Static processes, muscle fibrosis or overacting muscle groups are anatomic alterations of the end organ.

Nonsurgical treatment is directed primarily to the sensory defects and the dynamic aspects of the motor misalignment. The prescription of plus lenses for accommodative esotropia may completely manage the motor misalignment. Occlusion therapy for amblyopia or orthoptic treatment of anomalous retinal correspondence addresses important sensory defects but usually has little effect on the angle of strabismus. Eye muscle surgery as an "orthopedic" exercise can be expected to alter static and anatomic abnormalities. It less predictably affects the dynamic innervational processes.

Surgical and nonsurgical treatment modalities often overlap in certain patients. Nonsurgical treatment sometimes serves a therapeutic and a diagnostic purpose. It can segregate into two groups those patients for whom surgery is inappropriate and those patients for whom surgery is indicated. For some patients however, "nonsurgical" actually is "pre-surgical" treatment of strabismus.

This chapter presents our personal approach to the nonsurgical modalities of strabismus treatment. Proper application of these techniques can eliminate the need for surgery in some patients and increase the chance of successful and enduring surgical results in others.

The Doctor-Parent Relationship

A child with strabismus is often brought to an ophthalmologist because his parents or his pediatrician notice an obvious misalignment. Correction of the visible defect may be foremost in the parents' minds and they may bring pressure on the ophthalmologist to "straighten the eyes" of their child. It is important at the first office consultation that the ophthalmologist and the parents share a common set of treatment goals. Parents can be therapeutic allies or adversaries. If they as primary caretakers of the patient are not extensions of the ophthalmologist, the young patient will be the loser.

One important goal in the treatment of strabismus is to make children appear cosmetically normal. Ocular misalignment can be an aesthetically disturbing defect and the ophthalmologist must identify with the parents' desire to normalize the eye position. Sadly, however, the eyes can be straightened and remain or become deeply amblyopic. Parents must be made to appreciate the sensory alterations which may be the cause or the result of the ocular misalignment. The ophthalmologist must educate them to these unseen forces which must be effectively countered in order to achieve a satisfactory result.

At the first office visit it is a good idea to present the parents with a prioritized list of treatment goals. The same list of goals will have to be repeated several times throughout the course of the treatment as the emphasis shifts from one goal to another. When a goal is identified, the short-term and long-term treatment plan must be stated as clearly as possible. The goals for children with strabismus are equal vision, straight eyes and the ability to use the eyes together.

Knowing how much to tell parents is basic to the art of medicine. It is learned by trial and error, and relearned and modified by successes and failures.

The ophthalmologist should make his explanations simple, logical, concise and sequential. It is useful when embarking on a given course of treatment to restate the goal and perhaps cite alternative treatments that might become necessary. This avoids "dropping a bomb" at a later date when more aggressive treatment is required.

Preprinted handouts can be a two-edged sword. On the one hand, they make it easier for the physician to dispense a great deal of information and for the parents to retain this information. On the other hand, they often bring forth a flood of questions which invariably are peripheral to the important issues at hand. Forms can be very useful and timesaving for specific purposes such as the administration of eye drops, teaching the E-game, or explaining certain general topics such as amblyopia or refractive errors. In some ways, the limitation of time and the frailty of memory insures that only important ideas will be communicated and, with repetition, that core concepts will be remembered.

In the nonsurgical treatment of strabismus, the single most important therapeutic consideration is parental cooperation. The ophthalmologist often asks parents to perform difficult and apparently unrewarding tasks. Compliance is unlikely unless the physician and the parents share the same resolve and set of goals.

Optical Correction

In the treatment of strabismus, the refractive error is corrected in order to provide a clear retinal image and to control accommodative convergence. The value of a precise refraction can not be overestimated. There are few procedures in medicine which carry such little risk and which promise so much benefit.

Refraction can be both diagnostic and therapeutic. A child with a sensory esotropia from unilateral high myopia will require treatment that is different from the undercorrected hyperope with refractive accommodative esotropia. The technique of refraction and the prescribing philosophy is quite different when comparing strabismic children to their normal adult parents. The ophthalologist who refracts young children must often rely entirely on his objective retinoscopy.

This demands that there be clear media, adequate cycloplegia, and that the retinoscopy be performed "on axis." With some experience, the examiner can detect qualities in the retinoscopic reflex which indicate residual accommodation or "off axis" measurement. Corneal irregularities and lenticular or vitreous opacities in children can be diagnosed quite easily with the retinoscopy.

Refractive Accommodative Esotropia

Refractive accommodative esotropia is an esodeviation that occurs as a natural result of the normal amount of the accommodative convergence which accompanies accommodation in uncorrected hyperopia. When the accommodative convergence exceeds the fusional divergence, esotropia occurs. In these cases, the accommodative convergence/accommodation (AC/A) ratio is said to be normal. Refractive accommodative esotropia has its peak occurrence between the ages of 2 and 3 in patients with moderate to high hyperopia in the range of +4.00 diopters or more. We have seen patients with pure accommodative esotropia having its onset as early as 1 year of age and as late as 7 years of age. "Mixed mechanism" or partially accommodative esotropia can be seen both in the older and younger age groups.

In pure refractive accommodative esotropia, the deviation may be intermittent, or in the case of a totally decompensated fusional mechanism, the deviation may be constant. These patients often report diplopia or they become clumsy or tentative in their childhood activities. In a very short time, the second image may be suppressed with either free alternation or suppression amblyopia setting in. The timely prescription of the full hyperopic refractive correction usually results in the realignment of the eyes and in equal binocular vision. Depending on how long the deviation was present prior to treatment or whether a small angle esotropia existed prior to the onset of the cosmetically obvious deviation determines the sensory result. If glasses are not provided soon enough or if the hyperopia is undercorrected, secondary sensory and anatomic changes occur which compromise the eventual result. If glasses are worn faithfully and strong fusional patterns are established early, good fusional results are possible. The most frequent mistakes that we observe are in the refractive undercorrection of patients with strabismus and amblyopia. This can be avoided by adhering to the aforementioned recommendations regarding refraction. It goes without saying that one should never underplus patients unless there is a compelling reason to do so. Children are extremely tolerant of their full cycloplegic refractive error.

Nonrefractive Accommodative Esotropia

The patient with nonrefractive accommodative esotropia is unique in that his typically low hyperopia or even myopia is combined with a high AC/A ratio. These patients have straight eyes or a moderate esotropia at distance fixation, with a much larger esotropia at near. Amblyopia is frequently present if the condition remains untreated. As with refractive accommodative esotropia, this condition ordinarily becomes evident in early childhood with a peak incidence between ages 2 and 3 years. The treatment consists of full correction for the distance refractive error, with the addition of bifocals for near (Figure 4-1). Ideally, one should prescribe as little bifocal as is required to give the patients a manageable phoria or a small angle esotropia at near fixation (Figure 4-2). In practice, however, this nearly always means the prescription of a +3.00 bifocal. Our choice is for an executive bifocal which bisects the pupil. The need for a bifocal segment at this height is obvious when one considers the needs of the pediatric

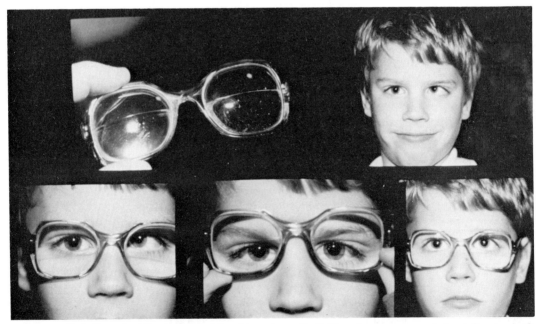

Figure 4-1A-E. A. Executive bifocal set at a height to bisect the pupils. B. Nonrefractive accommodatiave left esotropia. C. Persistent left esotropia while viewing a near target through the distance segment. D. Orthophoria at near fixation through the bifocal segments. E. Orthophoria at distance fixation through distance segments. This represents a good response to optical treatment.

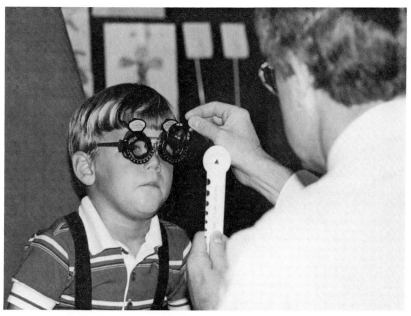

Figure 4-2. In attempting to determine the proper bifocal, alternate cover testing is performed at near fixation while increasing the strength of the optical aid. The use of Halberg clips over the patient's own glasses facilitates this process. Similarly, one can utilize minus lenses over a bifocal segment to assess the effect of reduction of bifocal strength on a given near deviation. This is particularly useful when attempting to wean older children out of bifocals.

patient. Unlike a presbyope who is bothered by blurred vision at near, the nonrefractive accommodative esotropic child is usually asymptomatic. The deviating eye is often suppressed and the patient enjoys good vision out of the fixating eye. One must therefore place the bifocal in a position that the patient cannot avoid. The ophthalmologist must explain to the patient in advance the reasons for these unusual appearing lenses. The parents can perform the important role of quality control inspector prior to accepting glasses from the optician. It is crucial that bifocal glasses be fitted properly in these children.

Refraction

The technique of refracting strabismic children is decidedly different from that employed with normal adults. In most cases the child in a darkened room will naturally look at the retinoscopic light. Provided the cycloplegia is adequate, this is the easiest and most accurate way of refracting. In the case of alternating strabismus it is a simple matter to select the eye to be refracted by occluding the fellow eye with the hand which is holding the trial lens. Refracting densely amblyopic eyes becomes a more difficult task, although it can be accomplished with patience and persistence. We recommend refracting with loose lenses and a battery-powered retinoscope. This gives the examiner the greatest mobility and increases the chances for an accurate refraction on a squirming child. It is easiest to rapidly identify the most plus and least plus meridians using spherical lenses. The axis of astigmatism can also be accurately determined with this method. The refraction can then be further refined with cylindrical lenses in a pediatric trial frame (Figures 4-3 and 4-4). Phoroptors are more of a hindrance than a help and should not be used with these young patients.

An automatic refractor which employs entirely objective techniques can be useful in pediatric practice. We have used successfully the NIDEK AR 3000 Refractor on pediatric patients for the past two years. With this instrument, we have obtained 90% agreement with retinoscopy done after cycloplegia in patients three years of age and older. The instrument will not give a reading if the refraction was done off axis or if excess movement on the part of the patient occurs. In patients without cycloplegia, retinoscopy was more likely to be reliable. Patients who continued to accommodate tended to experience excess "machine accommodation" when using the automatic refractor. Another advantage of the automatic refractor is that results obtained after examinations done by orthoptists and technicians were equally reliable to those done by the ophthalmologist.

Although the ophthalmologist rarely is involved in frame selection, it is a good idea to advise parents to choose a sensible frame, preferably plastic,

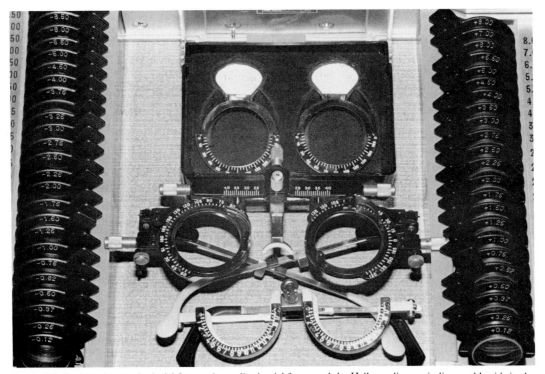

Figure 4-3. Besides the standard trial frame, the pediatric trial frame and the Halberg clips are indispensable aids in the refracting of children and patients with strabismus.

INSTRUCTIONS FOR ATROPINE REFRACTION

These drops are 1/2% Atropine. Keep them refrigerated. They permit accurate refraction (determination of need for glasses) and examination of the inside of the eye.

Some children react to these drops by becoming flushed and developing a fever. If the temperature rises above 100°F (oral), stop using the drops. If the child shows any reaction other than a flushing of the face, stop the drops.

These drops will cause the pupil to enlarge and may temporarily blur near vision. On bright days sun glasses may be helpful in reducing the glare caused by the large pupil; nothing need be done for the near blur.

PLACE DROPS AS FOLLOWS: (Important: Use only One Drop)

3 days prior to appointment: 1 drop right eye morning
                               1 drop left eye afternoon

2 days prior to appointment: 1 drop right eye morning
                               1 drop left eye afternoon

1 day prior to appointment: 1 drop right eye morning
                               1 drop left eye afternoon

Day of appointment: 1 drop right eye and left
                               eye together in morning
                               on awakening

These drops should be used only in the eyes of the person for whom they were prescribed. Nobody else should use them and they should be discarded after the above routine has been completed.

Like many common medicines such as aspirin, these drops can be extremely dangerous, possibly even fatal, to a small child if swallowed. Be sure to keep these drops out of the reach of all children. They are safe if used as directed.

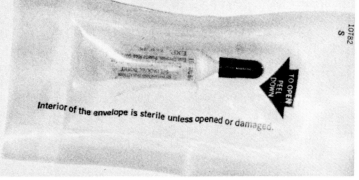

Figure 4-4. When an atropine refraction is desired, we provide our patients with a 1 ml dropperette of atropine ½% drops and a detailed instruction sheet for administration of the drops. Utilizing one drop of ½% atropine per eye per day has yielded excellent compliance and cycloplegia with rare pharmacologic adverse effects. Single dose dropperettes of atropine ½% are available through Cooper Vision Pharmaceuticals Inc.

with a lens size which is principally functional and secondarily fashionable. Polycarbonate lenses provide the best combination of safety, lightweight comfort and scratch resistance.

Pharmacologic Therapy

The pharmacologic agents which alter the relationship between accommodation and accommodative convergence have definite value in the treatment of some forms of esotropia. Providing a pharmacologic accommodative stimulus allows for less accommodative effort by the patient and consequently less accommodative convergence. Pilocarpine, eserine, and other short-acting parasympathomimetics are less convenient than the more popular longer-acting anticholinesterase agents echothiophate (phospholine iodide), and diisopropyl fluorophosphate (DFP). The anticholinesterase drugs exert their effect on the eye by interfering with the enzymatic inactivation of the parasympathetic neurotransmitter acetylcholine. Acetylcholine is inactivated by high concentrations of acetocholinesterase found at the synaptic cleft of the neuromuscular junction. This enzyme rapidly degrades acetylcholine which restores the membrane permeability to its resting state. Anticholinesterase drugs prevent inactivation of the neurotransmitter acetylcholine. This therefore causes a prolongation of the effect of the neurotransmitter.[2]

Anticholinesterase agents affect ciliary body and iris sphincter tone. The resultant miosis may provide a greater depth of field and this induced ciliary body spasm results in the reduction of accommodative effort needed to produce a given amount of accommodation, and a lowering of the accommodative convergence/accommodatio (AC/A) ratio. These drugs may be indicated as diagnostic agents to help identify the accommodative component in a given case of esotropia. Any pharmacologic reduction of the near deviation suggests that additional plus lenses will reduce the deviation at that fixation distance. This may result in the prescription of glasses. If there is no change in the angle of deviation but if an accommodative component is suspected glasses are prescribed anyway. Because this diagnostic test has the potential for false-negative results, we do not rely on a "trial of P.I. (phospholine iodide)."

Therapeutically, these drugs enjoy their widest use in the treatment of nonrefractive accommodative esotropia. Prolonged treatment is indicated if binocularity can be restored. If the drug reduces the near deviation to 10 prism diopters or less and at least peripheral fusion is maintained, we advocate continuation of the treatment. Partial reduction of the near deviation is of little or no value unless it is accompanied by improvement in binocular functions. The rationale for treatment is to create circumstances suitable for the development of fusion. Treatment can then be gradually tapered after the deviation has been converted from a tropia to a phoria.

The major advantage of topical pharmacologic treatment is that many patients can avoid expensive and cumbersome and cosmetically objectionable bifocal spectacles. The main disadvantages are the need for daily installation of drops in small children and adverse drug affects.

Anterior subcapsular cataract formation is associated with chronic anticholinesterase use in glaucomatous adults. This finding has not been confirmed in children. Likewise, canalicular concretions are an uncommon side-effect to this treatment. Iris cysts are by far the most common adverse drug effect and they occur frequently with prolonged treatment. These cysts are located in the iris pigment epithelium at the pupillary border. They consist of a proliferation of iris neuroepithelium containing large cystic spaces. These cysts can become so large as to totally occlude the pupil. Discontinuing the drug causes regression of the cysts, however it is common to see vestigial tags of redundant iris pigment epithelium years after treatment has been stopped.[3] The concurrent use of Phenylephrine 2½% drops reduces the incidence and severity of iris cysts.

The most serious complication of anticholinesterase agents is systemic poisoning. This can occur as a generalized parasympathetic crisis characterized by gastrointestinal distress, weakness and cold sweats. A more subtle form of poisoning is the occult depression of the endogenous cholinesterase system. This subtle abnormality becomes obvious only when the body is challenged by a neuromuscular relaxant such as succinylcholine. This drug is commonly used for endotracheal intubation during general anesthesia induction. If the endogenous cholinesterase system is depressed the effect of the succinylcholine blockage may endure for days. The resultant need for mechanical ventilation, pulmonary toilet, decubitus precautions, etc., illustrate the wisdom in discontinuing the use of anticholinesterase drops at least six weeks prior to anticipated general anesthesia. This potential complication should always be explained to parents whenever these drugs are prescribed. If a child requires emergency surgery for any reason, a forewarned anesthesiologist will simply choose a different induction method and avert a serious problem.

Our approach is to prescribe 0.06% echothiophate (phospholine iodide), one drop in each eye at bedtime. Some ophthalmologists prefer use of the drops in the morning to insure that the greatest therapeutic effect occurs during waking hours. The treatment is tapered by decreasing the frequency of the installation to every other day, every third day, etc. We use pharmacologic treatment for high AC/A esotropia as an adjunct to spectacle and surgical treatment. Occasionally we employ anticholinesterase drops on a long-term basis when spectacle or surgery are unmanageable or contraindicated.

Amblyopia

Amblyopia has been defined by von Noorden as "a unilateral or bilateral decrease of visual acuity caused by form deprivation, abnormal binocular interaction, or both, for which no organic cause can be detected by physical examination of the eye and which, in appropriate cases, is reversible by therapeutic means."[4]

The functional visual decrease which occurs in susceptible individuals is brought on by an extraneural stimulus such as cataract, astigmatism, uncorrected unilateral or bilateral refractive error, lid abnormalities, or strabismus. The decrease in vision results from unequal visual input leading to suppression during a critical state of development. The decreased vision usually persists even after the amblyopiagenic factor has been removed. In addition to the elimination of the factor causing the amblyopia, active antisuppression treatment must be carried out. Strabismic amblyopia can be treated successfully with or without straightening the eye.

The incidence of amblyopia is between 1 and 2% of the population. The variation in incidence results from variations in the definition of amblyopia. Because the potential increase liability to injury of the better eye, an amblyopic individual may find his employment opportunities are limited. If for no other reason than the socioeconomic importance of relatively equal visual acuity, amblyopia identification and treatment must be foremost in the minds of ophthalmologists who treat strabismus.

The extent of visual loss and amblyopia varies. Minimal loss as little as one or two lines may be easily reversible. On the other hand, functional amblyopia may produce a visual acuity loss of 20/400 or worse which may be difficult or impossible to reverse.

Strabismic amblyopia occurs in an individual with strabismus who habitually suppresses the same eye on a subconscious level in order to avoid diplopia. Cross fixation, that is the use of the left eye for right gaze and the right eye for left gaze, and free alternation usually coexist with some form of suppressions; however, because each eye is stimulated, amblyopia does not occur. Strabismic amblyopia results from an abnormal binocular interaction between the two eyes. Each eye views a different object in the environment and transmits this image to the occipital cortex. Only one image is the object of regard; the other object is suppressed in order to deal with the confusion and diplopia.

The diagnosis of amblyopia requires both the demonstration of a visual acuity loss and the absence of an organic cause. Visual acuity loss can be diagnosed from the objective evaluation of the fixation pattern of a preverbal infant. The more unsteady the fixation and the more preferred the fellow eye, the poorer is the vision in the nonpreferred eye. The further from the fovea that the nonpreferred eye fixates, the poorer will be the visual acuity. In some cases, however, amblyopia is present in spite of central fixation.

Full-line standardized visual acuity is the only accurate and reproducible method for determining vision in functional amblyopia. The "crowding phenomenon" may produce erroneously good visual acuity in an amblyopic eye due to the presentation of single optotypes, whereas presenting the amblyopic eye with a full-line of optotypes significantly decreases the acuity. Acuity in the amblyopic eye is also relatively better in reduced illumination. The neutral density filter test may be used to differentiate functional amblyopia from organic amblyopia. With filters of increasing density a normal eye or an eye with an organic visual defect will show a gradually reduced visual acuity response. On the other hand a functionally amblyopic eye will have vision that remains the same or is reduced less when compared with a normal eye.

A graded neutral density filter has been employed to produce change of fixation from the normal to the amblyopic eye. The visual acuity of the normal eye through the graded filter will probably be slightly less than the acuity of the amblyopic eye as it takes up fixation. This technique can be used as a rough estimate of acuity in an amblyopic eye in a preverbal child.

Amblyopia Treatment

In general, the younger the patient, the more rapidly he will develop amblyopia from any cause and the more rapidly he may be treated successfully by appropriate methods. If amblyopia remains untreated until after the age of 6 to 9 years, the visual defect may be irreversible. The precise cutoff age for susceptibility and treatment cannot be established with certainty. There may be individual variations of neurophysiology and there are, no doubt, many unknown factors which affect this condition. Similarly, the precise age of the onset of amblyopia cannot always be determined.

The single most effective treatment for amblyopia is occlusion of the preferred eye. This may be accomplished in a complete, incomplete, constant or intermittent fashion. Complete, constant occlusion with an opaque skin patch is the best treatment for dense amblyopia provided the amblyopiagenic stimulus has been removed (refractive errors, cataracts, etc.) or advisedly disregarded (strabismus requiring surgery).

With complete, constant occlusion, the nonpreferred eye is forced to become the fixating eye. In most cases, if treatment is instituted early enough, the functional vision defect can be reversed.

Patching Routine

When the diagnosis of strabismic amblyopia is made in children under the age of 1, treatment should begin as soon as the diagnosis is made. Depending on the depth of amblyopia, one should begin with constant complete occlusion of the preferred eye using an opaque skin patch. Depending on the age of the child and the ability to closely follow a patient, one can intermittently occlude the amblyopic eye to prevent the development of "patch amblyopia." von Noorden suggests that children under 1 year of age should have the preferred eye patched for three days and the amblyopic eye patched for one day as a beginning routine. He then suggests that the physician alter the intensity of occlusion therapy based on treatment response. The importance fact to realize is that severe patch amblyopia can develop in an infant and that during the patching routine, one eye should always remain patched to avoid recurrence of suppression.

When strabismic amblyopia is present in children older than 1 year of age, the preferred eye is patched constantly. The patient must then be followed at an interval appropriate for his age. A good rule of thumb is to follow-up total occlusion at an interval equal to one week per year of patient age. A 3-year-old child would be reexamined three weeks after full-time occlusion therapy is instituted.

Determining the end point of patching is simple when patching is successful and vision in the amblyopic eye returns to normal. In some cases, however, there will be improvement but not complete restoration of normal vision. If there is no improvement after three months of full-time occlusion, we do not expect patching or any other amblyopia treatment to be effective. Frequently a patient may have an initial visual acuity of 20/200 which can be improved to 20/40 with occlusion therapy. If there is no further improvement after three months of treatment then we would recommend stopping treatment. In the case of an older child, we would discontinue occlusion and reexamine him three months later. If the vision in the amblyopic eye has deteriorated then part-time patching would be reinstituted. It is relatively easy to regain former levels of vision with part-time patching. In a younger child with a definite fixation preference, we would recommend decreasing the duration of occlusion each day until one reaches the least amount required to maintain the best level of visual acuity.

A more difficult situation arises not uncommonly when a child is referred with a suspicion of amblyopia from a school screening examination. Often these children are 6 or 7 years of age and the prognosis is poor. Still, we believe that these children should be given a trial of occlusion to attempt to regain function in the amblyopic eye. Usually there is anisometropia or some other amblyopiagenic factor which requires attention. Again, if there is no improvement after three months of full-time treatment, none can be expected.

Penalization

Amblyopia may be treated successfully by providing the preferred eye with a blurred image and the amblyopic eye with a clear image. This is best done by fully atropinizing the preferred eye and withholding its hyperopic correction. At the same time the amblyopic eye is given the full distance correction and in some cases a bifocal to enhance the near visual acuity. In this instance, penalization is carried out in the preferred eye both for distance and for near. The effectiveness of penalization is enhanced if some hyperopia exists in the preferred eye. If the preferred eye is not hyperopic, a minus lens may be placed in front of this fully atropinized eye to accomplish distance penalization. This also enhances near penalization in the atropinized eye. Other more complicated schemes have been devised for penalization but they do not seem to add much to the picture of amblyopia treatment. Penalization seems to work best when acuity has been improved by other means to the 20/80 level or better.

A very simple test has been devised by Dr. David Guyton which fairly accurately predicts which patients will respond to penalization. Our variation on this test is to place one drop of Cyclogyl 1% (cyclopentolate) in the preferred eye followed by a second drop 10 minutes later. The patient is then examined 30 to 40 minutes after the second drop and his fixation pattern is assessed. If the patient prefers to fixate with the amblyopic eye, one is fairly safe in assuming that penalization treatment will be effective. On the other hand, if the patient still prefers to fixate with the eye which has accommodation paralyzed, penalization is likely to be less effective. If after prolonged cycloplegia the patient does not fixate with the amblyopic eye, penalization will be totally ineffective. In practice, however, some patients do switch fixation early in penalization treatment so that a negative response with Cyclogyl drops in the office may lead one to predict erroneously pessimistic results.

Partial Occlusion

On-glass spectacle occlusion may be carried out in a variety of ways. An opaque clip may be used over the lens. Scotch tape in the form of "Magic-Mending" tape may be used to frost the glass. Clear contact paper on the back of a spectacle lens will provide a cosmetically acceptable, clear-appearing pitted glass which blurs images. All these on-glass occlusion techniques have the same inherent weakness which is that the patient can easily look around the occluder if he wishes to see better. On-glass occlusion has few indications as patching can be fairly easily performed with proper motivation. Strip or segmental on-glass occlusion is an exercise in artistry and craftsmanship, however it has no place whatsoever in the treatment of amblyopia. Some more aggressive and risky maneuvers include a high plus or opaque contact lens for occlusion of the preferred eye. Some ophthalmologists have advocated a Frost suture in the lids of the preferred eye and others have suggested gluing the eyelashes together with tissue adhesive. This is analogous to protecting a cornfield with microwaves instead of using a scarecrow. We have never used any of these more aggressive modalities. Finally the black cloth pirate patch is preferred by many parents, probably because it is well tolerated by children. Unfortunately the ease with which patients can peek around this form of occluder renders it ineffective in most cases.

A variety of techniques have been employed to provide partial on-glass occlusion. Binasal occlusion, homonogous occlusion, strip occlusion, etc., have been suggested to treat suppression in strabismics as well as amblyopic patients. While these techniques have advocates, partial on-glass occlusion has not been shown to be an effective anti-amblyopia measure.

Twenty-four hour occlusion has some distinct advantages over patching that is conducted during "all waking hours." The first advantage is that the amblyopic eye is constantly occluded. The visual stimulation that occurs during the nonpatched time certainly is detrimental to the goals of aggressive treatment. Similarly, if a child expects to have a patch on "all the time," changing the patch becomes less of a "negotiations time" and the amount of patient fussing and fuming may be reduced.

A homemade eye patch (Figure 4-5) compares favorably to the store-

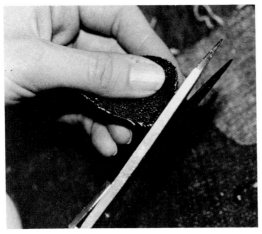

Figure 4-5A.

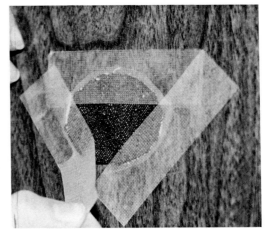

Figure 4-5B.

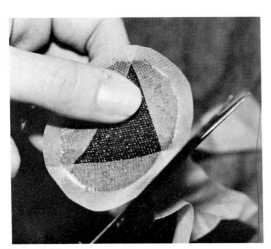

Figure 4-5C.

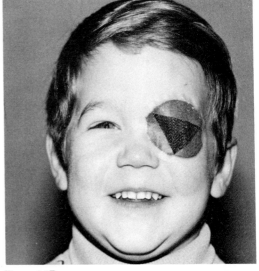

Figure 4-5D.

Figure 4-5A-D. The homemade eye patch. A. An oval of 100% cotton denim is cut with scissors. B. A triangle of hypoallergenic adhesive tape is applied to the denim on a counter-top. C. Excess adhesive is trimmed. D. A comfortable light-occlusive patch is shown in place.

bought variety. Besides being far less expensive, the homemade variety can be fabricated from better materials (cotton cloth, hypoallergenic tape, etc.) and can be varied in size and shape so that the skin which contacts the adhesive can be allowed to recover by changing the size and shape of the patch. In addition, this gets the parents slightly more involved in the regimen, which has some beneficial side-effects for compliance.

Pleoptics

Designed to reestablish the superiority of the fovea, pleoptics is the technique specifically applied to the treatment of eccentric fixation. Of course, eccentric fixation is always accompanied by amblyopia. With pleoptics the fovea is stimulated either actively by afterimages or passively by parafoveal dazzling. The treatment technique originated in Europe and was popular in the early 1950's. It has recently been determined that pleoptics offers no clear-cut advantage over standard occlusion techniques in the treatment of amblyopia with or without eccentric fixation. Inverse occlusion or occlusion of the amblyopic eye in order to reduce some of the adaptation that occurs in eccentric fixation is also probably of little value. A red filter placed before the amblyopic eye in cases of eccentric fixation likewise has little established value. If pleoptics has any value it is in the adult patient with long-standing amblyopia and eccentric fixation who loses his good eye. Perhaps pleoptics will in these instances hasten the recovery period of the amblyopic eye.

Orthoptics

As emphasized by vonNoorden, all nonsurgical therapies aimed to provide comfortable binocularity can be called "orthoptics." In this country, "orthoptics" generally refers to those activities supervised by a Certified Orthoptist. They usually include convergence exercises, fusional amplitude training and treatment designed to correct abnormal sensory adaptations to strabismus.

We regard the orthoptist as a member of the health care team which is directed by the physician. Often orthoptics is employed preoperatively to sensorially prepare patients for a new motor alignment. Postoperatively orthoptics can enhance the stability of surgical results. In successful cases, orthoptic training can convert a decompensated strabismus into a well compensated deviation. It is important however to remember that the patient still has strabismus, albeit better controlled.

Convergence insufficiency is usually best treated by means of orthoptics. First, we recommend "pencil push-ups" in which a patient fixates an accommodative target (an ordinary pencil with a star or face drawn on the eraser) while moving the target toward the bridge of the nose. The effect of this exercise can be increased by adding base-out prism against which the patient must converge. Conversely, base-in prism will make it possible for a patient with a remote near point of convergence to begin doing this exercise. When convergence tone improves, the base-in prism can be discarded and later reversed to base-out.

Deficient fusional amplitudes can be easily detected based on symptoms and by measuring the amount of prism against which a vergence can be maintained. Prescription of a loose prism or fresnel of a strength equal to the maximum vergence amplitude (the maximum prism still permitting fusion) for part-time wear results in the tonic stimulations of the deficient vergence. The amount of prism can be increased until normal fusional amplitudes are achieved and comfortable binocularity is possible.

The most frequent antisuppression method used in our practices is part-time occlusion therapy for intermittent exotropia. Patients with this condition typically experience no diplopia or confusion during the heterotopic phase of the deviation. Occlusion presumably allows the covered eye to be exotropic while depriving it of visual stimulation. While patched, suppression is rendered unnecessary and it can be eroded by judicious application of occlusion. With suppression reduced after occlusion is discontinued, the deviation is held in check by fusional amplitudes. Whatever the mechanism, part-time occlusion can sometimes result in improved control of intermittent exotropia.

Red filters have been employed as a therapeutic adjunct in amblyopia by forcing use of the fovea which has relinquished its normal dominance to extrafoveal retina. One combats the eccentric fixation by occluding the better eye and covering the amblyopic eye with a red filter. Because the highest concentration of cones is found in the fovea, specific tasks done through a red filter have the greatest theoretical possibility of "waking up" these suppressed receptors.

The number and variety of orthoptic therapeutic regimens is a reflection of the level of creativity of physicians and orthoptists who treat strabismic patients. Like all treatments however, orthoptics can be extremely helpful or grossly inappropriate. Convergence exercises can contribute to surgical overcorrections of exotropia and antisuppression can convert a comfortable nonfusing patient into a miserable diplopic one. The physician bears the ultimate responsibility for patient care and if he refers patients to orthoptists he must have an adequate understanding of orthoptic management. This decision must be subjected to the same risk-benefit analysis required for any therapy. Proper indications and reasonable expectations are prerequisites to having satisfied patients.

CAM Stimulator

In 1978 a group of investigators from Cambridge, England reported spectacular results with a new form of treatment of functional amblyopia. The treatment consisted of exposing the treated eye to a contrast grating which was rotated at one revolution per minute. The sessions were 7 minutes long and the patients received no treatment between sessions, which were as infrequent as once a week. This therapy is based on the theory that central nervous system cells respond best to stimulation of retinal receptors which are organized with specific spatial frequency and orientation. This new simple treatment of amblyopia resulted in 73% of their subjects achieving a visual acuity of 20/40 or better.[5]

Unfortunately, no other investigators were able to duplicate these results. A collaborative study was undertaken in the United States to investigate the efficacy of the CAM stimulator. This study concluded that the CAM stimulator did not work as advertised. We do not employ CAM stimulation as part of our amblyopia treatment.

Prisms

Sometimes the distinction between diagnosis and therapy becomes unclear. Such is the case when one discusses the use of prisms in strabismus. Clearly, the placement of a prism before a deviating eye during a cover test is diagnostic. Similarly, the therapeutic value of ground-in vertical prism to restore binocularity in a comitant hyperdeviation is obvious. A gray zone exists, however, when one uses membrane prisms to alter the sensory state prior to anticipated eye muscle surgery. Recognizing the duality of purpose of prisms, we will restrict our comments to their uses which primarily "make people better."

The introduction of membrane prisms by Woodward in 1965 provided ophthalmologists with the ability to create "prism orthotropia" and sensorially simulate any deviation desired (Figure 4-6). Theoretically, an esotropic patient could be given a sensory exotropia by spectacle correction of base-out prism in excess of his deviation. Suppression and anomalous retinal correspondence could be eliminated, thereby increasing the chances of sensory restoration after surgery. Likewise, strabismus and amblyopia could be managed with greater effectiveness by the use of these devices. In fact, press-on membrane prisms have been extremely useful, however experience has shown that they have significant limitations.

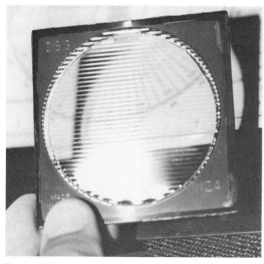

Figure 4-6A.

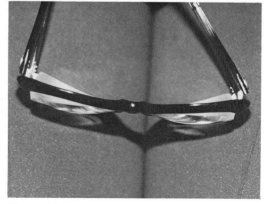

Figure 4-6B.

Figure 4-6A & B. A. A Fresnel membrane prism of 12 diopters. This can be easily applied to a pair of spectacles without increasing the weight of the glasses. B. 12 diopters base-out in each lens as a ground-in prism. The weight of these glasses was intolerable for this patient.

We use prism therapy as a substitute for and an adjunct to eye muscle surgery. In cases of small comitant deviations, the incorporation of prism into spectacles can provide patients with comfortable single binocular vision, thus avoiding the need for surgery. Comitant hyperdeviations are particularly receptive to prism therapy. Quite often these deviations are combined horizontal and vertical problems. In these cases, correcting the vertical deviation frees the patient to use his horizontal fusional amplitudes. The presence of significant incomitance or torsion are poor prognostic signs for the success of prism therapy. Fresnel-type membrane prisms have the advantage of modest cost, easy replaceability and lightness of weight. They are readily available in powers up to 30 prism diopters. Once it is determined that prism therapy is successful, the fresnel prism is discarded and the prismatic power is ground into the spectacles, usually divided between the two eyes.

Our most common use of prisms is in the postoperative period. Overcorrections and undercorrections can be effectively managed with the strategic use of press-on prisms. In the case of overcorrected exotropia, one can place base-out prism in front of the dominant eye to achieve fusion. The prism can then be reduced as the patient's functional amplitudes increase. Overcorrected esotropia with anticipated good fusion potential also responds well to prism therapy.

A particularly gratifying use of membrane prisms is in the management of sensory exotropia in adults following visual deprivation by cataract or corneal opacity. Following the cataract extraction or keratoplasty, the crossed diplopia can be eliminated with base-in prisms. It is surprising how rapidly these prisms can be reduced and eventually removed as the patient recovers former fusional ability. In cases of surgical undercorrection where the fusion drive is weak, press-on prisms generally add little to improve the eventual final alignment.

Intramuscular Injections

Direct injection of pharmacologic agents into extraocular muscles is an alternative to incisional surgery. Botulinum toxin injection of eye muscles, pioneered by Dr. Alan Scott and his associates at the Smith-Kettlewell Institute of Visual Sciences, is currently an investigational procedure used by us and by dozens of ophthalmologists worldwide.[6] It has become an accepted primary and adjunctive treatment modality for strabismus.

If one accepts the notion that all drugs are poison, depending on the dose, it is easier to counsel perfectly healthy patients to have an injection of a deadly toxin for what is essentially a benign disease. Botulinum A toxin (Oculinum) is a neuromuscular blocking agent which is injected into extraocular muscles under electromyographic (EMG) control in a dilution which delivers approximately one billionth of a gram of toxin. The tip of the needle records electrical activity in the muscle and the ophthalmologist guides the needle into the center of the muscle belly based on the amplified EMG signal. The procedure is performed under topical anesthesia and the entire treatment takes 5 to 10 minutes to perform (Figure 4-7).

The mechanism responsible for strabismus correction involves the creation of an iatrogenic temporary paralysis of a relatively overacting extraocular muscle. In the case of esotropia, the medial rectus is injected with Botulinum A toxin. Within a few days a medial rectus palsy is evident. The eye assumes a relatively exotropic position due to the unopposed action of the lateral rectus muscle. Stretching of the medial rectus and contracture of the lateral rectus occurs. As the effect of the injection diminishes, the paralyzed medial rectus muscle gradually recovers function. The lengthening of the muscle during the paralysis phase of the treatment combined with the contracture of the antagonist lateral rectus muscle accounts for the straightening effect on the eye.

The duration of paralysis depends upon the dose of Botulinum toxin injected. The dose is calculated based on the size of the ocular deviation. In general, a more prolonged period of weakness yields a greater amount of correction. For this reason, small to moderate angle strabismus is more likely to respond to a single injection. Repeat injections in larger doses are most often required for large angles of strabismus. The initial dose of Botulinum A toxin varies between 5×10^{-4} and 2×10^{-3} micrograms.

Dr. Scott estimates that 40% of his patients will be treated by a single injection with 40% requiring a second treatment. The remaining 20% will require a series of injections or will be treatment failures.

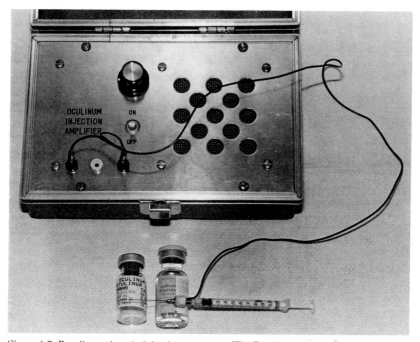

Figure 4-7. Botulinum A toxin injection apparatus. The Botulinum A toxin is supplied in the crystalline form for reconstitution with normal saline solution. The syringe containing the toxin is attached to the bipolar injection needle which is attached to the EMG amplifier. An audible signal is emitted when the needle tip comes in contact with recruited motor units.

Because a temporary overcorrection is desired, patients may experience uncomfortable diplopia until the injected muscle recovers function. Patching may be required for diplopia avoidance.

This technique is theoretically applicable to nearly all forms of strabismus. Vertical deviations are somewhat less well suited to this form of treatment since injection of the superior rectus muscle is associated with a disturbing although transient blepharoptosis. The inferior rectus muscle is technically more difficult to identify because the adjacent inferior oblique muscle also provides an electromyographic signal. To date there have been no complications arising from systemic absorption of the Botulinum A toxin.

Paretic strabismus is ideally suited to this technique. In the case of an abducens nerve palsy, one could inject the medial rectus and prevent its secondary contracture and subsequent esotropia. The treatment could be titrated according to the rate of recovery of the lateral rectus function.

We have successfully injected extraocular muscles of patients who had prior unsuccessful incisional surgery. A major limitation of this technique is that it affects muscle tone and has no direct effect on extramuscular mechanical factors such as fibrosis, scarring, and alterations in Tenon's capsule. Still, the alteration of the muscle forces has yielded surprisingly good results in these multiply operated individuals.

The ultimate application of Botulinum A toxin injection is in the primary treatment of childhood strabismus. The need for general anesthesia, the necessity of multiple injections and the lack of long-term follow-up are major drawbacks. One important unanswered question is whether pretreatment with Botulinum A toxin alters the effect of future incisional extraocular muscle surgery.

As more experience is gained with injection of pharmacologic agents into the extraocular muscles, the indications, methods, and expected results will become available to all ophthalmologists. The exact place of this technique in the armamentarium of the ophthalmologist who treats strabismus has yet to be determined.

Summary

The goals of strabismus treatment are equal vision, ocular alignment and improved binocularity. Surgical, nonsurgical, or both modalities may be necessary to achieve these goals. Uncorrected refractive errors must be recognized and corrected. Suppression amblyopia must be recognized and treated preoperatively. Orthoptics may convert a decompensated strabismus into a well compensated deviation and remains the best method for treatment of convergence insufficiency. Pre- and postoperative orthoptics can enhance the stability of the surgical result. Judicious use of both surgical and nonsurgical treatment modalities help both clinician and patient attain the goals of strabismus therapy.

(Editor)

References
1. Burian HM: Pathophysiology of exodeviations. In: Manley DR (ed): Symposium on horizontal ocular deviations. St. Louis: C.V. Mosby Co., 1971, p 119.
2. Havener WH: Ocular Pharmacology. St. Louis: C.V. Mosby Co., 1970, p 228.
3. ibid., p 241.
4. von Noorden GK: Binocular vision and ocular motility. St. Louis: C.V. Mosby Co., 1980, p 220.
5. Campbell FW et al: Preliminary results of a physiologically based treatment of amblyopia, Brit J Ophthal, 62(11):748-755, November 1978.
6. Scott AB: Botulinum toxin injection of eye muscles to correct strabismus. Trans Am Ophth Soc, 79:734-770, 1981.

Chapter 5

Diplopia and Cranial Nerve Palsies

James A. Rush, MD

DIPLOPIA AND CRANIAL NERVE PALSIES

Introduction

Patients with diplopia are among the most frequent referrals to neuro-ophthalmologists and constitute a large proportion of neuro-ophthalmic diagnosis. True neuro-ophthalmic double vision is characterized by being binocular and hence absent with either eye occluded. In contrast, monocular diplopia, caused by refractive aberrations due to corneal or lenticular disease, persists in the affected eye when the contralateral eye is occluded. This diplopia is monocular and may be bilateral, and is usually due to incipient cataract formation. It is never due to imbalance of the extraocular muscles or nerves serving them and will not be further discussed.

Diplopia due to neuro-ophthalmic causes can be conveniently classified into three categories according to cause: neural disease (palsy of cranial nerves III, IV, or VI), neuromuscular disease (myasthenia gravis), and myopathy (dysthyroid myopathy and others).

Palsy of Cranial Nerves III, IV, VI

The most common cause of diplopia is interference of normal function of cranial nerves III, IV, and VI. Three consecutive series analyzing the causes of involvement of these cranial nerves have been reported from the Mayo Clinic.[1-3] These reports indicate that paralysis of the sixth cranial nerve and consequent lateral rectus muscle dysfunction is consistently the most common cause of diplopia. Except for the small proportion of cases caused by intracranial aneurysm, the causes of sixth nerve palsies were fairly evenly distributed among the major categories of head trauma, neoplasm, vascular (hypertension, diabetes mellitus, atherosclerosis), and miscellaneous causes listed in Table 5-1.[3]

Of great interest was the finding that, even in the present CT scan era, most causes of paralysis of cranial nerves III, IV or VI remained elusive; approximately 25% of all cases remain undiagnosed.[3] It is important to remember that patients with paralysis of cranial nerve VI may have an underlying, otherwise clinically silent, intracranial neoplasm.[4] These patients should be referred to a neurologist for complete neurological examination and computed tomography, particularly if the sixth nerve paralysis is chronic.[4] Not all isolated chronic sixth nerve palsies are caused by intracranial neoplasm however,[5] but they remain a frequent cause of sixth cranial nerve involvement, more so than neoplasm-induced paralysis of cranial nerves III and IV.

Table 5-2 describes the causes of paralysis of cranial nerves III, IV and VI. It should be noted that head trauma is the most common single cause of

Table 5-1
Causes of Paralysis of the Sixth Cranial Nerve

N = 419

CAUSE	No. (%)
Undetermined	124 (29.6)
Head trauma	70 (26.7)
Neoplasm	61 (14.6)
Vascular*	74 (17.7)
Aneurysm†	15 (3.6)
Other	75 (17.9)
TOTAL	419 (100.0)

*Twenty-four patients had diabetes mellitus, 22 had hypertension, 9 had atherosclerosis, and 19 had more than one condition.

† Includes 11 cases of subarachnoid hemorrhage.

fourth cranial nerve palsy, aneurysms cause a much higher percentage of third cranial nerve palsies than fourth or sixth cranial nerve palsies, and neoplasms are responsible for a significant percentage of third and sixth nerve palsies.

The so-called vascular causes of cranial nerve palsy are those occurring usually in the elderly population who have a history of diabetes mellitus, hypertension, or systemic atherosclerosis. The mechanism in these cases is ischemia. It is fortunate for the patient who suffers from a "vascular" palsy that improvement is very common.[3] Symptomatic improvement is a useful clinical sign that the palsy is most likely not due to a structural intracranial lesion, either aneurysm or neoplasm. If clinical improvement does not occur within the first three to four weeks after the onset of a third, fourth or

Table 5-2
Causes of Paralysis of Cranial Nerves III, IV, or VI

	CN III	CN IV	CN VI
Undetermined	23%	36%	30%
Head trauma	16%	32%	17%
Neoplasm	12%	4%	15%
Vascular	21%	19%	18%
Aneurysm	14%	2%	4%
Other	14%	8%	18%

sixth nerve palsy, then neuroradiological investigation should be performed.

Diabetes mellitus is a frequent cause of paralysis of cranial nerves III, IV and VI, and all patients manifesting such a cranial nerve palsy should receive an oral glucose tolerance test. Diabetes mellitus is most often associated with paralysis of the third cranial nerve, but is nearly equally common in palsies of cranial nerve IV and VI.[3] If an oral glucose tolerance test shows signs of previously undiagnosed diabetes mellitus, then the patient can be safely observed for signs of improvement. Because diabetes mellitus does not protect against the unrelated development of intracranial neoplasm or aneurysm, neuroradiological testing should be performed if improvement does not begin within the first month after development of symptoms.

Because diabetes mellitus is such a common cause of neurological diplopia, it is worthwhile to review the clinical profile of a patient with a diabetic third nerve palsy. A classical third nerve palsy due to diabetes mellitus is typically painless, occurs acutely causing incomplete paralysis of all the extraocular muscles innervated by the third nerve, and spares the pupil. However, periorbital pain may occur in diabetic third nerve palsies[6] and, on rare occasions, partial pupillomotor palsy occurs.[6] Any papillary involvement should prompt further neuroradiologic studies including angiography. The pain of a diabetic third nerve palsy is short-lived and less intense than that caused by intracranial aneurysm, and the pupil is never "fixed and dilated" as is often the case with an intracranial aneurysm. Remission, either partial or complete, which usually begins within one month after the onset of symptoms, is usually complete three to four months later. It is important to know that a fasting blood sugar value may be normal in a patient who has a mildly abnormal glucose tolerance test. In such a patient the third cranial nerve palsy may be the initial manifestation of adult onset diabetes mellitus.

Diabetes mellitus is a less heralded cause of fourth cranial nerve palsy, but 5% of all fourth cranial nerve palsies are due to diabetes mellitus.[3] Hence, patients with a fourth nerve palsy and no obvious traumatic or congenital cause should have an oral glucose tolerance test. Similarly, an oral glucose tolerance test should be considered in patients having sixth cranial nerve palsies, although it is necessary to continually keep in mind that an abnormal glucose tolerance test may coexist in a patient with an underlying intracranial structural lesion that is responsible for the palsy. Careful observation for evidence of clinical improvement is particularly warranted in these patients. Any combination of III, IV, or VI cranial nerve palsies should prompt a vigorous neuroradiologic evaluation to rule out aneurysm or tumor.

Myasthenia Gravis

Myasthenia gravis is a disease affecting striated musculature, characterized by weakness and fatigability of voluntary muscles. The defect lies in the neuromuscular junction wherein postsynaptic receptor sites for the neurotransmitter acetylcholine are relatively unavailable for binding and effective muscular contraction. The etiology and pathogenesis of myasthenia gravis are still being elucidated, but it is becoming increasingly clear that the basic defect is autoimmune in origin. Circulating antibodies to receptor sites are present in the serum of many patients, indicating that myasthenia gravis is a disease of the immune system. Clinical and laboratory evidence for the concurrence of a variety of proven or suspected immune disorders, such as Hashimoto's thyroiditis,[7,8] thyrotoxicosis,[9] multiple sclerosis,[10,11] and systemic lupus erythematosus further suggest an autoimmune etiology for myasthenia gravis. Recently an increased percentage of circulating T-suppressor cells has been found in the peripheral blood, providing a possible explanation for the break in self-tolerance that production of the autoantibody to acetylcholine receptor sites implies.[12] Thymectomy has a role in treatment of both young[13] and old[14] patients, with or without thymomas, and strengthens the association of an autoimmune etiology. Recent evidence suggests that the HLA-B8 locus of the major histocompatibility complex is present in increased frequency in myasthenic patients.[15]

Since weakness of the extraocular muscles or eyelids is present at the onset of symptoms in up to 90% of patients[16] and is the only clinical sign in approximately 35% of patients,[17] the term ocular myasthenia is a useful appellation because it will heighten clinical suspicion by ophthalmologists and non-ophthalmologists alike. The diagnosis of ocular myasthenia should be suspected in any patient with a history of diplopia or blepharoptosis, occurring separately or in combination, with or without an established pattern of diurnal fatigue. A history of alternating ptosis is said to be pathognomonic of ocular myasthenia.[18]

Any combination of unilateral or bilateral involvement of levator palpebrae muscles or extraocular muscles, particularly if combined with orbicularis oculi muscle involvement, is virtually certain to be ocular myasthenia. The diagnosis can be verified with improvement in muscle strength of any one or combination of muscles following an intravenous injection of 10 mg Tensilon. Although false negative responses occasionally occur, the clinically suspect patient should receive subsequent testing after an initially negative result. Confirmatory clinical signs of ocular myasthenia are fatigue of the extraocular muscles on sustained lateral gaze[19] or continuously worsening blepharoptosis on sustained upgaze.[20] The so-called lid twitch sign, in which a ptotic upper eyelid momentarily twitches upward after the eye is moved from a position of downgaze to primary position, is highly suggestive of ocular myasthenia, occurring in about one-half of all patients, including those in whom blepharoptosis is the only clinical sign of disease.[21] Occasionally weakness of the superior oblique muscle causing vertical diplopia and a hypertropia, simulating a fourth nerve palsy, may be the initial sign of ocular myasthenia.[22]

If a clinical diagnosis of ocular myasthenia is made, a complete blood count, erythrocyte sedimentation rate, serum ANA assay, and thyroid function tests should be performed because of the increased incidence of lupus erythematosus and thyroid disease in myasthenic patients. Since thymomas occur in at least 8% of patients with myasthenia gravis, computed tomography of the anterior mediastinum is recommended for patients older than 40 years of age.[23] Because thymomas occur less frequently in younger patients, and because of the dramatic sensitivity of computed tomography in defining mediastinal masses which may merely be thymic hyperplasia, linear tomography in younger patients is recommended to complement computed tomography.[24]

Treatment of ocular myasthenia as well as systemic myasthenia gravis is best left to the neurologist who may administer Mestinon or prednisone, either alone or in combination. Alternate day oral corticosteroid therapy, beginning in small doses to avoid the possibility of inducing severe generalized weakness including respiratory paralysis, is effective in most patients with ocular myasthenia, resulting in stable remission in many.[19] Thymectomy has been proven to be effective therapy in myasthenia gravis among patients of all age groups,[25] but may be less effective among patients with juvenile myasthenia gravis.[13] Late onset myasthenia gravis, in which symptoms first occur in patients 55 years of age or older, has also been effectively treated with thymectomy.[14]

Extraocular Muscle Myopathy

Ophthalmoplegia due to direct involvement of the extraocular muscles is the least frequent cause of impaired ocular motility, and if bilaterally symmetrical (as in chronic progressive external ophthalmoplegia), diplopia may not even occur. Among the less common causes of myopathic disease are amyloid infiltration associated with multiple myeloma,[26] carcinoma metastatic to the extraocular muscles,[27] and idiopathic orbital inflammation with[28] or without[29] primary extraocular muscle infiltration.

By far the most common myopathic cause of acquired diplopia is that due to infiltration of the extraocular muscles consequent to thyroid disease. It is interesting that this dysthyroid myopathy can occur in patients with neither prior history of nor current clinical or laboratory evidence for thyroid gland dysfunction. Most commonly, however, there is a previous history of treated hyperthyroidism, which renders the patient either euthyroid or hypothyroid. Months to years following successful treatment, the patient is seen by the ophthalmologist for complaint of diplopia due to an infiltrative myopathy of obscure pathogenesis but of presumed autoimmune etiology.[30] Any or all the extraocular muscles in one or both orbits can be affected, but the usual clinical presentation of acquired diplopia in dysthyroid myopathy is due to selective or predominantly unilateral inferior rectus involvement. Although the medial recti muscles are a common foci of dysthyroid myopathy, their involvement tends to be bilateral, resulting in symmetric limitation of lateral gaze without diplopia.

Diagnosis of infiltrative inferior rectus myopathy is facilitated by other common features of dysthyroid ophthalmopathy such as proptosis, lid retraction, ocular injection, etc. These features are not always present in the patient who clinically has solitary inferior rectus muscle involvement.

In these cases a TRH test, in which abnormalities of the hypothalmic-pituitary-thyroid axis are demonstrated, may be necessary to secure the diagnosis.[31] Once the disease has stabilized and there are no further changes in the ocular muscle imbalance between orbits, then careful extraocular muscle surgery can be performed to ameliorate the diplopia.

Summary

Acquired diplopia is symptomatically a problem for the patient and diagnostically a challenge for the physician. Keeping in mind the three general categories of causes of acquired diplopia: neurologic, neuromuscular junction, and myopathic, the physician can systematically approach diagnosis and plan effective therapy.

References

1. Rucker CW: Paralysis of the third, fourth, and sixth cranial nerves. *Am J Ophthalmol* 46:787-794, 1958.
2. Rucker CW: The causes of paralysis of the third, fourth, and sixth cranial nerves. *Am J Ophthalmol* 61:1293-1298, 1966.
3. Rush JA, Younge BR: Paralysis of cranial nerves III, IV, and VI. *Arch Ophthalmol* 99:76-79, 1981.
4. Sakalas R, Harbison JW, Vines FS, et al: Chronic sixth nerve palsy. *Arch Ophthalmol* 93:186-190, 1975.
5. Savino PJ, Hilliker, JK, Casell GH, et al: Chronic sixth nerve palsies: Are they really harbingers of serious intracranial disease? *Arch Ophthalmol* 100:1442-1444, 1982.
6. Goldstein JE, Cogan DG: Diabetic ophthalmoplegia with special reference to the pupil. *Arch Ophthalmol* 64:592-600, 1969.
7. Krol TC: Myasthenia gravis, pernicious anemia, and Hashimoto's thyroiditis. *Arch Neurol* 36:594-595, 1979.
8. Osher RH, Smith JL: Ocular myasthenia gravis and Hashimoto's thyroiditis. *Am J Ophthalmol* 79:1038-1043, 1975.
9. Kiessling WR, Pflughaupt KW, Ricker K, et al: Thyroid function and circulating antithyroid antibodies in myasthenia gravis. *Neurology* 31:771-774, 1981.
10. Aita JF, Snyder DH, Reichl W: Myasthenia gravis and multiple sclerosis: An unusual combination of diseases. *Neurology* 72-75, 1974.
11. Achari AN, Trontelj JV, Campos RJ: Multiple sclerosis and myasthenia gravis: A case report with single fiber electromyography. *Neurology* 26:544-546, 1976.
12. Miller AE, Hudson J, Tindall RSA: Immune regulation in myasthenia gravis: Evidence for an increased suppressor T-cell population. *Ann Neurol* 12:341-347, 1982.
13. Snead OC, Benton JW, Dwyer D, et al: Juvenile myasthenia gravis. *Neurology* 30:732-739, 1980.
14. Olanow CW, Lane RJM, Roses AD: Thymectomy in late-onset myasthenia gravis. *Arch Neurol* 39:82-83, 1982.
15. Keesey J, Naiem F, Lindstrom J, et al: Acetylcholine receptor antibody titer and HLA-B8 antigen in myasthenia gravis. *Arch Neurol* 39:73-77, 1982.
16. Simpson JF, Westerberg MR, Magee, KR: Myasthenia gravis: An analysis of 295 cases. *Acta Neurol Scand* 42(S):23, 1966.
17. Bever CT, Aquino AV, Penn AS, et al: Prognosis of ocular myasthenia. *Ann Neurol* 14:516-519, 1983.
18. Daroff RB: Ocular myasthenia: diagnosis and therapy. *In:* Glaser J (ed): Neuro-ophthalmology, Hagerstown: Harper and Row, 1980.
19. Osher RH, Glaser JS: Myasthenic sustained gaze fatigue. *Am J Ophthalmol* 89:443-445, 1980.

20. Gorelick PB, Rosenberg M, Pagano RJ: Enhanced ptosis in myasthenia gravis. *Arch Neurol* 38:531, 1981.
21. Cogan DG: Myasthenia gravis. *Arch Ophthal* 74:217-221, 1965.
22. Rush JA, Shafrin F: Ocular myasthenia presenting as superior oblique weakness. *J Clin Neuro-ophthalmol* 2:125-127, 1982.
23. Fon GT, Bein ME, Mancuso AA, et al: Computed tomography of the anterior mediastinum in myasthenia gravis. *Radiology* 142:135-141, 1982.
24. Janssen RS, Kaye AD, Lisak RP, et al: Radiologic evaluation of the mediastinum in myasthenia gravis. *Neurology* 33:534-539, 1983.
25. Buckingham JM, Howard FM, Bernatz PE, et al: The value of thymectomy in myasthenia gravis: A computer-assisted matched study. *Ann Surg* 184:453-458, 1976.
26. Raflo GT, Farrell TA, Sioussat RS: Complete ophthalmoplegia secondary to amyloidosis associated with multiple myeloma. *Am J Ophthalmol* 92:221-224, 1981.
27. Divine RD, Anderson RL: Metastatic small cell carcinoma masquerading as orbital myositis. *Ophthalmic Surg* 13:483-487, 1981.
28. Weinstein GS, Dresner SC, Slamovitz TL, et al: Acute and subacute orbital myositis. *Am J Ophthalmol* 96:209-217, 1983.
29. Rush JA, Kennerdell JS, Donin JF: Acute periscleritis—a variant of idiopathic orbital inflammation. *Orbit* 1:221-230, 1982.
30. Sergott RC, Felberg NT, Savino PJ, et al: Graves' ophthalmopathy—immunologic parameters related to corticosteroid therapy. *Invest Ophthal Vis Sci* 20:173-182, 1981.
31. Rush JA, Older JJ: Graves' orbitopathy and the Thyrotropin-releasing hormone (TRH) test. *J Clin Neuro-ophthalmol* 1:219-224, 1981.

Section II

Ocular
Disorders

OCULAR DISORDERS

This section starts with a review of basic immunology and then applies these concepts to the evaluation and management of uveitis and external ocular diseases. Basic concepts of immunology are essential for understanding the pathogenesis of many ocular disorders as well as systemic diseases affecting the eye and adnexa. Webb and Friedlaender lead off this section with a review of general immunologic principles and their relationship to ocular diseases, especially uveitis. A practical approach to the diagnosis and treatment of uveitis concludes the chapter.

In the following chapter, Mondino details the diagnosis, pathogenesis and treatment of immunologic diseases of the cornea and conjunctiva. These may range from minor annoyances such as hay fever conjunctivitis to vision-threatening ocular pemphigoid and Mooren's ulcers. Understanding immunology facilitates the diagnosis and management of these disorders.

There is more to glaucoma control than laser trabeculoplasties and trabeculectomies. Medical management utilizes ocular hypotensive agents. Knowledge of their pharmacology, mode of action and side-effects facilitates the safe and appropriate treatment of the glaucoma patient. The chapter by Mosteller and Zimmerman accomplishes this as well as describes therapeutic regimens that encourage patient compliance. These principles will aid your medical management of glaucoma.

The final chapter reviews the diagnosis and treatment of retinal and choroidal diseases. Common disorders are emphasized, specifically: retinal artery and vein obstruction, diabetic retinopathy, preretinal macular gliosis and macular degeneration. Less common, but interesting, retinal disorders are also discussed in less detail.

(Editor)

Chapter 6

Immunology and Uveitis

Robert Webb, MD
Mitchell Friedlaender, MD

IMMUNOLOGY AND UVEITIS

Introduction

Immunology is undoubtedly the most rapidly growing field in all of medicine. A general working knowledge of immunology is extremely important to the ophthalmologist because an ever increasing number of ophthalmic diseases seem to have an immunologic basis. This is particularly true of uveitis, where advances in diagnosis and treatment have closely paralleled those in immunology.

This chapter reviews ocular immunology and uveitis, emphasizing certain important points for the practicing ophthalmologist.

(Editor)

Principles of General Immunology

Immunology is the study of immunity, a term derived from the Latin "immunis" meaning "free from burden." In one sense, immunity refers to the protection of the host from infection or reinfection by a microbial agent. The scope of immunity has been broadened, however, to include also the harmful or unpleasant effects resulting from the interaction of a foreign substance with the host's defenses.

The immune system has specificity. That is, it can recognize, in a highly selective way, those substances which it considers foreign. The immune system also has memory. It can, at some time after an initial exposure, interact quickly with a foreign substance it has already come in contact with. It also exhibits tolerance, the ability to tolerate its own components and to distinguish between "self" and "non-self."

Cell-Mediated and Humoral Immunity. Two different populations of small lymphocytes are known to exist, both derived from bone marrow stem cells. T lymphocytes are those that are under the influence of the thymus. They are responsible for cell-mediated immunity. T cells comprise 60-75% of all lymphocytes in the peripheral blood, spleen, and lymph nodes. A number of T lymphocyte "subsets" have been identified. The most important are the "helper" or "inducer" T cells and the "suppressor" T cells. These cells are important in the regulation of the immune response.

B lymphocytes comprise 20-30% of the lymphocytes and are dependent on the so-called bursa of Fabricius, a gut-associated lymphoid organ in birds. The equivalent in man is not definitely known but is probably in the bone marrow. B cells are responsible for antibody-mediated or humoral immunity. After stimulation by a foreign substance or antigen, B lymphocytes differentiate into plasma cells which produce antibody. Antibodies react specifically with the antigen that was responsible for their formation.

Most human T cells will form rosettes with sheep erythrocytes. B cells will not form rosettes unless the erythrocytes are first coated with antibody.

Antigens. In order for a molecule to immunize, it must appear foreign to the host. Although some smaller molecules may serve as antigens, larger molecules (with molecular weights over 10,000) are usually more antigenic. Antigens are generally proteins or combinations of proteins and polysaccharides.

Haptens are small molecules which induce an immune response only after combining with a protein. The hapten-protein complex may then function as a complete antigen and a specific immune response will be directed against the hapten or the hapten and carrier proteins.

Exogenous antigens are those which confront the host in the environment. They include microorganisms, drugs, airborne pollens, and pollutants. Antigens found within the host are known as endogenous antigens. Those antigens shared by phylogenetically unrelated species are known as heterologous antigens. Homologous antigens are genetically controlled determinants which are specific to a given species, and serve to differentiate one individual from another within that species. The histocompatibility antigens are examples of homologous antigens. Autologous antigens are the antigens of the host's own body constituents. These are usually recognized as "self" and will not normally induce an immune response. In autoimmune disease, these autologous antigens are in some way altered so that they appear foreign, and an immunological attack occurs on the host's own tissues.

Histocompatibility antigens are found on the surfaces of all nucleated cells. They form the basis for organ transplants and graft rejection. One system of histocompatibility antigens is known as the HLA system. It is determined by a series of four genes located on the short arm of chromosome 6. These gene loci are known as HLA-A, HLA-B, HLA-C, and HLA-D. In most transplant operations, an attempt is made to match the donor HLA antigens as closely as possible with those of the host. Certain HLA types have an increased frequency in certain diseases. The most important of these are HLA B27 (anterior uveitis, ankylosing spondylitis, Reiter's syndrome, psoriatic arthritis), HLA-B5 (Behcet's disease), HLA-BW22J (Vogt-Koyanagi-Harada disease), HLA-B7 (macular histoplasmosis), HLA-A29 (birdshot chorioretinopathy), and HLA-B8 (iridocyclitis in black Americans).

Antibodies. Antibodies are immunoglobulin, protein molecules produced by plasma cells. They have the ability to react specifically with the antigen responsible for their formation. In man, there are five known classes of antibodies, designated as IgG, IgA, IgM, IgD, and IgE. Each class has a specific chemical structure and biologic role.

All immunoglobulin molecules contain four polypeptide chains, two heavy chains and two light chains. There are five structurally distinct types of heavy chains, one for each class of immunoglobulin, but only two different types of light chain, known as kappa and lambda chains.

Heavy chains are attached to one another and to the light chains by disulfide bonds. Since there are five different kinds of heavy chains, and two different kinds of light chains, ten possible combinations of heavy and light chains may be found in any individual.

Antibody molecules are highly specific owing to the variations in the primary amino acid sequence at one end of the molecule. It is in this variable region that antigen binding occurs.

IgG. IgG, or immunoglobulin G, is the most abundant immunoglobulin in the serum, with a concentration of 1.0-1.4 g/100 ml. It is a symmetric structure having two heavy chains and two light chains joined together by disulfide bonds. IgG crosses the placenta, and is the main immunoglobulin that provides protection for the newborn infant during the first months of life. IgG accounts for most of the antibody directed against infectious agents.

IgA. IgA is the second most abundant class of immunoglobulin in the serum, having a concentration of 0.2-0.3 g/100 ml. It is important in the body's defense against viral infections, and is the principal immunoglobulin found in tears, saliva, nasal secretions and colostrum. In these external secretions, IgA is found in a dimeric form known as secretory IgA. The two components are bound together by a J chain and by a "secretory" or "T" piece. Secretory IgA is produced locally at mucosal surfaces. The secretory piece is synthesized by epithelial cells.

IgM. IgM is the largest of immunoglobulins, with a serum concentration of 0.04-0.15g/100 ml. It is restricted almost entirely to the intravascular space. IgM molecules contain five (5) monomeric units joined together by disulfide bonds in a pentameric structure.

IgM is an efficient agglutinator of particulate antigens such as red blood cells and bacteria.

IgD. This relatively unknown immunoglobulin is present in very low concentration in serum (approximately 0.003 g/100 ml), and is distributed mainly in the intravascular space. Its structure is similar to that of IgG. IgD has been found on the surfaces of human lymphocytes and may serve as some type of receptor for antigen. It is particularly prominent on the lymphocytes of newborn infants.

IgE. This immunoglobulin is present in trace amounts in the serum with concentrations in the range of 70 g/100 ml. It is structurally similar to IgG. Since IgE fixes to mast cells and basophils, it is known as homo-cytotropic or reaginic antibody. It is of great importance in patients with atopic allergy.

The Complement System.
The complement system consists of a number of serum proteins which react sequentially in antigen-antibody reactions and lead to cell lysis.

Activation of the complement system results in production of a number of pharmacologically active molecules. Some cause contraction of smooth muscle, increased vascular permeability, release of histamine, and chemotaxis of leukocytes.

The Ocular Immune Response

The events that occur when an antigen enters the body depend on a number of factors: the size and composition of the antigen, the portal of entry, and the body's previous exposure to the antigen. It is useful to view the immune process as having an afferent or sensitizing limb and an efferent or effector limb. The afferent limb is concerned with the uptake and processing of an antigen, the transfer of information to the lymphocytes, and the imprinting of information on the body's immune system. The efferent limb is concerned with responding to and eliminating the foreign material.

Upon repeat exposure to an antigen, the immune system produces a stronger and more rapid response. This secondary response, known as the anamnestic response, allows the immune system to respond in a quicker, stronger and more efficient way.

While the effector mechanisms are usually protective, they may respond in an exuberant way which is harmful to the host tissues. Such responses are known as hypersensitivity responses. There are four types of hypersensitivity responses[1]: Types 1, 2, and 3 are mediated by antibody (humoral immunity) and type 4 by sensitized lymphocytes (cell-mediated immunity).

Type I Hypersensitivity (Figure 6-1). IgE molecules attach to mast cells or basophils. When an antigen combines with cell-bound IgE, events are triggered at the cell surface which lead to the release of vasoactive substances contained in the cytoplasmic granules of the cell. These mediators produce dilation of small blood vessels, exudation of serum, smooth muscle constriction, and attraction of eosinophils.

A type 1 reaction in the skin or conjunctiva develops within seconds or minutes of antigen exposure. It is characterized clinically by erythema, edema, and itching. The conjunctiva becomes infiltrated by eosinophils which can be demonstrated in conjunctival scrapings.

A more generalized reaction may occur if antigen is introduced into the bloodstream. This response, known as anaphylaxis, is characterized by vascular collapse, falling body temperature, smooth muscle constriction, slow heart rate, and decreased serum complement. Death may result from circulatory collapse and respiratory distress.

There are several ocular disorders due to type 1 hypersensitivity mechanisms. These include allergic conjunctivitis associated with airborne pollens and animal dander, atopic keratoconjunctivitis seen in patients with atopic dermatitis, and vernal keratoconjunctivitis.

The first goal of therapy is avoidance of the offending allergen. If this is not possible, an attempt is made to desensitize an individual by repeated low dose injections of the offending substance.[2] The mechanism of desensitization is somewhat obscure. It may involve the production of blocking antibody, the consumption of IgE by repeated small doses of allergen, a decrease in IgE production (tolerance) or the production of nonspecific IgE that blocks effector cell receptors.

Drug therapy of allergic reactions is aimed at stabilizing the mast cell and preventing its degranulation, or blocking the target organ's receptors for histamine and other mediators. Disodium cromoglycate (cromolyn) stabilizes mast cells and prevents release of their mediators. Antihistamines block histamine receptors, thereby inhibiting histamine-induced vasodilation and smooth muscle constriction.

Type II Hypersensitivity (Figure 6-2). These reactions are cytotoxic or cytolytic reactions. Special antibody combines with cell membrane antigen (or antigens attached to the cell membrane) of a target cell. The antigen-antibody interaction causes target cell destruction by one or more mechanisms: (1) cell lysis or inactivation through the participation of

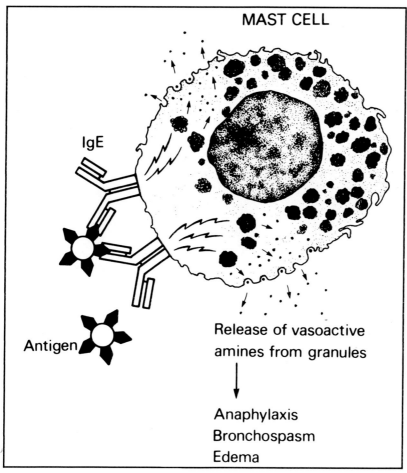

Figure 6-1. Type I hypersensitivity.

complement; (2) phagocytosis of target cells with or without the participation of complement; (3) inactivation or lysis of target cells in the presence of lymphoid cells (cell-dependent cytotoxicity).

Type II hypersensitivity reactions are important clinically in collagen-vascular and other autoimmune diseases, hematological disorders, and blood transfusion reactions. These mechanisms may also be important in cicatricial pemphigoid, in which a circulating antibody against basement membrane is found. Cytotoxic antibodies are also found in the serum of malignant melanoma patients. They may play a role in killing tumor cells.

Type III Hypersensitivity (Figure 6-3). When antigen combines with antibody, soluble antigen-antibody or immune complexes are formed. These circulating complexes can be deposited in tissues where they bind complement and create an inflammatory reaction.

Immune complex reactions are very important clinically. Microbial infections, malignancies, autoimmune diseases and drug reactions have been associated with immune complex tissue deposition. The Arthus reaction results from the deposition of antigen-antibody complexes in small blood vessels, leading to a vasculitis and local tissue inflammation. The reaction begins 1-2 hours after immune complex deposition, reaches a maximum intensity at 3-6 hours, and disappears after 10-12 hours. Histo-

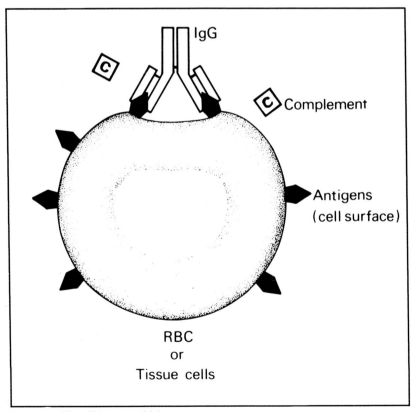

Figure 6-2. Type II hypersensitivity.

logically, neutrophils are the hallmark of the Arthus reaction, but they are replaced by mononuclear cells and eosinophils in later stages. The Arthus reaction provides an experimental model of immune complex deposition.

Serum sickness is a disease produced by immune complex formation. It is usually caused by injection of a foreign serum such as horse serum antitoxin. During the first phase, the serum level of antigen falls rapidly as the antigen equilibrates through the body. During the next phase the level of antigen declines because of the formation of immune complexes. When larger complexes are formed, they are deposited in tissues where they react with complement. Acute inflammatory lesions are produced at the site of deposition. The immune complexes are eventually removed by the reticuloendothelial system. By this stage, free antibody may be detected in the circulation.

Deposition of the immune complexes is influenced by their size and by properties of the affected tissues. For example, only relatively large complexes will be trapped in blood vessel walls and create a vasculitis.

Type IV Hypersensitivity (Figure 6-4). Also referred to as cell-mediated or cellular immunity, type 4 hypersensitivity is dependent on sensitized T lymphocytes rather than antibody. These reactions develop slowly, and reach their maximum intensity in 24-72 hours. The tuberculin reaction is the classic example of delayed hypersensitivity. We now know that cell-mediated immunity is important in the defense against many microbial agents, in tumor surveillance, transplant rejection, and contact allergy.

Delayed hypersensitivity reactions are characterized histologically by perivascular infiltration of mononuclear cells. Recently a specialized form of delayed hypersensitivity known as cutaneous basophil hypersensitivity has been studied in the skin and eye.[3] Both skin and corneal reactions

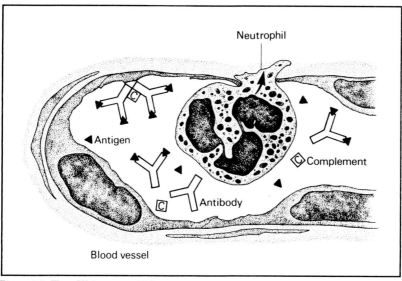

Figure 6-3. Type III hypersensitivity.

contain large numbers of basophils and eosinophils in addition to mono-nuclear cells. The cellular events that take place in a cell-mediated immune response depend on the release of certain mediators from lympho-cytes known as lymphokines. Lymphokines influence the behavior of other cells in the inflammatory response. For example, migration inhibition factor inhibits the migration of macrophages in vitro. Lymphokines that are chemotactic for neutrophils, monocytes, lymphocytes, eosinophils and basophils have also been demonstrated.

Cellular immune responses have considerable biological significance. The recovery from many viral, bacterial and fungal infections depends on an intact cellular immune system. If cellular immunity is suppressed by disease or therapy with immunosuppressive agents, an individual may develop an overwhelming infection. Allograft rejection, including the rejection of corneal transplants, is dependent on lymphocytes recognizing that the foreign graft is "non-self."

"Immunological surveillance," a host mechanism for detecting and eliminating potentially mutant cells, also seems to depend on the cellular immune system.

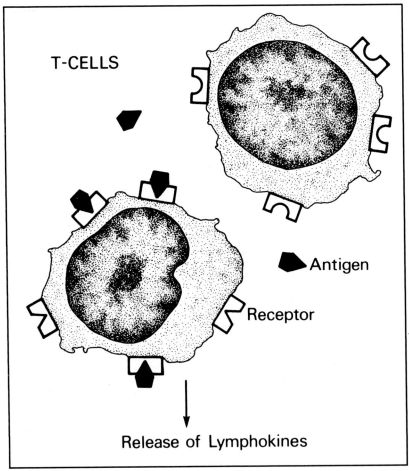

Figure 6-4. Type IV hypersensitivity.

Contact allergy is one of the unpleasant manifestations of cell-mediated immunity in which an individual reacts adversely to sensitizing substance. Contact sensitivity reactions usually are studied in the skin, but can be elicited in the eye as well. Many topical medications and their preservatives are excellent contact sensitizers. The treatment is the elimination of the offending antigen. Only rarely are steroids needed.

Uveitis

Uveitis is the term used to denote inflammation of the uveal tract, which consists of the iris, ciliary body and choroid. It is the field of ophthalmology that is most intimately associated with immunology. Recent advances in immunology have led to great advances in the diagnosis and treatment of the various uveitides. In the following section, a practical approach to the diagnosis and treatment of uveitis will be given, stressing the authors' personal preferences, with helpful, useful hints for the practicing ophthalmologist.

Uveitis History. A careful, thorough history is of paramount importance in evaluating a patient with uveitis. G. Richard O'Connor, M.D., an eminent authority in the field, believes that the history is by far the most important aspect in the diagnosis of uveitis.

History of Present Illness. The symptoms of the patient's uveitis give particular clues to its etiology. Pain, redness, and photophobia are the classical symptoms of acute anterior uveitis. There may or may not be an associated loss of vision. These acute symptoms are much less severe in chronic anterior uveitis, and in fact, may not be present at all. The patient may instead complain only of visual loss. Vitreous involvement is heralded by floating spots. When the retina and choroid are affected, there may be profound loss of vision sometimes accompanied by metamorphopsia and visual field defects. If the retinal periphery is affected, the patient may be totally asymptomatic. In such cases retinochoroiditis may be detected on a routine examination.

Past Medical History. Uveitis is often associated with systemic disease. Therefore, it is absolutely necessary to know what prior illness a patient has had, no matter how unimportant it may seem. This is especially true of prior infectious or inflammatory diseases. In many cases, a viral or flu-like syndrome will predate the attack of uveitis. Unless specifically asked for, a patient may ignore an important association between an infection and uveitis.

A detailed history of eye infections or inflammation, trauma, surgery and refractive error is mandatory. Special attention should be given to whether the previous condition was unilateral or bilateral.

Age, sex, and race are routinely recorded. The patient's sexual history should be discussed if an ocular manifestation of venereal disease is suspected. Intravenous drug abuse should be considered in certain forms of uveitis, such as Candida. Certain elements of the history should be discussed discretely with the patient, preferably with no one else in the room. Pets and exposure to animals should be noted especially if ocular toxoplasmosis or Toxocara are suspected.

Certain types of uveitis are found in specific areas of the country. Thus, a geographic history is important in diseases such as coccidiodomycosis (San Joaquin Valley), histoplasmosis (Missouri, Mississippi and Ohio River valleys), and sarcoidosis (Southeastern United States "Pine Tar Belt"). It is also important to know if the patient has traveled beyond the borders of the continental United States as there are a number of uveitides that are relatively rare in the United States but much more common elsewhere (i.e., leprosy, Behcet's syndrome, and certain parasitic diseases).

The dietary and nutritional habits of the patient should also be known. This is especially true when ruling out toxoplasma retinochoroiditis, as this disease entity is often associated with the ingestion of raw meat.

Family History. There are a number of uveitis entities in which hereditary factors have been implicated. This is especially true of conditions associated with certain HLA antigens. Of particular importance is a history of maternal infections such as toxoplasmosis, cytomegalovirus, or syphilis. Venereal disease serology is a helpful and often ignored part of the uveitis work-up.

Classification of Uveitis.
Much confusion has resulted from the many different classifications of uveitis.

A simple, yet inclusive approach used at the Uveitis Survey Unit of the Proctor Foundation and at Albany Medical Center Hospital is the "naming-meshing system," described by Smith and Nozik.[4]

In classifying uveitis, important points are gleaned from the history and physical examination. Then a "name" or "working diagnosis" is established. Uveitis may be acute or chronic; anterior, posterior, or diffuse; granulomatous or nongranulomatous; characterized by single or multiple attacks; stable or progressive; responsive or unresponsive to therapy; and having an insidious or a sudden onset. Thus, a "name" may carry many descriptive terms.

Example: a. chronic bilateral granulomatous iridocyclitis associated with pars planitis and retinal periphlebitis in a 23-year-old black male from Virginia.

In "meshing," one can match a "name" with a known uveitis entity. In the above example, sarcoid uveitis would be more likely than tuberculous uveitis. After "meshing," the "working diagnosis" is used to order laboratory tests and consultations tailored to fit the "working diagnosis." When all this information is assembled, a "final diagnosis" can usually be made. In the above example, if angiotensin converting enzyme (ACE) and serum lysozyme were elevated and a gallium scan and chest x-ray were consistent with sarcoid, a diagnosis of sarcoid uveitis could be made.

It goes without saying that a complete ophthalmological exam with dilated funduscopy and scleral depression is mandatory in any patient suspected of having uveitis. The following section will deal with those examination techniques and physical signs that should be particularly stressed in evaluating a patient with uveitis. The signs of uveitis will differ depending on which part of the uveal tract is affected.

Anterior Uveitis. The eye is diffusely injected and there may be a violaceous, perilimbal or ciliary flush. The ciliary flush is caused by involvement of the deep ciliary blood vessels.

The pupil is often miotic and may be poorly reactive to light if posterior synechia have formed. If the iris becomes adherent to the peripheral cornea (peripheral anterior synechia), the anterior chamber angle can become closed. In granulomatous uveitis, keratic precipitates may be large and greasy ("mutton fat"). In nongranulomatous uveitis, they may be small or medium in size. Pigment and fibrin "dusting" of the corneal endothelium and lens capsule may also be seen.

Anterior chamber "cell and flare" are a prominent feature of anterior uveitis. Flare and cells can be graded on a scale of 1-4+ using the short vertical and wide horizontal beam of the slit lamp.[5] Flare is caused by increased protein in the aqueous humor, and cells are inflammatory cells circulating through the anterior chamber.

The iris is often affected in uveitis, especially the granulomatous variety. Iris nodules are a hallmark of granulomatous anterior uveitis. Koeppe nodules occur at the pupillary margin. They may be clear or pigmented. Busacca nodules occur in the iris stroma and also may be clear or pigmented. Iris granulomas are much larger than either Koeppe or Busacca nodules. They may be seen at the pupillary margin or more peripherally and they are generally vascularized.

It is important to examine the substance and color of the iris in daylight as well as in the examining room. Heterochromia is an important diagnostic sign in Fuchs' heterochromic iridocyclitis. Iris atrophy and loss of iris crypts (due to edema) should be noted.

Pigment clumping on the anterior lens capsule may be a sign of previous posterior synechia. Lens opacities may be related either to inflammation or use of corticosteroids.

A severe anterior chamber reaction may lead to a hypopyon. Occasionally, a hyphema may be present, especially in herpes simplex and herpes zoster uveitis.

Intraocular pressure may be either high or low. In the early stages, pressure is often low because of decreased ciliary body secretion. As the inflammation persists, inflammatory cells and debris may block the trabecular meshwork and lead to glaucoma. If posterior synechia form, the pupil can become secluded, and an "iris bombé" can develop. The possibility of steroid-induced glaucoma should always be kept in mind.

Intermediate Uveitis. Cells in the anterior vitreous, which aggregate and gravitate inferiorly are referred to as "vitreous snowballs." They are usually associated with an inflammatory exudate or "snowbanking" at the pars plana of the ciliary body.

Posterior Uveitis. In posterior uveitis, the retina or choroid is the primary focus of involvement. When eye tissue is inflamed, the adjacent tissue may be secondarily affected. Vitreous cells may be present if inflammation is severe. A diffuse haze or aggregates of cells may be seen. A retinitis, choroiditis, or retinochoroiditis may either be focal or diffuse. Vasculitis may affect both the arterioles and venules. Hemorrhage, exudates and vascular "sheathing" may occur. Diffuse, retinal edema, or cystoid macular edema may be seen. Serous or traction retinal detachments are occasional complications of uveitis. Chorioretinal lesions become inactive and their borders may become pigmented with time. Bare sclera may be seen in the center of the lesion.

Laboratory Testing. Only after the history and physical examination has been completed and after the "naming-meshing" process has been performed, should laboratory testing be considered. A "shotgun" approach to laboratory investigation should never be used. It is expensive, wasteful, and time consuming, and most often unrewarding. A tailored, "bullet" laboratory approach, based on the results of the "naming-meshing" process, is much more effective.

Certain cases of uveitis are "relatively benign" and do not require laboratory investigation. These cases are generally unilateral, respond quickly to treatment, and do not recur. Uveitis following trauma, flu-like syndromes, and allergic reactions are in this category. They are almost always acute, anterior, nongranulomatous and very responsive to therapy. Cases which require laboratory investigation are often chronic and unresponsive to therapy. Recurrent and bilateral cases, granulomatous uveitis, and all cases of posterior uveitis, are good candidates for laboratory investigation.

Serologic Testing. Both the FTA-ABS and VDRL tests should be obtained in most cases of posterior uveitis. The VDRL test is an excellent indicator of disease activity, and a titer can be obtained. The FTA-ABS test is much more sensitive and specific. The VDRL test can be modified by antibiotic treatment. It becomes negative about six months after treatment. If syphilis is strongly suspected, the laboratory should be asked to report the test in undiluted serum since any positive titer is significant. The FTA-ABS test is not modified by prior treatment. Once it becomes positive it remains so for life. False positives may occur in systemic lupus erythematosus. If there is any question of a false positive or laboratory error these important tests should be repeated.

Tests for Toxoplasmosis. A number of tests are used to diagnose toxoplasmosis. They include the indirect fluorescent antibody test, precipitin test, agglutination test and the toxoplasma dye test. The dye test is now performed less often because it requires live toxoplasma organisms. The enzyme linked immunosorbent assay test (ELISA) is rapidly replacing the other tests for toxoplasmosis. It is as sensitive and as specific as the dye test. As with syphilis, any antibody titer is significant when considering a diagnosis of toxoplasmosis.

Of special significance is the issue of toxoplasmosis during pregnancy. This is important not only for women with a history of ocular toxoplasmosis but also for women who may acquire the disease during pregnancy. If a woman's dye test is positive before pregnancy, the fetus will be protected by maternal antibodies even if the mother has a reactivation of her ocular disease during pregnancy. If the dye test results are not known, a test for both IgG and IgM toxoplasma antibodies should be performed. IgM antibodies may indicate a newly acquired infection which could affect the fetus as often as 40% of the time.

Additional Tests. Radiographic studies, ultrasonography, fluorescein angiography, CT scanning, electrophysiologic testing, and visual field examinations may be performed when indicated.

Anterior chamber and vitreous aspirations and uveal tissue biopsies are occasionally performed. They should be reserved only for diagnostic dilemmas and/or therapeutic failures.

Consultations.
Selective consultations for certain uveitis patients are often valuable. The ophthalmologist should guide the consultant in a specific direction and should provide as much information about the patient as possible. The ophthalmologist should never lose control of the patient or transfer the patient to an internist or general practitioner.

Surgery in the Uveitis Patient.
It is beyond the scope of this chapter to discuss surgical principles and techniques. However certain guidelines should be followed when considering surgery in patients with uveitis. Inflammation should be as well-controlled as possible. If surgery is urgent, as it may be in secondary glaucoma and lens-induced uveitis, corticosteroids should be used judiciously to minimize postoperative inflammation. Such inflammation is almost always more severe than in non-uveitis patients. For medical-legal reasons, the patient should always be warned of the greater surgical risk and the possibility of increased postoperative inflammation.

Medical Treatment of Uveitis

Mydriatic-cycloplegic drugs. During the acute stages of uveitis, when pain and photophobia are severe and the pupil is miotic, 1% atropine drops can be given every twelve hours. The duration of action is much less in the acutely inflamed eye than in the normal eye. Atropine dilates the pupil, relieves ciliary spasm, decreases the production of aqueous humor by the ciliary body and prevents formation of posterior synechia. The combined effect is a dramatic relief of symptoms. The patient can then be placed on a short acting mydriatic/cycloplegic drop to keep the pupil moving and prevent permanent mydriasis and synechiae. Homatropine 5% one to four times daily is useful for this purpose.

When synechiae formation is already present, an attempt should be made to lyse them as soon as possible. If frequent dilating drops are unsuccessful, a pledget soaked in Neo-Synephrine, tropicamide or cocaine should be placed in the cul-de-sac adjacent to the synechia. This treatment may not appear to be effective initially, but after 24 hours, an effect may be obvious. If this regimen is still unsuccessful, a subconjunctival injection of "blasting mixture" may be given adjacent to the synechia. A mixture containing equal parts of cocaine 4-10%, atropine 1-4% and epinephrine 1:1000 is very effective. The solution should be freshly made under sterile conditions. No more than .25 ml is usually necessary. The patient's vital signs should be observed in order to monitor any systemic effect of the drugs.

Corticosteroids. In the management of patients with uveitis, steroids are particularly useful for their anti-inflammatory and immunosuppressive effects. But because they are potent agents with significant local and systemic side-effects, they should be used with caution. The ophthalmologist should be quick to recognize and deal with these side-effects.

The actions of corticosteroids are of two types: 1) their effect on the traffic, circulation, and availability of cells in various sites or compartments of the body, and 2) their effect on the function of cells.

After a single large dose of corticosteroids, a transient reduction of blood lymphocytes occurs. A maximal effect is seen in 4-6 hours. While T and B lymphocytes are both reduced, T cell reduction is considerably greater. The lymphopenia is not the result of cell lysis, but rather a redistribution of blood lymphocytes. T cells may be temporarily sequestered in the bone marrow.[6] Blood lymphocytes return to normal in about 24 hours.

Corticosteroids also affect the distribution of other leukocytes. There is a temporary increase in neutrophils 4-6 hours after steroids are given.[7] This granulocytosis is due to two factors: increased release of cells from the bone marrow, and reduced granulocyte adherence to vascular endothelium.[8] Steroids also induce eosinopenia and monocytopenia by redistributing cells.[9]

The exact mechanism by which corticosteroids alter the circulation of leukocytes still is unclear. They may affect the endothelium of small vessels, creating a change in the cells passing through these vessels. There is also reason to believe that steroids alter the lymphocyte surface in some way that redistributes the cells in other body compartments.[9]

In vitro studies have shown that in very high concentrations, steroids suppress phagocytosis and antibacterial activity of neutrophils. They also may reduce inflammation and fever by stabilizing granulocyte lysosomes and reducing leukocyte pyrogen production. In addition to stabilizing lysosomes, steroids inhibit allergic reaction by stabilizing the intracellular membranes of mast cells and basophils. This stabilization prevents the release of vasoactive mediators and decreases the inflammatory response.

The effect of steroids on antibody production is not yet completely defined. These agents produce a modest decrease in serum immunoglobulin concentrations, mainly IgG. This may be due to inhibition of IgG synthesis or to increased immunoglobulin metabolism.

Steroids are known to impair cell-mediated immune responses, and several mechanisms have been postulated to explain this phenomenon. Steroids seem to inhibit the migration of T cells to sites of antigen deposition. They also prevent lymphocytes from releasing lymphokines, which are needed to recruit additional cells that can participate in inflammation. Steroids interfere with lymphocyte-induced target cell lysis and reduce the number of monocytes available to participate in such responses. In addition, they block the local interaction between the lymphocyte and the monocyte. Inhibition of cell-mediated immunity can lead to overwhelming infection by opportunistic organisms that normally are controlled by cell-mediated immunity.

Corticosteroid Side-effects.

Ocular

- Posterior subcapsular cataract—depends on the amount and duration of therapy
- Increased intraocular pressure—occurs in susceptible individuals after prolonged topical or periocular therapy. It may take three to four weeks to develop and is usually reversible on cessation of treatment.
- Infection—secondary bacterial, viral and fungal infections have been reported but are rare.
- Mydriasis and ptosis—following topical administration may be caused by preservatives.

Systemic

- Cushing's syndrome
- Peptic ulcer
- Osteoporosis
- Electrolyte imbalance
- Mental changes
- Exacerbation of diabetes and hypertension
- Infection, particularly reactivation of tuberculosis
- Adrenal suppression
- Hyperglycemic non-ketotic coma

Corticosteroid Mode of Delivery. The effectiveness of a given preparation depends on its penetration into the eye. This is determined by the lipid and water solubility of the drugs. Compounds which are both lipid and water soluble (biphasic) are preferred because they penetrate both corneal epithelium (lipophilic) and stroma (hydrophilic). Prednisolone acetate 1%, a biphasic suspension, remains the topical drug of choice in anterior uveitis. It is important to instruct the patient to shake the bottle approximately 30 times before instillation to fully suspend the drug. It must be remembered that topically applied drugs do not penetrate to the posterior part of the eye in high enough concentrations to be effective in treating posterior uveitis.

It would be unrealistic to expect a patient to instill a drop of medication more than once per hour without hospitalization. Therefore, with compliance in mind, a regimen of one drop of 1% prednisolone acetate every hour while awake is the most realistic regimen for acute anterior uveitis. As the inflammatory reaction improves, the medication is slowly tapered over 2-3 weeks until the reaction has completely subsided. In cases of chronic anterior uveitis, long-term maintenance doses of topical steroids may be necessary to control inflammation. Each patient's dose must be individualized.

Periocular injections of corticosteroids can provide a sustained anti-inflammatory effect for as long as four weeks. The anterior and posterior sub-Tenon's root of administration may be used depending on the location of pathology. Aqueous Kenalog (triamcinolone acetonide) 40 mg/ml is a useful agent. This may be injected through a 25 or 27 gauge 5/8 inch needle after topical application of 4-10% cocaine or 4% Xylocaine at the injection site. The bevel of the needle should be directed toward the globe at all times to minimize the possibility of perforating the eye.

Repository injection of steroids may be used in a noncompliant patient, or when uveitis fails to respond to topically-applied preparations. Except in rare circumstances, they should not be used until an infectious cause of uveitis has been ruled out.

Prednisone is the oral preparation of choice for treating uveitis. Systemic steroids are rarely used in the treatment of anterior uveitis but are highly effective in treating posterior uveitis. It still remains the least favorable method of administration because of their many side-effects. Systemic corticosteroids are used only when other, more targeted forms of steroid therapy have proven unsuitable.

There is some controversy over the proper way to administer oral corticosteroids. In order to provide a prolonged, sustained effect, we begin therapy with 80-100 mg of prednisone in four equally divided doses. We then slowly taper the medication over three to four weeks. If continued steroid use is necessary, the patient may take the prescribed dose once a day or once every other day. These schedules minimize systemic side-effects without diminishing the anti-inflammatory effects of the drug. When inflammation is under control, medication should be tapered to the lowest possible level.

When systemic steroids are used, it is sound medical practice to have the patient seen by an internist or family practitioner on a regular basis.

Immunosuppressive Agents—Nonsteroidal. These potent, cytotoxic drugs are useful in certain forms of uveitis (i.e., Behcet's syndrome) but should be reserved for severe cases that have not responded to routine therapy. They should be reserved for those types of uveitis which are known to respond to these agents. Patients receiving immunosuppressive agents should be followed by their ophthalmologist and an internist skilled in their use.

Other Agents. Anti-prostaglandin agents such as aspirin, indomethacine, phenylbutazone and oxyphenbutazone have been widely used in the treatment of uveitis. Unfortunately, the effects are minimal in most cases. They are much more effective in the treatment of scleritis and may have some effect on cystoid macular edema.

Other Treatment Guidelines. When uveitis is associated with a systemic disease, treatment of the systemic disease will often lead to improvement of the ocular component. Therefore, every attempt should be made to recognize and treat any systemic disease which accompanies uveitis.

Secondary glaucoma should be recognized and treated immediately. Pilocarpine and related compounds which constrict the pupil should be avoided since they will aggravate the signs and symptoms of uveitis. Timoptic, propine, epinephrine and carbonic anhydrase inhibitors are useful in controlling the pressure of uveitis patients.

Summary

Basic concepts of immunology, hypersensitivity reactions and their clinical implications are reviewed for the ophthalmologist.

This background elucidates the diagnosis and management of uveitis, the area of ophthalmology most intimately associated with immunology.

The importance of history in evaluating the uveitis patient is paramount. Associated diseases, i.e., syphilis, tuberculosis and ankylosing spondylitis, are examples. The uveitides are then classified, confusion being somewhat obviated by the "naming-meshing system." Appropriate laboratory and ancillary studies should be obtained as indicated. Treatment is reviewed in detail with appropriate emphasis on the use, mode of administration and side-effects of corticosteroids. The ophthalmologist should not lose control of the management of the uveitis patient regardless of the consultations obtained.

References

1. Gell PGH, Coombs RRA: Clinical Aspects of Immunology, Oxford: Blackwell, 1968, pp
2. Bloch-Michel E, Dry J, Campinchi R, Vallery-Radot C, Borst M, Mugnier M-P: La Conjunctivite Printantiere, rev., fr. allergol. 17:157, 1977.
3. Friedlaender MH, Dvorak H: Morphology of delayed type hypersensitivity reactions in the guinea pig cornea. *J Immunol 118:1558*, 1977.
4. Smith RE, Nozik RA: Uveitis: A Clinical Approach to Diagnosis and Management. Baltimore: Williams and Wilkins, pp 23-24.
5. Kimura SJ, Thygeson P, Hogan MJ: Signs and symptoms of uveitis. I. Anterior Uveitis. *Am J Ophthalmol* 47:155, 1959.
6. Cohen JJ: Thymus derived lymphocytes sequestered in the bone marrow of hydrocortisone-treated mice. *J Immunol* 108:841, 1972.
7. Ebert RH, Barclay WR: Changes in connective tissue reaction induced by cortisone. *Ann Intern Med* 37:506, 1952.
8. Fauci AS, Dale DC: The effect of in vitro hydrocortisone on subpopulations of human lymphocytes. *J Clin Invest* 53:240, 1974.
9. Woodruff J, Gesner BM: Lymphocytes: Circulation altered by trypsin. *Science* 1961:176 1968.

Chapter 7

Immunologic Diseases of the External Eye

Bartly J. Mondino, MD

IMMUNOLOGIC DISEASES
OF THE EXTERNAL EYE

Immunologic disorders represent an important and expanding segment of external ocular disease. These diseases cause problems for patients that range from a minor nuisance in some cases of hay fever conjunctivitis to severe destruction of the eye in cases of Mooren's ulcer or ocular cicatricial pemphigoid. In this chapter, the diagnosis, pathogenesis and treatment of suspected immunologic diseases of the external eye are detailed. For convenience, these diseases have been listed under conjunctiva or cornea, depending upon the predominant site of involvement.

Conjunctiva

Contact Dermatoconjunctivitis. Contact allergy of the eyelids and conjunctiva is a common allergic reaction encountered in ophthalmic practice.[1] It may be caused by drugs, cosmetics, jewelry, plastics or chemicals. If the conjunctiva is the focal point of contact, the allergic reaction usually begins as a conjunctivitis and soon involves the adjacent skin of the eyelids in a typical dermatitis (contact dermatoconjunctivitis). If the skin of the eyelid is the primary site of contact, dermatitis occurs and conjunctivitis plays little or no role. The symptoms of contact dermatitis include redness, swelling, and mild to moderate itching. The signs of contact dermatitis include erythematous, edematous skin on which vesicles and papules may be found. The involved skin may develop cracking and weeping. The conjunctivitis causes symptoms of itching and tearing. Slit-lamp examination discloses conjunctival hyperemia, edema and papillae.

Cell-mediated immunity (type IV hypersensitivity mediated by sensitized T lymphocytes) is the basis of contact dermatoconjunctivitis. This type of hypersensitivity is transferred by means of lymphocytes and not serum. The dermal route of inoculation tends to favor the development of a T-cell response, and delayed-type hypersensitivity reactions are often produced by foreign materials capable of binding to body constituents to form new antigens. In other words, a chemical agent (hapten) in combination with a body protein (serum or soluble epithelial component) is necessary for the formation of a complete antigen and the development of an allergic reaction.

Contact allergy can be simply and easily demonstrated by patch tests. A small amount of the suspected substance or a small piece of gauze saturated with a suspected liquid is applied to the normal skin of the patient and covered with impermeable tape. The patch is removed at 48 hours and the site of the skin test examined at that time and 24 hours later for the development of erythema, edema, vesicles and papules.

The treatment of contact dermatoconjunctivitis involves the elimination of the offending antigen. Topical corticosteroids may be applied to the conjunctiva or skin to hasten elimination of signs and symptoms.

Atopic Ocular Disorders. Anaphylactic or type I hypersensitivity is the immunologic mechanism responsible for atopic disease. Patients with atopy have an hereditary background of allergic disease and show immediate wheal-and-flare skin reactivity to allergens that are injected intradermally. These allergens react with specific IgE antibodies attached to mast cells or basophils. This skin reactivity can be transferred by an injection of serum IgE from an atopic patient into the skin of a normal patient so that the subsequent application of the appropriate allergen is followed by the immediate development of wheal-and-flare (Prausnitz-Küstner reaction). Approximately 15% of the population have atopic disorders, the most common of which are hay fever, bronchial asthma and atopic dermatitis.

Hay Fever Conjunctivitis. Hay fever conjunctivitis is a recurrent inflammation of the conjunctiva that is associated with airborne allergens such as pollens, molds, dusts and danders.[2] The symptoms of hay fever conjunctivitis include itching, tearing and burning. The signs include lid swelling and conjunctival hyperemia and edema. The palpebral conjunctiva may show papillae. The cornea is usually normal.

The immunopathogenesis of hay fever conjunctivitis involves the interaction of airborne allergens with IgE molecules that are bound to the surface of tissue mast cells. This binding causes the release of pharmacologically active mediators that include histamine, slow-reacting substance of anaphylaxis, eosinophil chemotactic factor of anaphylaxis, platelet activating factor, and heparin. These mediators cause vasodilation and an increase in vascular permeability. Elevated levels of cyclic AMP inhibit the release of these mediators. Stimulators of the beta-adrenergic system (epinephrine, isoproterenol) as well as phosphodiesterase inhibitors (aminophylline, theophylline, caffeine) increase levels of cyclic AMP. The release of histamine apparently stimulates H-1 receptors (responsible for itching) and H-2 receptors (responsible for redness), both of which are found in the conjunctiva.[3]

The treatment of hay fever conjunctivitis includes eliminating or minimizing exposure to the offending allergen, topical vasoconstrictors such as naphazoline hydrochloride and topical antihistamines such as antazoline phosphate that block H-1 receptors. Topical disodium cromoglycate 4% (an inhibitor of mast cell degranulation) may be effective and is applied 4-5 times each day.[4] In some cases, it may be necessary to use topical corticosteroids in the lowest anti-inflammatory dose that is effective. The prolonged use of topical corticosteroids has side-effects that include glaucoma and cataracts. Specific desensitization has been found to be of value for some patients with allergic rhinitis or asthma. The development of IgG-blocking antibodies has been used to explain the effectiveness of this treatment. It has also been suggested that antigen-specific suppressor cells, probably bearing histamine receptors, are generated during allergic desensitization and may be partly responsible for the efficacy of this therapy.[5]

Conjunctivitis Associated with Atopic Dermatitis. The cutaneous lesions of atopic dermatitis are persistent and symmetrical. The skin is thick and dry with scales. The sites of involvement include the antecubital and popliteal areas, the sides and back of the neck, face, head, axillae, shoulders, thorax and retroauricular area. Patients with atopic dermatitis may develop atopic keratoconjunctivitis in the teenage years up to the fifth decade. The symptoms of itching, burning and tearing are associated with inflamed and thickened lid margins and conjunctival hyperemia, edema and papillae. Conjunctival scarring may develop in some cases. The corneal changes include punctate epithelial keratitis, pannus, ulceration and scarring.[6] Anterior subcapsular or posterior subcapsular cataracts are found in 10% of atopic dermatitis cases. Corticosteroids may aggravate the cataracts that are associated with this disease.

Conjunctival scrapings may contain eosinophils, and serum and tear IgE levels may be elevated. In addition to anaphylactic or type I hypersensitivity, cutaneous basophilic hypersensitivity may play a role in this condition.[2] Cellular immune mechanisms are usually deficient in atopic patients. Delayed hypersensitivity skin tests to Candida and streptokinase-streptodornase antigens are depressed, and patients may be unable to be sensitized to topical dinitrochlorobenzene.[7] Defective T-cell function and decreased percentages of peripheral blood T-cells have been found.[8] Atopic patients may be more susceptible to fungal and viral diseases because of suppressed cell-mediated immune function. Ocular infections with staphylococci may be a recurrent problem.

The treatment of atopic keratoconjunctivitis includes disodium cromoglycate 4% applied topically 5 times each day.[9] Topical corticosteroids in as low a concentration and frequency as possible may also be necessary. Long-term corticosteroid therapy is risky because of complications that include not only cataracts and glaucoma but also infections in these patients with depressed cellular immunity.

Vernal Conjunctivitis. Vernal conjunctivitis is a recurrent, bilateral inflammation of the conjunctiva that is aggravated by warm weather. It is a childhood disease, usually occurring from age 4 to 20. More boys are affected than girls until puberty when the incidence is about equal in both sexes. A family history of atopy is generally found, and the majority of patients with vernal conjunctivitis have other atopic diseases such as hay fever, asthma, atopic dermatitis and allergies to food, dust and molds.

Vernal conjunctivitis is considered to be an allergic disease with the responsible allergens most probably airborne pollens of grass and weeds.[2] Type I hypersensitivity (IgE-mediated) probably plays a role, and patients with vernal conjunctivitis have been shown to have both specific IgE and IgG antibodies in the tears to pollen allergens.[10] Increased levels of histamine have also been found in tears.[11] The presence of basophils in the conjunctival epithelium and stroma suggests that cutaneous basophil hypersensitivity may also play a role.[2]

The dominant symptom of vernal conjunctivitis is itching. Photophobia and tearing are also frequent complaints. Vernal conjunctivitis is always bilateral. It presents in three forms: 1) palpebral, 2) limbal, and 3) a mixed type. The palpebral form is characterized by large papillae predominantly of the upper lid (Figure 7-1). In severe and long-standing cases, the papillae may become cobblestone vegetations. The limbal lesions of vernal appear as yellow-gray gelatinous elevations. Trantas' dots, which are composed of eosinophils, are white points which sometimes cap the limbal excrescences and are diagnostic of vernal conjunctivitis. The diagnosis of vernal is rarely a problem, and conjunctival scrapings reveal massive eosinophilia that is rarely found in other allergic diseases. As differentiated from phlyctenules, vernal lesions do not stain with fluorescein, have less inflammatory reaction and are associated with conjunctival eosinophilia.

Vernal conjunctivitis is characterized by a marked and continuously increasing formation of hyalinized connective tissue in the conjunctival stroma. The palpebral conjunctiva may be covered by a thick, tenacious pseudomembrane which may be peeled off without bleeding.

The most frequent and characteristic corneal lesion of vernal is a superficial epithelial keratitis which stains in a punctate fashion and which is usually located in the upper one-half of the cornea. Noninfectious, transversely oval corneal ulcerations predominantly in the upper one-half of the cornea may be found in vernal and may be associated with plaques of calcific material.

Vernal conjunctivitis generally disappears when the patients reach adulthood. Exceptions to this are found, and in these cases the sex incidence is equal.

The removal of a patient to a cool environment may be helpful but is usually impractical. Topical corticosteroids are effective in the treatment of vernal, but systemic corticosteroids may occasionally be necessary. Cold compresses may also be useful. Topical disodium cromoglycate 4% may be used as a substitute for topical corticosteroids once the patient is well-controlled.[12] Disodium cromoglycate is better in this type of situation than in suppressing the acute manifestations of vernal which probably require topical corticosteroids. Oral aspirin (an inhibitor of prostaglandin synthesis) has been recommended as adjunctive therapy for difficult cases of vernal because prostaglandins may be involved in its pathogenesis.[13]

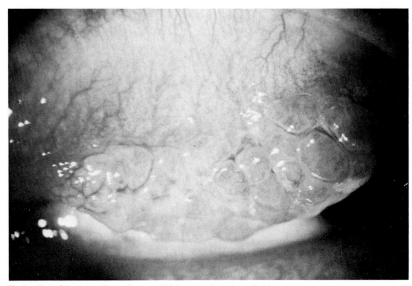

Figure 7-1. Giant papillae of upper lid in vernal conjunctivitis.

Giant Papillary Conjunctivitis (GPC). In 1974, Spring described an allergy-like reaction of the tarsal plate with mucus, discomfort and wearing difficulty in 78 of 170 long-term soft lens wearers.[14] Allansmith and co-workers described many features of this entity and labeled it giant papillary conjunctivitis (GPC).[15] GPC develops in soft contact lens wearers after as few as 3 weeks and as long as 4 years of daily successful wear. It can also develop in hard lens wearers but the minimum time was 14 months. It is characterized by excess mucus, mild itching and diminished tolerance to lens wear. Papillae that may be greater than 1 mm in diameter are noted in the upper tarsal conjunctiva.

Conjunctival scrapings show eosinophils but fewer than found with vernal. Histopathologic examination of the conjunctiva shows an irregular thickening of the epithelium with infiltration of mast cells, as well as eosinophils, basophils, polymorphonuclear leukocytes and an occasional lymphocyte.[15] The conjunctival stroma shows lymphocytes, plasma cells, mast cells, eosinophils and basophils. Conjunctival tissue from control subjects shows no eosinophils but mast cells, lymphocytes, plasma cells and polymorphonuclear leukocytes can be observed in the stroma.

Although not all patients with deposits on their lenses develop GPC, soft lens deposits are found in this syndrome and are a constant feature of it. This syndrome may have two components: an allergic reaction to contact lens protein deposits and mechanical trauma of the lens itself.[2] In fact, GPC has been reported with exposed interrupted nylon sutures[16] and ocular prostheses.[17]

GPC may be treated by discontinuing the lenses. The signs and symptoms of GPC gradually disappear. In the early stages of GPC with mild disease, decreasing wearing time, switching to new lenses or cleaning the lenses thoroughly with papain may interrupt the syndrome and permit lens use. Topical disodium cromoglycate 4% may be of value in mild cases. Topical corticosteroids may hasten the disappearance of symptoms when the lenses have been discontinued.

GPC has features which are similar to vernal keratoconjunctivitis. However, vernal keratoconjunctivitis is associated with more itching and with more eosinophils in conjunctival scrapings, and is more prominent in hot weather and in adolescent males. Patients with vernal keratoconjunctivitis are not wearing contact lenses and are more difficult to treat.

Ocular Cicatricial Pemphigoid (OCP). Cicatricial pemphigoid is characterized by recurrent blisters or bullae of the mucous membranes and skin with a tendency for scar formation. Ocular involvement is characterized by progressive shrinkage of the conjunctiva, entropion, trichiasis, xerosis and finally reduced vision from corneal opacification.[18,19] OCP affects more women than men and is essentially a disease of late life with the average age of onset being 58 years.[20]

The skin develops vesicles and bullae less frequently than the mucous membranes and is affected in approximately 25% of cases (Figure 7-2). Mucous membrane involvement includes the mouth, conjunctiva, nose, pharynx, larynx, esophagus, anus and vagina. Rupture of vesicles and bullae of the mucous membranes may lead to scarring.

OPC eventually involves both eyes. The first symptoms are those of any chronic nonspecific conjunctivitis, with irritation, burning and tearing. Later, corneal involvement leads to foreign body sensation, photophobia and finally reduced vision.

The essential and destructive process in OCP is fibrosis beneath the conjunctival epithelium.[18,19] Symblepharon passing from the palpebral to the bulbar conjunctiva develop with the inferior fornix involved first (Figure 7-3). The conjunctival shrinkage increases in extent until the entire conjunctival sac is obliterated.

OCP is associated with a diminished and unstable tear film. Fibrous occlusion of the ducts of the lacrimal and accessory lacrimal glands leads to decreased aqueous tear secretion. Destruction of the conjunctival goblet cells may result in a mucin deficient and unstable tear film.[21] Conjunctival scarring and symblepharon cause entropion with trichiasis and lagophthalmos with abnormal blinking and exposure. Because of the decreased aqueous tear secretion, decreased mucous production and lid problems, the integrity of the tear film is disturbed, resulting in a dry eye with breakdown and eventual keratinization of the ocular surface epithelium.

Smears of the conjunctiva in OCP reveal neutrophils, keratinized squamous cells and eosinophils.[18,22] Patients with OCP are more likely to show potential pathogens on the lids and/or conjunctiva than controls.[19]

Blisters or bullae are found in a subepithelial location. Blisters of the conjunctiva probably rupture readily in this location and are only rarely observed. The conjunctiva shows a metaplasia of the normal columnar epithelium into squamous epithelium with parakeratinization and keratinization.[23] Mucous-producing goblet cells are scarce or absent.[21] The early stages show granulation tissue beneath the conjunctival epithelium with an infiltration predominantly of lymphocytes, plasma cells, occasional

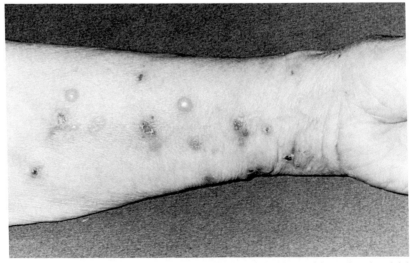

Figure 7-2. Intact and ruptured blisters of forearm in patient with ocular cicatricial pemphigoid.

eosinophils and relatively few neutrophils.[22,23] Later, pronounced fibrosis takes place in the conjunctival stroma and is responsible for the conjunctival shrinkage which characterizes this disease. Patients with acute manifestations of OCP show numerous neutrophils within and beneath the conjunctival epithelium in addition to the chronic inflammatory cells typically found in this disease.[24]

In cicatricial pemphigoid, immunoglobulins and components of both the classical and alternative complement pathways are found bound to the basement membrane zone of skin and oral mucosa.[25,26] Immunoglobulins and complement are also found bound to the conjunctival epithelium and its basement membrane.[27-30] Circulating antibodies which bind to the conjunctival and corneal epithelium but rarely to the conjunctival basement membrane have been demonstrated.[29,30] Approximately one-half of patients with OCP have elevated IgA levels[27,30] and HLA-B12.[31] Patients with OCP have decreased numbers of circulating T-cells.[32]

Radiation, severe chemical burns, particularly with alkali, adenovirus 8 and 19, primary herpes simplex keratoconjunctivitis, diphtheria, beta-hemolytic streptococcus and erythema multiforme may all cause conjunctival scarring.[18,28,33] The acute, self-limited nature of these conditions contrasts with the chronic, progressive conjunctival shrinkage found with OCP. Symblepharon and conjunctival shrinkage has been associated with the use of systemic practolol[34] and topical epinephrine,[35] echothiophate iodide[36] and pilocarpine.[34] Symblepharon has also been reported with Sjögren's syndrome[37] and sarcoidosis.[38] Trachoma causes conjunctival scarring but this usually begins and predominates in the superior fornix and on the upper tarsus. Bullous pemphigoid and pemphigus rarely cause conjunctival shrinkage.

OCP is generally described as a chronic disease characterized by progressive shrinkage of the conjunctiva. Episodes of acute disease activity may interrupt this course and result in rapid shrinkage of the conjunctiva.[24] Surgical procedures on the eye may entail a risk of setting off acute disease activity. The acute manifestations consist of diffuse and intense conjunctival hyperemia and edema and localized, ulcerated conjunctival mounds (Figure 7-4).

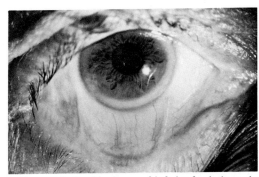

Figure 7-3. Symblepharon of inferior fornix in ocular cicatricial pemphigoid best demonstrated by drawing lower lid down and having patient look up.

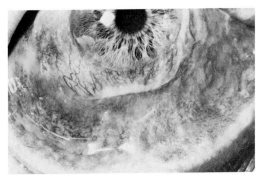

Figure 7-4. Diffuse conjunctival hyperemia and edema as acute manifestation of ocular cicatricial pemphigoid.

A prospective study of progression in OCP has shown that the majority of patients with OCP progress.[19] However, the disease has a variable course because there are patients with either mild or severe conjunctival shrinkage that do not necessarily progress. Moreover, progression is more likely to occur in the advanced stages.

The treatment of OCP must be directed at all the factors that complicate this devastating disease. Artificial tears may alleviate to some extent the aqueous tear deficiency which develops. In addition to the basic disease process, secondary bacterial infections may complicate and aggravate OCP. Antibiotics should be prescribed on the basis of specific antibiotic sensitivity testing. The staphylococcal blepharitis which frequently accompanies this condition may be treated effectively with lid scrubs followed by an antibiotic ointment.

Entropion with trichiasis may be corrected early in the disease by ocular plastic surgical techniques. Electrolysis, cryotherapy and hyfrecation may be used to eliminate trichiasis. When the fornices are sufficiently deep, therapeutic soft contact lenses may be used to protect the cornea from trichiasis and drying.

Systemic corticosteroids are of definite value in the treatment of the acute manifestations of OCP.[24] Systemic immunosuppressives including corticosteroids may be useful in the management of OCP.[39,40] Cyclophosphamide or azathioprine with or without prednisone reduce conjunctival inflammation and may inhibit progression of conjunctival shrinkage. In the final stages of OCP with ankyloblepharon and a keratinized ocular surface, a keratoprosthesis may be useful in restoring some sight to these unfortunate patients.[41]

Erythema Multiforme (EM).

Erythema multiforme is an acute, generally self-limited inflammatory disorder of the skin and mucous membranes with a variable recurrent pattern. The minor form of EM primarily involves the skin. The major form (the Stevens-Johnson syndrome) is characterized by mucosal as well as cutaneous lesions, toxemia with fever and prostration and ocular involvement. The minor variant of the disease may last two or three weeks while the major form may last six weeks. This disease may be seen at almost any age but peaks in the second and third decades and occurs only rarely in infancy and old age. There is no racial or geographic predilection.

EM may develop as a reaction to a wide variety of precipitating factors: herpes simplex, mycoplasmal pneumonia, recurrent bacterial infections, radiation therapy, malignancy, collagen-vascular diseases, and drugs, notably sulfonamides, penicillin, barbiturates, salicylates, mercurials, arsenic, phenylbutazone and diphenylhydantoin.[42] EM has been reported following the use of topical ophthalmic scopolamine, tropicamide and sulfonamides.[43]

The prodromal symptoms of EM include malaise, fever, symptoms of upper respiratory tract infection, prostration and headache. Mucous membrane and skin involvement follow. The cutaneous lesions are found most frequently on the extremities and except for the more severe cases spare the trunk. The skin lesions develop in crops that are symmetrically dis-

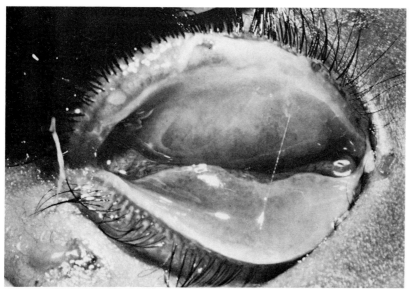

Figure 7-5. Pseudomembranes of tarsal conjunctiva in patient with erythema multiforme.

tributed. They begin as erythematous macules and papules, progress to become vesicles and bullae and resolve leaving residual hyperpigmentation. The characteristic lesion of EM is the target lesion. This consists of a red center surrounded by a pale zone with another red ring peripheral to the pale zone. Tense bullae develop from these lesions.

The mouth and eyes are the most frequently and severely affected mucous membranes. The lips may be swollen and crusted. Oral lesions begin as macules that develop into bullae which eventually rupture. Except for the conjunctiva, mucosal and cutaneous lesions usually disappear without scarring.

The acute phase of ocular disease lasts two to three weeks. The lids are swollen, ulcerated and crusted. Conjunctival involvement ranges from a mild catarrhal conjunctivitis which terminates without sequelae, to pseudomembranous or membranous conjunctivitis (Figure 7-5). The conjunctival surfaces may heal with scarring and symblepharon and may even progress to ankyloblepharon. Conjunctival scarring may result in entropion with trichiasis and lagophthalmos with exposure. Obliteration of the lacrimal puncta and canaliculi by fibrosis may cause epiphora in some patients. Destruction of conjunctival goblet cells and fibrotic obstruction of the ducts of the lacrimal and accessory lacrimal glands may result in a dry eye condition similar to OCP. In severe cases, keratinization of the conjunctival and corneal epithelium may be found. The dry eye condition and entropion with trichiasis result in corneal complications that include punctate erosions, pannus, ulcers, opacification and even perforation.

EM leaves conjunctival shrinkage and symblepharon in its wake, but progressive scarring does not occur once the acute stage has subsided, unlike the chronic progressive course of ocular cicatricial pemphigoid. Further destruction of the eye depends upon complications resulting from the acute event.

The bullae of EM are subepithelial with adjacent lymphocytes, histiocytes and a few neutrophils or eosinophils. A similar cellular infiltrate is found in a perivascular location in the dermis. Recent studies have demonstrated circulating immune complexes in the sera of patients with EM.[44-46] In addition, direct immunofluorescent studies of the involved skin of patients with EM have shown deposition of C3, IgM, fibrin and occasionally IgG in the blood vessel walls of the dermis.[44,46] Patients with EM with ocular involvement have an increased prevalence of HLA-Bw 44.[47]

Any suspected etiological factors such as nonessential drugs should be eliminated. Wet dressings may be used to debride crusted erosions, and baths may minimize discomfort. With severe and extensive cutaneous and mucosal involvement, hydration may be necessary to maintain fluid balance. The systemic administration of antibiotics is indicated for underlying infection. Systemic corticosteroids have been recommended for the general manifestations of EM. A typical regimen consists of an initial dose of 60 to 80 mg of prednisone daily until improvement is noted, with gradual tapering over 3 to 4 weeks. The value of systemic corticosteroids has not been proven by a well-controlled, prospective study and has been challenged.[48]

Local treatment appears to have little influence on the severity of ophthalmic complications.[49] Early lysis of symblepharon should be attempted. Secondary bacterial infections of the conjunctiva should be treated by appropriate antibiotics. The dry, scarred eye resulting from EM may require artificial tears, closure of the lacrimal puncta, destruction of aberrant lashes, soft contact lenses to protect the cornea from drying and trichiasis, and lid scrubs followed by antibiotic ointment for the chronic blepharitis that may be found with this disease.

Cornea

Corneal Infiltrates and Soft Contact Lenses. Anterior stromal infiltrates of the cornea in patients wearing soft contact lenses have been shown to be a manifestation of delayed hypersensitivity to thimerosal, the preservative used in chemical disinfectants.[50] The patients complained of itching, redness, irritation and photophobia. These patients showed conjunctival hyperemia and edema without a prominent papillary reaction of the upper lids. The corneal changes included anterior stromal infiltrates with occasional extension to mid-stroma (Figure 7-6). The infiltrates were 1 to 2 mm in diameter and showed no overlying staining with fluorescein. Bacterial cultures of the conjunctiva, lids, lens cases, lens solutions and eye cosmetics were not helpful in these cases. Conjunctival cultures for adenovirus and chlamydial titers were negative. Giemsa stain of conjunctival scrapings showed a few mononuclear leukocytes and rare eosinophils but no inclusion bodies. Results of occlusive patch tests and intradermal tests suggested that these patients showed delayed hypersensitivity to thimerosal. Using heat disinfection and saline without preservatives, all patients were able to wear their soft contact lenses without signs and symptoms of inflammation.

Another study described patients with redness, irritation and corneal changes related to soft contact lens wear and also suggested that this represented a hypersensitivity to thimerosal with the thiosalicylate moiety being the culprit.[51]

Occlusive patch tests with .004% thimerosal or chemical disinfectants are easily performed by placing the solutions on 1 cm gauze pads which are then applied to the forearm and covered by impermeable tape. The patches are removed at 48 hours, and the sites are examined then and 24 hours later. A positive patch test will show erythema and edema and perhaps even papules and vesicles.

Thimerosal has also been implicated in patients wearing soft contact lenses that developed ocular irritation and a keratoconjunctivitis with features resembling superior limbic keratoconjunctivitis.[52] Positive skin and ocular sensitivity reactions to thimerosal were present in one-third (5/15) of patients tested. All patients had used contact lens solutions containing thimerosal as a preservative and could resume contact lens wear without difficulty if thermal disinfection using preservative-free solutions was employed.

Other reports have indicated that corneal infiltrates associated with the use of soft contact lenses may be related to chlamydial keratoconjunctivitis,[53] anoxia or an immunological reaction to staphylococcal antigens,[54] or a reaction to the lens itself.[55]

Corneal infiltrates in soft contact lens wearers may also represent a direct bacterial or fungal infection of the cornea. The management of these dense, yellow-white infiltrates of the cornea that stain with fluorescein is strikingly different from the corneal infiltrates described above. Corneal scrapings must be obtained for Gram stain as well as bacterial and fungal cultures. These patients should be admitted for intensive topical antibiotic therapy. These patients may be inadequately disinfecting their lenses and may have contaminated lens cases and solutions.[56,57] Pseudomonas aeruginosa is a common and serious cause of these corneal infiltrates. Early Pseudomonas corneal infiltrates in these patients typically have an elevated gelatinous appearance and stain with fluorescein.

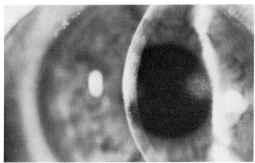

Figure 7-6. Anterior stromal infiltrates of cornea shown in slit-beam in patient with contact lens intolerance related to thimerosal.

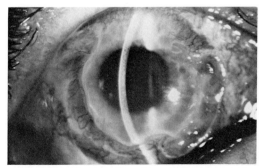

Figure 7-7. Mooren's ulcer with peripheral corneal thinning and steep central border indicated by slit-beam.

Interstitial Keratitis. Interstitial keratitis denotes an inflammation of the corneal stroma not primarily involving the anterior or posterior surfaces.[58] Inflammatory cells and then vessels invade the corneal stroma. An immunologic mechanism offers the best explanation for the two major types of interstitial keratitis encountered clinically: syphilitic and tuberculous. Syphilis is the most common cause of interstitial keratitis. In the majority of cases the disease is congenital. Syphilitic interstitial keratitis results in a widespread infiltrative inflammation of the corneal stroma, particularly of its deeper layers.[58] It is associated with an anterior uveitis with keratic precipitates. The residual corneal changes include stromal opacification and blood vessels. Congenital interstitial keratitis is usually bilateral, while acquired syphilis is unilateral in most cases. Interstitial keratitis is a late manifestation of congenital syphilis, with most cases being recognized in the age range of 5 to 20 years. Other stigmata of syphilis may be present. Interstitial keratitis, Hutchinson's teeth and deafness are commonly referred to as Hutchinson's triad.

Evidence for an allergic etiology is based on the ineffectiveness of specific antisyphilitic therapy, effectiveness of corticosteroids and onset of interstitial keratitis during the course of systemic arsenic therapy. The treatment of syphilitic interstitial keratitis includes topical cycloplegics and corticosteroids.

Tuberculous interstitial keratitis is rare, often unilateral, involves the middle or deeper layers of the cornea and is frequently limited to a sector usually in the inferior cornea. The treatment of tuberculous interstitial keratitis includes topical cycloplegics and treatment of the general disease with systemic antibiotics. Topical corticosteroids should be used cautiously if local infection is suspected.

Interstitial keratitis has also been described in association with viral infections such as mumps, herpes, influenza and lymphogranuloma venereum. It can also be seen as a complication of trypanosomiasis. Nonsyphilitic interstitial keratitis associated with vestibuloauditory symptoms was described by Cogan.[59] An interstitial keratitis with no proven etiology or association may respond dramatically to topical corticosteroids.

Disciform Keratitis. The commonest cause of disciform keratitis is herpes simplex. A history of a preceding dendrite is not invariably obtained, and the dendrite may subsequently appear after the disciform keratitis. The symptoms of disciform keratitis include pain, tearing and photophobia. Disciform keratitis generally appears as a disk-like area of both stromal and epithelial edema. The disc-shaped area of edema may be found not only in the central cornea but also in the peripheral cornea and for that matter may involve the entire cornea. Striate keratopathy may also be found in this area. Anterior uveitis and KP on the endothelium in the area of the disciform keratitis are usually found.

The mechanism of herpes disciform keratitis is felt to be primarily immunologic. The host mounts a cell-mediated immune response to viral antigens in the corneal stroma or a viral antigen integrated into the stromal fibroblasts, manifesting itself clinically as disciform corneal edema.[60]

Disciform keratitis responds well to low doses of corticosteroids such as fluoromethalone. Coverage with antiviral agents such as idoxuridine or trifluridine should be given. A central disciform keratitis with reduction in vision requires treatment, while a peripheral lesion may be observed. Disciform keratitis may be caused by other organisms including mumps, infectious mononucleosis, herpes zoster and vaccinia.

Catarrhal Infiltrates and Ulcers.
The catarrhal infiltrate and ulcer is usually a complication of long-standing staphylococcal blepharoconjunctivitis.[61-63] Cultures of the lid margins yield many colonies of mannitol-positive, coagulase-positive S. aureus or in rare instances coagulase-positive S. albus.

Catarrhal ulcers are common in adults but rare in children. These peripheral corneal infiltrates and ulcers are separated by a distinct lucid interval of approximately 2 mm from the limbus. The direction of spread of the corneal ulcers is concentric with the limbus with little tendency to spread centrally. The infiltrate appears first and is followed by fluorescein staining of the surface as ulceration develops. This course differs from peripheral herpetic keratitis which begins with an epithelial defect that is followed by an infiltrate. Corneal sensation is diminished in peripheral herpetic keratitis but is normal or very slightly diminished over catarrhal infiltrates. Blood vessels may eventually bridge the lucid interval, and after healing there may be a peripheral pannus directed to the ulcer site. The ulcer shows a marked tendency to recur. There are reports of these marginal ulcers coalescing to form ring ulcers.

Gram and Giemsa stains of corneal scrapings may reveal polymorphonuclear leukocytes, but no bacteria. Corneal cultures of the ulcers are negative for bacteria. The lesion is thought to represent an antigen-antibody reaction with complement activation and polymorphonuclear leukocyte infiltration in patients sensitized with staphylococcal antigens.[63] In fact, antibodies and C3 complement have been demonstrated in the catarrhal ulcer.[64] Rabbits immunized with phenol-inactivated S. aureus[65] or a preparation of their cell walls mixed with complete Freund's adjuvant[66] develop peripheral infiltrates of the cornea with features resembling catarrhal infiltrates in humans after topical challenge with viable S. aureus. These infiltrates in rabbits are separated from the limbus by approximately 2 mm and are composed of lipid and sparse numbers of acute and chronic inflammatory cells and vessels.

Although marginal or catarrhal ulcers are associated with staphylococcal blepharoconjunctivitis in the overwhelming majority of cases, they have also been found in association with positive conjunctival cultures for the diplobacillus of Morax-Axenfeld and Koch-Weeks bacillus. Catarrhal ulcers have been reported recently in association with acute beta hemolytic streptococcal conjunctivitis and chronic dacryocystitis (lacrimal conjunctivitis of Morax).[67]

The treatment of catarrhal infiltrates and ulcers should include treatment of the lids with lid scrubs followed by the application of an antibiotic ointment such as erythromycin. In addition to topical antibiotics, topical corticosteroids such as fluoromethalone are dramatically effective in healing these lesions.

Phlyctenulosis. Phlyctenular keratoconjunctivitis is characterized by nodules of the conjunctiva and cornea occurring mainly in children.[63,68,69] These nodules appear first at the limbus and then spread to the bulbar conjunctiva and cornea. The nodules last approximately ten days to two weeks. The phlyctenule occasionally resolves spontaneously but usually undergoes necrosis with the formation of an ulcer.

Phlyctenular ulcers of the cornea may appear as marginal ulcers. These marginal ulcers differ from catarrhal ulcers in that they leave no clear space between the ulcer and the limbus, and their axes are frequently perpendicular rather than parallel to the circumference of the cornea. The marginal ulcers may remain stationary but may also spread centrally as fascicular ulcers or wandering phlyctenules, which are perhaps the most characteristic of the phlyctenular corneal lesions. The peripheral area of the ulcer may heal while the central margin remains active and progresses across the cornea preceded by gray infiltration. Vessels run in a straight course from the limbus and follow the ulcer centrally. Scars are formed only on the cornea and are triangular with the base at the limbus. A rarely seen type of corneal involvement is miliary phlyctenulosis, in which there are minute phlyctenules that cover the corneal surface. Other manifestations of corneal phlyctenulosis include superficial and deep diffuse central infiltrates without ulceration, seen most commonly in recurrent phlyctenulosis of long duration, and phlyctenular pannus, that is characteristically irregular and inferior in location.

Phlyctenules are subepithelial inflammatory nodules composed of leukocytes and blood vessels. The inflammatory cells include macrophages, lymphocytes, plasma cells and polymorphonuclear leukocytes. The nodule may resolve or ulcerate.

Phlyctenulosis has been related to tuberculosis in the Eskimo and Indian populations in the U.S.[68] It has been suggested that the eye is sensitive to tuberculoprotein at an early age and that an attack of phlyctenulosis is precipitated by the presentation of tuberculoprotein to the sensitized eye either by the blood stream or by inoculation into the conjunctival sac.[63] Spontaneous desensitization seems to occur in adult life. Vitamin deficiency, malnutrition, blepharitis and acute bacterial conjunctivitis contribute to the disease and may act as trigger mechanisms.

At present most cases of phlyctenulosis are being related to staphylococcal blepharitis.[63] Photophobia and tearing are less severe and corneal perforations are rarer in phlyctenular disease associated with staphylococci than with tuberculosis. Phlyctenulosis has also been related to Candida albicans, Coccidioides immitis, the agent of lymphogranuloma venereum and nematodes.

A rabbit model of phlyctenulosis has been developed.[65] Rabbits immunized with phenol-inactivated S. aureus or a preparation of their cell wall mixed with complete Freund's adjuvant[66] developed vascularized, elevated nodular infiltrates of the cornea resembling phlyctenules in humans after topical challenge with viable S. aureus. The nodular corneal infiltrates were found in a subepithelial location and were composed of vessels, polymorphonuclear leukocytes and mononuclear cells including lymphocytes, plasma cells and macrophages. Results of skin tests and antibody tests suggested that the development of phlyctenules in rabbits was an antibody-mediated phenomenon to ribitol teichoic acid, a component of the cell wall of S. aureus.[70] This hypothesis was confirmed by showing that rabbits immunized intravenously by ribitol teichoic acid attached to sheep red blood cells developed phlyctenules after topical challenge with viable S. aureus.[71] Hypersensitivity to ribitol teichoic acid of S. aureus may be the mechanism of development of phlyctenules associated with S. aureus.

Topical corticosteroids adequately control phlyctenular keratoconjunctivitis. Systemic and subconjunctival corticosteroids are generally not necessary. Any secondary bacterial infection should be treated with antibiotics. An associated staphylococcal blepharitis should be treated with lid scrubs followed by an antibiotic ointment such as erythromycin. Cycloplegics should be used when a secondary iritis is present. Orally administered tetracycline has been recommended for phlyctenular keratoconjunctivitis.[72] Six patients who had recurrent episodes of nontuberculous phlyctenular keratoconjunctivitis and progressive corneal vascularization and scarring were treated with oral tetracycline. This treatment resulted in rapid relief of symptoms and the apparent arrest of the disease. Oral tetracycline is a safe and effective treatment for resistant and recurrent nontuberculous phlyctenular keratoconjunctivitis and an alternative to topical corticosteroid treatment in those patients suffering from corticosteroid-induced complications.

Mooren's Ulcer.

Mooren's ulcer is a chronic, painful ulceration of the cornea which begins in the periphery with a steep, undermined and occasionally infiltrated leading border. The ulcer advances both centripetally and circumferentially, leaving in its wake a thinned, vascularized cornea. It is a rare disease that is bilateral in approximately 25% of cases. It does not necessarily develop simultaneously in both eyes and an interval of several years may lapse between involvement of the first eye and the second.

Mooren's ulcer may begin as infiltrates near the margin of the cornea which slowly spread, coalesce and eventually break down to form a shallow furrow. The ulcer spreads slowly, undermining the corneal epithelium and the superficial lamellae at its advancing border so that a gray, infiltrated, overhanging edge is formed, which in some cases can be lifted up. Swelling and hyperemia of the limbus adjacent to the ulcer is found. The ulcer may undergo remissions and exacerbations, spread slowly and remorselessly or may be self-limited (Figure 7-7).

Mooren's ulcer spreads around the periphery of the cornea, toward the center of the cornea and occasionally into the sclera. Behind the active border of the ulcer, healing takes place from the periphery with the development of new vessels, but the healed area remains permanently clouded. In most cases there is little tendency for fibrous tissue formation as a reparative response so that the remaining cornea consists of Descemet's membrane and the most posterior corneal lamellae covered by conjunctival epithelium.

A mild iritis is found, and a secondary cataract may develop, but hypopyon or perforation are usually not found.[73]

During the stages of advancing disease, patients usually experience severe pain, photophobia and lacrimation. Visual acuity is decreased because of extension of the ulcer into the pupillary area or because of the development of irregular astigmatism.

In 1971, Wood and Kaufman[74] suggested that there were two different types of Mooren's ulcer, a unilateral limited type, occurring in older patients and responding to relatively conservative surgery, and a relentlessly progressive type occurring most commonly in younger patients, frequently involving the sclera as well as the peripheral cornea and not responding to any therapy.

Histopathologic examination of the conjunctiva adjacent to Mooren's ulcer shows plasma cells and lymphocytes with an occasional neutrophil.[75] The leading edge of the ulcer is infiltrated with leukocytes. In the ulcerated area, Bowman's membrane and the corneal stroma are destroyed except for the most posterior lamellae. Descemet's membrane and the endothelium are not damaged.

An unequivocal etiology has not been established for Mooren's ulcer. It has been related to previous ocular trauma, with many cases having either physical or chemical injuries antedating the development of the ulcer. Mooren's-like ulcers have been reported following intracapsular cataract extraction[76] and also following herpes zoster ophthalmicus.[77]

In recent years an autoimmune etiology has been suggested for Mooren's ulcer because of the demonstration of plasma cells in the conjunctiva adjacent to the ulcer,[75] the finding of immunoglobulins and complement bound to the conjunctival epithelium and basement membrane adjacent to the ulcer,[30,78,79] the presence of circulating antibodies to conjunctival and corneal epithelium[30,78] and the demonstration that the lymphocytes of patients with Mooren's ulcer are sensitized to corneal antigens.[80] It may be that Mooren's ulcer represents a final common pathway to a variety of insults to the cornea in susceptible patients. The cornea may be altered in such a way that autoimmune phenomena develop that are either intimately involved in the pathogenesis of the ulcer or are responsible for aggravating and perpetuating the basic disease process, whatever it may be.

The limited, unilateral form of Mooren's ulcer may respond to topical corticosteroids in some cases. If unsuccessful, a resection of 3 to 4 mm of the conjunctiva adjacent to the ulcer may be performed. This is generally successful in the limited, unilateral variety but may have to be repeated. Because the adjacent conjunctiva produces proteoglycanase and collagenase and contains plasma cells that may be producing autoantibodies,[75] its excision may facilitate healing.[81]

There is no consistently effective treatment for the bilateral, relentlessly progressive type of Mooren's ulcer. Topical corticosteroids are generally unsuccessful. Lamellar and penetrating keratoplasties performed in a setting of acute disease activity are generally unsuccessful and may be invaded by the disease process. Following the destruction of all but the most posterior corneal lamellae, ulceration and the associated inflammatory activity subside. This end stage of Mooren's ulcer may be hastened by lamellar keratectomy of the remaining central island of cornea as suggested by Maumenee.[82] The epithelium rapidly heals over the area of the excised corneal tissue with subsidence of ulceration, inflammation and pain. When these eyes have been quiet for several months, penetrating keratoplasty may be successful in some cases and provide useful vision.[83]

Treatment with subconjunctival heparin adjacent to the ulcer has been recommended to improve the primary ischemic process that has been postulated to exist in this condition.[84] Collagenase inhibitors applied topically and systemic corticosteroids are ineffective. Systemic immunosuppressives have been recommended but are not consistently effective. Soft contact lenses may relieve pain but probably have little effect on the ulcerative process.[84]

Marginal Corneal Ulcers Associated with Systemic Diseases.

Wegener's granulomatosis and periarteritis nodosa may be associated with marginal corneal ulcers, with features that resemble the early stages of Mooren's ulcer.[85] These peripheral corneal ulcers are associated with moderate infiltrate and vascularization and may be accompanied by scleritis. The peripheral corneal ulcers associated with Wegener's granulomatosis may respond to systemic immunosuppressives[86] and resections of the adjacent conjunctiva. Ring infiltrates and ulcers have been associated with systemic diseases that include bacillary dysentery, influenza, acute leukemia, periarteritis nodosa, scleroderma and lupus erythematosus.[87] The infiltrate and eventually the ulcer form a continuous ring in the periphery of the cornea. Topical corticosteroids have been used to treat ring infiltrates and ulcers.[87]

Scleritis is a well-recognized complication of rheumatoid arthritis.[88] The scleritis can spread into and involve the adjacent cornea as a sclerokeratitis, and this may be associated with marginal thinning. Characteristic marginal corneal ulcers have been described in patients having rheumatoid arthritis without scleritis.[89] The marginal furrows are located approximately 1 mm within the limbus and usually in the inferior cornea. The marginal thinning can be superficial and nonprogressive, or it can progress to epithelial breakdown, marked stromal thinning and finally perforation. These furrows are usually associated with minimal gross inflammation and vascularization unless perforation occurs. The marginal furrows may encircle the cornea and may be bilateral. Central corneal melting without any noteworthy infiltration and Mooren's-like ulcers may also be associated with rheumatoid arthritis. Topical corticosteroids must be used with extreme caution in patients having rheumatoid arthritis and associated peripheral corneal ulcers. Resection of the conjunctiva adjacent to these marginal ulcers may halt the ulcerative process.[90,91] The conjunctiva adjacent to peripheral corneal ulcers associated with rheumatoid arthritis has been shown to produce collagenase, and this may provide the basis for the beneficial effects of conjunctival resection.[91] Immunosuppressives including corticosteroids used to treat the underlying rheumatoid disease can also have a beneficial effect on inflammation of the sclera and cornea.

Corneal Graft Rejection.

The cornea is an immunologically privileged site because of its avascularity and absence of lymphatic drainage. It has been shown in rabbits that donor epithelium, stroma and endothelium may be rejected individually.[92] An epithelial rejection line begins in the vicinity of congested limbal vessels and consists of an opaque line of inflammatory cells as well as dead and dying epithelial cells of the donor which are replaced by host epithelium. A stromal rejection line is manifested as an advancing band of haziness which consists of neutrophils, lymphocytes and plasma cells. An endothelial rejection line usually has its origin near invading vessels and is composed of KP advancing across the graft with destruction of the donor endothelium. Donor endothelial cell destruction is mediated by lymphocytes[93] that reach the endothelium from the limbal vessels through an unhealed Descemet's membrane or from the iris or ciliary body vessels through the aqueous humor. Retrocorneal membranes form after endothelial cell rejection and destruction.

Corneal grafts show an increased susceptibility to immunological rejection if there is preexisting vascularization of the host, anterior synechia or previous episodes of graft rejection. The clinical diagnosis of specific allograft rejection consists of 1) a preceding period of at least two weeks after transplantation during which the graft was technically successful and clear, 2) opaque rejection lines of the epithelium, stroma or endothelium, 3) subepithelial infiltrates of the graft,[94] and 4) stromal and epithelial edema or KP primarily confined to the donor tissue and beginning in proximity to the nearest blood vessels. Approximately 25% of penetrating keratoplasties have immunological rejection episodes. Graft failure in the first two weeks after surgery may result from 1) poor donor endothelium, 2) surgical trauma to the endothelium, 3) defective wound closure, 4) secondary infection or reactivation of host-infection such as herpes simplex, or 5) secondary glaucoma. Because the cornea is an immunologically privileged site, corneal transplantation is highly successful. In cases of previous sensitization or neovascularization, HLA matching has been suggested.[95]

The treatment of corneal graft rejection includes the use of hourly topical corticosteroids such as prednisolone acetate 1%. Topical corticosteroids have a lympholytic effect on killer lymphocytes that are attacking the donor endothelium.[93] In severe cases, it may be necessary to inject corticosteroids beneath the conjunctiva or in the sub-Tenon space. Triamcinolone diacetate 40 mg is recommended because it lasts several days. Oral prednisone 60 to 80 mg daily for several days is probably necessary only for the most severe cases of graft rejection. Cyclosporin A is a safe, potent immunosuppressive agent that has been shown to suppress corneal allograft rejection in animals but not humans.[96]

Summary

Immune related diseases of the external eye are common. Ocular sequelae range from minor irritation due to conjunctivitis to severe loss of vision in cases of ocular cicatricial pemphigoid or corneal graft rejection.

Conjunctival manifestations range from minor and reversible with appropriate treatment (hay fever conjunctivitis, giant papillary and vernal conjunctivitis) to severe disruption of conjunctival function resulting in visual loss from corneal opacification (ocular cicatricial pemphigoid and Stevens-Johnson syndrome).

Corneal involvement may be secondary to conjunctival disease or the cornea may be primarily involved. Examples of primary corneal involvement include interstitial and disciform keratitis, marginal ulcers and infiltrates, Mooren's ulcers and corneal graft rejection. The external eye may serve as a paradigm for immunologic disease processes.

References

1. Theodore FH, Bloomfield SE, Mondino BJ: Clinical Allergy and Immunology of the Eye. Baltimore: Williams and Wilkins, 1983, pp 36-71.
2. Allansmith MR, Abelson MB: Immunologic Diseases. Ocular Allergies. Chapter 6. *In:* Smolin G, Thoft RA (eds): Cornea. Boston: Little, Brown and Co., 1983, pp 231-243.
3. Abelson MB, Udell IJ: H2-receptors in the human ocular surface. *Arch Ophthalmol* 99:302-304, 1981.
4. Friday GA, Biglan AW, Hiles DA, Murphey SM, Miller DL, Rothbach C, Rand S: Treatment of ragweed allergic conjunctivitis with cromolyn sodium 4% ophthalmic solution. *Am J Ophthalmol* 95:169-174, 1983.
5. Rocklin RE, Sheffer AL, Greineder DK, Melmon KI: Generation of antigen-specific suppressor cells during allergy desensitization. *New Engl J Med* 302:1213-1218, 1980.
6. Hogan MJ: Atopic keratoconjunctivitis. *Am J Ophthalmol 36:937*, 1953.
7. McGeady SJ, Buckley RH: Depression of cell-mediated immunity in atopic eczema. *J Allergy Clin Immunol* 56:393, 1975.
8. Rachelefsky GS, et al: Defective T cell function in atopic dermatitis. *J Allergy Clin Immunol* 57:569, 1976.
9. Jay JL: Clinical features and diagnosis of adult atopic keratoconjunctivitis and the effect of treatment with sodium cromoglycate. *Brit J Ophthalmol* 65:335-340, 1981.
10. Ballow M, Donshik PC, Mendelson L, Rapacz P, Sparks K: IgG specific antibodies to rye grass and ragweed pollen antigens in the tear secretions of patients with vernal conjunctivitis. *Am J Ophthalmol* 95:161-168, 1983.
11. Abelson MB, Soter NA, Simon MA, Dohlman J, Allansmith MR: Histamine in human tears. *Am J Ophthalmol* 83:417, 1977.
12. Easty DL, Rice NSC, Jones BR: Disodium cromoglycate in the treatment of vernal conjunctivitis. *Trans Ophthalmol Soc UK 91:491*, 1971.
13. Abelson MB, Butrus SI, Weston JH: Aspirin therapy in vernal conjunctivitis. *Am J Ophthalmol* 95:502-505, 1983.
14. Spring TF: Reaction to hydrophilic lenses. *Med J Aust* 1:499, 1974.
15. Allansmith MR, Korb DR, Greiner JV, Henriguez AS, Simon MA, Finnemore VM: Giant papillary conjunctivitis in contact lens wearers. *Am J Ophthalmol* 83:697-708, 1977.
16. Sugar A, Meyer RF: Giant papillary conjunctivitis after keratoplasty. *Am J Ophthalmol* 91:239-242, 1981.
17. Srinivasan BD, Jakobiec FA, Iwamoto T, DeVoe AG: Giant papillary conjunctivitis with ocular prostheses. *Arch Ophthalmol* 97:892, 1979.
18. Mondino BJ: Bullous diseases of the skin and mucous membranes. *In:* Duane T (ed): Clinical Ophthalmology. Philadelphia: Harper and Row, 1980, Vol 4, Chap 12, pp 1-16.
19. Mondino BJ, Brown SI: Ocular cicatricial pemphigoid. *Ophthalmol* 88:95, 1981.
20. Hardy KM, Perry HO, Pingree GC, Kirby TJ: Benign mucous membrane pemphigoid. *Arch Dermatol* 104:467, 1971.
21. Ralph RA: Conjunctival goblet cell density in normal subjects and in dry eye syndromes. *Invest Ophthalmol* 14:299, 1975.
22. Norn MS, Kristensen EB: Benign mucous membrane pemphigoid. II. Cytology. *Acta Ophthalmol* 52:282, 1974.
23. Andersen SR, Jensen OA, Kristensen EB, Norn MS: Benign mucous membrane pemphigoid. III. Biopsy. *Acta Ophthalmol* 52:455, 1974.

24. Mondino BJ, Brown SI, Lempert S, Jenkins MS: The acute manifestations of ocular cicatricial pemphigoid: diagnosis and treatment. *Ophthalmol* 86:543, 1979.

25. Griffith MR, Fukuyama K, Tuffanelli D, Silverman S: Immunofluorescent studies in mucous membrane pemphigoid. *Arch Dermatol* 109:195, 1974.

26. Rogers RS, Perry HO, Bean SF, Jordan RE: Immunopathology of cicatricial pemphigoid. Studies of complement deposition. *J Invest Dermatol* 68:39, 1977.

27. Bean SF, Furey N, West CE, Andrews T, Easterly NB: Ocular cicatricial pemphigoid. *Trans Am Acad Ophthalmol Otolaryngol* 81:106, 1976.

28. Furey N, West C, Andrews T, Paul PD, Bean SF: Immunofluorescence studies of ocular cicatricial pemphigoid. *Am J Ophthalmol* 80:825, 1975.

29. Mondino BJ, Ross AN, Rabin BS, Brown SI: Autoimmune phenomena in ocular cicatricial pemphigoid. *Am J Ophthalmol* 83:443, 1977.

30. Mondino BJ, Brown SI, Rabin BS: Autoimmune phenomena of the external eye. *Ophthalmol* 85:801, 1978.

31. Mondino BJ, Brown SI, Rabin BS: HLA antigens in ocular cicatricial pemphigoid. *Arch Ophthalmol* 97:479, 1979.

32. Mondino BJ, Rao H, Brown SI: T and B lymphocyte enumerations in ocular cicatricial pemphigoid. *Am J Ophthalmol* 92:536-542, 1981.

33. Darougar S, Quinlan MP, Gibson JA, Jones BR, McSwiggan DA: Epidemic keratoconjunctivitis and chronic papillary conjunctivitis in London due to Adenovirus type 19. *Brit J Ophthalmol* 61:76, 1977.

34. Jones DB: Prospects in the management of tear deficiency states. *Trans Am Acad Ophthalmol Otolaryngol* 83:693, 1977.

35. Christensen EB, Norn MS: Benign mucous membrane pemphigoid. 1. Secretion of mucus in tears. *Acta Ophthalmol* 52:266, 1974.

36. Patten JR, Cavanagh HD, Allansmith MR: Induced ocular pseudopemphigoid. *Am J Ophthalmol* 82:272, 1976.

37. Jones BR: Ocular diagnosis of benign mucous membrane pemphigoid. *Proc R Soc Med* 54:109, 1961.

38. Flach A: Symblepharon in sarcoidosis. *Am J Ophthalmol* 85:210, 1978.

39. Foster CS, Wilson LA, Ekins MB: Immunosuppressive therapy for progressive ocular cicatricial pemphigoid. 89:340-352, 1982.

40. Mondino BJ, Brown SI: Immunosuppressive therapy in ocular cicatricial pemphigoid. *Am J Ophthalmol* (in press).

41. Rao GN, Bladt HL, Aquavella JV: Results of keratoprosthesis. *Am J Ophthalmol* 88:190, 1979.

42. Yetiv JZ, Bianchine JR, Rowen JA: Etiologic factors of the Stevens-Johnson syndrome. *South Med J* 73:599, 1980.

43. Guill MA, Goette DK, Knight CG, Peck CC, Lupton GP: Erythema multiforme and urticaria. *Arch Dermatol* 115:742, 1979.

44. Boskell LL, Mackel SE, Jordan RE: Erythema multiforme: Direct immunofluorescence studies and detection of circulating immune complexes. *J Invest Dermatol* 74:372, 1980.

45. Wuepper KD, Watson PA, Kazmierowski JA: Immune complexes in erythema multiforme and the Stevens-Johnson syndrome. *J Invest Dermatol* 74:368, 1980.

46. Imamura S, Uanase K, Taniguchi S, Ofuji S, Mangaoil L: Erythema multiforme: demonstration of immune complexes in the sera and skin lesions. *Brit J Dermatol* 102:161, 1980.

47. Mondino BJ, Brown SI, Biglan A: HLA antigens in the Stevens-Johnson syndrome with ocular involvement. *Arch Ophthalmol* 100:1453-1454, 1982.

48. Rasmussen JE: Erythema multiforme in children. Response to treatment with systemic corticosteroids. *Brit J Dermatol* 95:181, 1976.

49. Arstikaitis MJ: Ocular aftermath of Stevens-Johnson syndrome. *Arch Ophthalmol* 90:376, 1973.

50. Mondino BJ, Groden LR: Conjunctival hyperemia and corneal infiltrates with chemically disinfected soft contact lenses. *Arch Ophthalmol* 98:1767-1770, 1980.

51. Wilson LA, McNath J, Reitshel R: Delayed hypersensitivity to thimerosal in soft contact lens wearers. *Ophthalmology* 88:804-809, 1981.

52. Sendele DD, Kenyon KR, Mobilia EF, Rosenthal P, Steinert R, Hanninen LA: Superior limbic keratoconjunctivitis in contact lens wearers. *Ophthalmology* 90:616-622, 1983.

53. Gassett AR: Contact Lenses and Corneal Disease. New York: Appleton-Century-Crofts, 1979, pp 254-257.

54. Smolin G, Okumoto M, Nozik R: The microbial flora in extended-wear soft contact-lens wearers. *Am J Ophthalmol* 88:543-547, 1979.

55. Bernstein HN, Lemp MA: An unusual keratoconjunctivitis occurring after long time wearing of the AO softcon (formerly Griffin or Bionite) hydrophilic contact lens. *Ann Ophthalmol* 7:97-106, 1975.

56. Cooper RL, Constable IJ: Infective keratitis in soft contact wearers. *Brit J Ophthalmol* 61:250-254, 1977.

57. Pitts RE, Krachmer JH: Evaluation of soft contact lens disinfection in the home environment. *Arch Ophthalmol* 97:470-472, 1979.

58. Duke-Elder S: Diseases of the outer eye. Part II. Cornea and Sclera. *In:* System of Ophthalmology. St. Louis: C.V. Mosby, 1965, Vol 8,pp 815-839.

59. Cogan DG: Syndrome of nonsyphilitic interstitial keratitis and vestibuloauditory symptoms. *Arch Ophthalmol* 33:144, 1945.

60. Metcalf JF, Kaufman HE: Herpetic stromal keratitis: Evidence for cell-mediated immunopathogenesis. *Am J Ophthalmol* 82:527, 1976.

61. Thygeson P: Complications of staphylococcic blepharitis. *Am J Ophthalmol* 68:446, 1969.

62. Thygeson P: Marginal corneal infiltrates and ulcers. *Trans Am Acad Ophthalmol Otolaryngol* 51:198, 1947.

63. Smolin G, Okumoto M: Staphylococcal blepharitis. *Arch Ophthalmol* 95:812, 1977.

64. Mondino BJ, Brown SI, Rabin BS: The role of complement in corneal diseases. *Trans Ophthalmol Soc UK* 98:363, 1978.

65. Mondino BJ, Kowalski R, Ratajczak HV, Peters J, Cutler SB, Brown SI: Rabbit model of phlyctenulosis and catarrhal infiltrates. *Arch Ophthalmol* 99:891-895, 1981.

66. Mondino BJ, Kowalski RP: Phlyctenulae and catarrhal infiltrates. Occurrence in rabbits immunized with staphylococcal cell walls. *Arch Ophthalmol* 100:1968-1971, 1982.

67. Cohn H, Mondino BJ, Brown SI, Hall GD: Marginal corneal ulcers with beta streptococcal conjunctivitis and chronic dacryocystitis. *Am J Ophthalmol* 87:541-543, 1979.

68. Thygeson P: The etiology and treatment of phlyctenular keratoconjunctivitis. *Am J Ophthalmol* 34:1217-1236, 1951.

69. Sorsby AP: The etiology of phlyctenular ophthalmia. *Brit J Ophthalmol* 26:159, 1942.

70. Mondino BJ, Cruz TA, Kowalski RP: Immune responses of rabbits that develop phlyctenules and catarrhal infiltrates. *Arch Ophthalmol* 101:1275-1277, 1983.

71. Mondino BJ, Dethlefs B: Occurrence of phlyctenules after immunization with ribitol teichoic acid of Staphylococcus aureus. *Arch Ophthalmol* (in press).

72. Zaidman GW, Brown SI: Orally administered tetracycline for phlyctenular keratoconjunctivitis. *Am J Ophthalmol* 92:173-182, 1981.

73. Duke-Elder S: Diseases of the outer eye. Part II. Cornea and Sclera. *In:* System of Ophthalmology. St. Louis: C.V. Mosby, 1965, Vol 8, pp 914-920.

74. Wood TO, Kaufman HE: Mooren's ulcer. *Am J Ophthalmol* 71:417, 1971.

75. Brown SI: Mooren's ulcer. Histopathology and proteolytic enzymes of adjacent conjunctiva. *Brit J Ophthalmol* 59:670, 1975.

76. Arentsen JJ, Christiansen JM, Maumenee AE: Marginal ulceration after intracapsular cataract extraction. *Am J Ophthalmol* 81:194, 1976.

77. Mondino BJ, Brown SI, Mondzelewski JB: Peripheral corneal ulcers with herpes zoster ophthalmicus. *Am J Ophthalmol* 86:611, 1978.

78. Brown SI, Mondino BJ, Rabin BS: Autoimmune phenomenon in Mooren's ulcer. *Am J Ophthalmol* 82:835, 1976.

79. Eiferman RA, Hyndiuk RA: IgE in limbal conjunctiva in Mooren's ulcer. *Can J Ophthalmol* 12:234, 1977.

80. Mondino BJ, Brown SI and Rabin BS: Cellular immunity in Mooren's ulcer. *Am J Ophthalmol* 85:788, 1978.

81. Brown SI: Mooren's ulcer. Treatment by conjunctival excision. *Brit J Ophthalmol* 59:675, 1975.

82. Maumenee AE: Lecture at University of California. San Francisco, 1972.

83. Brown SI, Mondino BJ: Penetrating keratoplasty in Mooren's ulcer. *Am J Ophthalmol* 89:255-258, 1980.

84. Aronson SB, Elliott JH, Moore TE, O'Day DM: Pathogenetic approach to therapy of peripheral corneal inflammatory disease. *Am J Ophthalmol* 70:65, 1970.

85. Cogan DG: Corneoscleral lesions in periarteritis nodosa and Wegener's granulomatosis. *Trans Am Ophthalmol* 53:321, 1955.

86. Jampol LM, West C, Goldberg MF: Therapy of scleritis with cytotoxin agents. *Am J Ophthalmol* 82:266, 1978.

87. Wood WJ, Nicholson DH: Corneal ring ulcer as a presenting manifestation of acute monocytic leukemia. *Am J Ophthalmol* 76:69, 1973.

88. Jayson MIV, Easty DL: Ulceration of the cornea in rheumatoid arthritis. *Ann Rheum Dis* 36:428, 1977.

89. Brown SI, Grayson M: Marginal furrows, a characteristic corneal lesion of rheumatoid arthritis. *Arch Ophthalmol* 79:563, 1968.

90. Wilson FM, Grayson M, Ellis FD: Treatment of peripheral corneal ulcers by limbal conjunctivectomy. *Brit J Ophthalmol* 60:713, 1976.

91. Eiferman RA, Carothers DJ, Yankeelow JA: Peripheral rheumatoid ulceration and evidence for conjunctival collagenase production. *Am J Ophthalmol* 87:703, 1979.

92. Khodadoust AA, Silverstein AM: Transplantation and rejection of individual cell layers of the cornea. *Invest Ophthalmology* 8:180-195, 1969.

93. Polack FM: Lymphocyte destruction during corneal homograft reaction. *Arch Ophthalmol* 89:413-416, 1973.

94. Krachmer JH, Alldredge OC: Subepithelial infiltrates. A probable sign of corneal transplant rejection. *Arch Ophthalmol* 96:2234-2237, 1978.

95. Stark WJ, Taylor AR, Bias WB, Maumenee AE: HLA antigen and keratoplasty. *Am J Ophthalmol* 86:595, 1978.

96. Salisbury JD, Gebhardt BM: Suppression of corneal allograft rejection by cyclosporin A. *Arch Ophthalmol* 99:1640-1643, 1981.

Chapter 8

The Medical Management of Glaucoma

Matthew W. Mosteller, MD
Thom J. Zimmerman, MD

THE MEDICAL MANAGEMENT
OF GLAUCOMA

Glaucoma is an ocular disease in which the intraocular pressure is too high to maintain normal optic nerve function. The disease is characterized by optic disc pallor and excavation secondary to pressure-induced nerve fiber bundle damage. The prevention of this nerve fiber damage and the associated visual field loss is the goal of glaucoma therapy.

The medical management of glaucoma is approached through use of the ocular hypotensive agents. Knowledge of the pharmacology, mode of action, and potential side-effects of these agents facilitates proper therapeutic decisions in the treatment of glaucomatous patients. First, this chapter will present essential pharmacologic aspects of each group of ocular hypotensive agents available to the clinician. Second, we discuss application of this knowledge to a therapeutic regimen that encourages patient compliance and proper use of medications. This information should guide the clinician toward a more successful use of ocular hypotensive agents in the medical management of glaucoma.

Parasympathomimetic Agents

One branch of the peripheral autonomic nervous system is the parasympathetic. The neurotransmitter of all parasympathetic fibers is acetylcholine and thus the term "cholinergic" is used to describe neurons that release this neurotransmitter. There are two types of parasympathetic agents used in glaucoma therapy: the direct acting cholinomimetics or "false transmitters" (pilocarpine, carbachol) which mimic acetylcholine at the postsynaptic receptor, and anticholinesterase agents (echothiophate iodide) that indirectly potentiate acetylcholine at the receptor sites by inhibiting the enzyme breakdown of the natural neurotransmitter.[1]

In the eye, parasympathomimetic drugs cause the cholinoceptive pupillary sphincter and ciliary muscle to respond, resulting in miosis, increased accomodation, and a decrease in intraocular pressure; it is felt that the decrease in pressure is secondary to an inward pull of the ciliary muscle which increases the facility of outflow of the aqueous humor by its mechanical change in the trabecular meshwork.[2]

Pilocarpine. Pilocarpine has been the foundation of glaucoma medical management for decades. Its related chemical structure to acetylcholine allows the drug to directly stimulate the smooth muscle cholinergic receptors in the eye. It is available in 0.5% to 10% topical solutions but most commonly is used in the 1% to 4% range. The initial decrease in intraocular pressure begins one hour after topical instillation with a maximum effect at 75 minutes. The duration of a single dose is approximately six hours, thus the dosage frequency needs to be four times a day.[3] The duration of action seems to be potentiated in darkly pigmented eyes secondary to drug absorption by the iris and ciliary body pigment. However, the ocular hypotensive effect of pilocarpine in these heavily pigmented eyes is decreased due to the decreased availablity of the drug to intended ciliary body receptor sites.[34]

The pilocarpine-induced miosis begin 15 to 30 minutes after installation and lasts 4 to 8 hours. There is no association between miosis and the control of intraocular pressure. The miosis and induced accommodative spasm are the major disadvantages of this drug. Patients with lens opacities have difficulty with miotic agents in general, and those younger patients with strong accommodative ability have problems adjusting to the ever fluctuating myopia.

Other ocular effects induced by this class of drugs include shallowing of the anterior chamber, increased lacrimation, vasodilatation, breakdown of blood aqueous barrier, orbital muscle spasm, and allergic reaction. Systemic cholinergic effects of pilocarpine can include stimulation of any smooth muscle with muscarinic cholinergic receptors, especially those in the gastrointestinal, pulmonary, and genitourinary system. Side-effects of toxic dosage can include nausea, vomiting, and diarrhea, as well as bronchospasm, salivation, and sweating.[5]

A major advance in the delivery of pilocarpine has been the membrane delivery system, the Ocusert.® The flat oval membrane inserts into the

TABLE 8-1.
OCULAR HYPOTENSIVE AGENTS

Class Agent	Mode of Action	Example
Parasympathomimetics Direct acting cholinergics	Increase aqueous outflow facility	Pilocarpine Carbachol
Indirect acting cholinergics (anticholinesterage agents)		Echotheophate iodide
		Demecarium bromide
Sympathomimetics	Increase uveal-sceral outflow	Epinephrine Dipivalyl epinephrine
Beta-adrenergic blockers maleate	Decrease aqueous humor production	Timolol
Carbonic anhydrase inhibitors	Decrease aqueous humor production	Acetazolamide
Hyperosmotics	Decrease volume of fluid in the eye by a diffusion gradient	1) Glycerin 2) Isosorbide 3) Mannitol

conjunctiva cul-de-sac and releases a constant therapeutic dose of pilocarpine without the peak-trough cycle of a traditional topical medication.[6] There are two levels of dose release: P20 at 20 microgram per hour, and P40 at 40 microgram per hour. These dosages are equivalent to pilocarpine 2% and 4% drops, respectively. Each insert decreases intraocular pressure for a five-to-seven-day period.[7]

The Ocusert's major advantage is seen in the patient who is visually handicapped secondary to the fluctuating myopia of topically instilled parasympathomimetics. The induced accommodation of the insert is fairly constant, thus glasses can be prescribed for this stable refractive error. Because of a decrease in the overall amount of drug delivered, the risk of systemic side-effects and allergic reactions is also decreased with the Ocusert.® The convenience of a once-a-week delivery system as opposed to a four-times-a-day application is evident. The Ocusert4RS is more expensive than topical pilocarpine and requires manual dexterity and patience to insert and keep in place. However, many motivated patients for whom a miotic is indicated have tolerated the membrane delivery system well.

Carbachol.

Carbachol. The second major parasympathomimetic ocular hypotensive agent is the direct-acting drug, carbachol. It is a cholinester similar to acetylcholine and stimulates both muscarinic and nicotinic receptors of the parasympathetic autonomic nervous system.[1]

It is available in 0.75% to 3% topical drops and is administered every 8 hours for the diurnal control of intraocular pressure. The magnitude of the decrease in intraocular pressure caused by carbachol and pilocarpine is proportional to the level of the pretreated intraocular pressure. Considering the similar mode of pharmacologic action, the comparable ocular and systemic effects of pilocarpine and carbachol are easily understood.[8]

Because of its polar charge induced by the quaternary nitrogen group, carbachol does not penetrate the cornea or decrease the intraocular pressure as consistently as pilocarpine. However, carbachol has been shown to decrease the pressur in some patients who have become refractile to the hypotensive effects of topical pilocarpine. The benefits of the three-times-a-day installation as opposed to a four-times-a-day regime will help to encourage patient compliance.

The clinical use of N-dimethyllated carbachol (DMC) or a similarly altered cholinergic drug is a possiblity in the future. This drug was developed in an effort to obtain a cholinester with enhanced corneal permeability. Early studies have indicated that a 9% concentration can lower the intraocular pressure comparable to that of 3% carbachol. Surprisingly, this drug did not seem to have the accommodative and miotic side-effects of the other parasympathomimetics.[9] Investigative work has shown that the cholinergic effect of the pupil and ciliary body can be separated, thus explaining the lack of miosis. However, the decrease in intraocular pressure without an increase in accommodation is contradictory to the present beliefs regarding the mechanism of action of the cholinergic drugs in general. This drug and others similar in nature are excellent research tools into the investigation of aqueous dynamics and are potentially important drugs in the medical management of glaucoma.

Anticholinesterase Agents. The enzyme acetylcholinesterase terminates the transmitter action of acetylcholine at the junction of the cholinergic nerve endings. Drugs which inhibit or inactivate this enzyme are called anticholinesterase agents. These agents cause acetylcholine to accumulate at the receptor site, thus potentiating the neurotransmitter stimulation effect.[1] Echothiophate iodide (Phospholine Iodine®) and demecarium bromide (Humorsol®) are the two agents in this group of drugs that are most widely used in the control of glaucoma. The indicated twice-a-day instillation is very convenient, but their systemic and ocular side-effects are more frequent than the other parasympathomimetic agents. With the present clinical drugs available, a direct-acting cholinergic like pilocarpine should not be given simultaneously with one of the anticholinesterase agents because of the potential deleterious effect on efforts to control the intraocular pressure.

Problems with this class of miotics include the miosis and strong accommodative spasm and also a cataractogenic property.[10] Due to the drug's strong contractive stimulation of the ciliary body, there is a tractional force exerted on the vitreous base and peripheral retina, thus increasing the risk of retinal detachment.[11] A thorough fundus examination should be performed before initiating miotic therapy, especially the anticholinesterase drugs.

Iris cysts have a tendency to form at the pupillary margin with anticholinesterase agents but usually regress when the drug is stopped. The propensity for cyst formation may be decreased by the addition of topical phenylephrine.[12]

Nasolacrimal absorption of the anticholinesterase agents can lead to a high incidence of systemic side-effects. One of the serious complications is seen when there is concomitant use with succinylcholine, a neuromuscular blocking agent used frequently as a rapidly reversible paralysing agent in general anesthesia. This paralyzing depolarization of the skeletal muscles by succinylcholine is inactivated by thesame cholinesterase enzymes which inactivate acetylcholine. This action by the anticholinesterase drug can prolong the postoperative paralysis induced by succinylcholine and thus should not be used for several weeks prior to the use of succinylcholine-induced general anesthesia.

Sympathomimetic Agents

The next important class of ocular hypertensive agents is the sympathomimetics. The sympathetic outflow is a major division of the peripheral autonomic nervous system with norepinephrine as the major neurotransmitter. Norepinephrine, epinephrine, and other structurally-related catecholamines can produce the "adrenergic" sympathetic response by an inhibitory or excitatory effect on the smooth muscle of the adrenoreceptive end-organ sites. These sites are divided into alpha- and beta-receptors, depending upon their response to certain sympathomimetic agents.[1]

In the eye, there are both alpha- and beta-receptors of the sympathetic nervous system that when stimulated are responsbile for changes in aqueous production, facility of aqueous outflow, pupillary size, and tonicity of the vasculature.

Epinephrine. Epinephrine is the prototype drug in the ocular sympathomimetic class. It stimulates both alpha- and beta-receptors with a secondary increase in the aqueous outflow facility and a subclinical change in the production of aqueous.[13] Epinephrine is available in 0.25% to 2% dosage strengths with maximal ocular hypotensive activity at one hour after instillation. The twice-a-day frequency of instillation is consistent with the 12-hour duration of action of the drug.

Ocular side-effects of epinephrine include adrenochrome pigmentation on the eye and nasolacrimal system, a reversible cystoid macular edema in aphakic patients, conjunctival vasodilatation and allergic rection.[14,15] There can be pupillary dilatation in one-third of patients using this drug, thus it should be used with caution in patients with narrow angles.

Due to the adrenoreceptive sites in the heart and vasculature of the body, the systemically-absorbed topical epinephrine can cause heart rate, blood pressure, and peripheral circulatory changes that could be deleterious to a patient with a compromised cardiovascular system.[16]

Dipivefrin Hydrochloride. In an effort to improve absorption and obtain a site-selective ocular effect, the prodrug dipivefrin hydrochloride (Propine®) was developed and is now in clinical use. A prodrug is a therapeutic agent that must undergo biotransformation into its active form before producing its effect. DPE is an epinephrine analog with added organic side chains. This lipophilic addition to epinephrine increases its corneal penetration 17 times,[17] and thus the clinically available 0.1% dose of DPE is equivalent in ocular hypotensive effect to the 2% standard topical epinephrine.[18]

This product exerts adrenergic effect only after the drug has penetrated the eye and the side chains have been hydrolyzed off the epinephrine. The fact that the active epinephrine is only intraocularly available decreases the possibility of systemic adrenergic side-effects secondary to nasal lacrimal system absorption. The topical effects of the active epinephrine on the eye, such as the pigmentation, burning, and vasodilatation, are also decreased. The problem of aphakic cystoid macular edema, which is felt to be releated to the intraocular concentration of epinephrine, is predicted to be of the same magnitude with this drug. The development of this first clinically available ocular prodrug is an advance toward better drug delivery systems for glaucoma.

Carbonic Anhydrase Inhibitors (CAI)

Carbonic anhydrase is an enzyme found in many sites of the body including the ciliary body, retina, and lens. In addition to its involvement in systemic acid-base physiology, the enzyme is important in the control of the production of aqueous humor. When more than 90% of this enzyme is inhibited, a suppressed production of aqueous humor is manifested with a decrease in the intraocular pressure in the glaucoma patient. This ocular effect seems to be independent of the systemic diuretic effect. There are many theories regarding the ocular hypotensive mode of action, but most center on the central theme of decreased aqueous production.[19] Furthermore, excellent evidence and proposed mechanism for the decrease in aqueous production exist.[20]

The two carbonic anhydrase inhibitors we most frequently use in the treatment of glaucoma are acetazolamide and methazolamide. Due to its pharmaoclogic properties, methazolamine (Naptazone®) should be given in a twice-a-day regimen of 25 mg to 50 mg orally. The higher the dose, the more systemic side-effects the patient will encounter. Most glaucoma patients will have a 4 mm to 5 mm decrease in intraocular pressure with this regimen without incapacitating side-effects.[21]

If the intraocular pressure is still in the unacceptable range after a regimen of appropriate topical medications and methazolamide, then this carbonic anhydrase inhibitor should be replaced with acetazolamide (Diamox®). With the 500 mg oral sequels given twice a day, the maximum ocular hypotensive effect of the CAI will be obtained. However, the systemic side-effects will also increase as compared to the comparable dosage of methazolamide. With both carbonic anhydrase inhibitors, the maximal effect in intraocular pressure is attained in two to four hours after oral administration and one to two hours after I.V. administration of the commercially-available parenteral acetazolamide.

Paresthesias, malaise, and GI symptoms are the side-effects most commonly responsible for discontinuance of this drug. Other potential side-effects include renal calculi, acid-base abnormalities, impotence, confusion and depression, as well as Stevens-Johnson syndrome, and bone marrow suppression.[19] The use of potassium supplementation has not been shown to be beneficial in reducing the CAI side-effects unless the patient is frankly hypokalemic from other reasons (concomitant thiazide diuretic administration). Controlled studies have failed to show that administering the medication with meals or with oral sodium bicarbonate contributes to a decrease in side-effects.

Finding the right pharmacologic preparation, in the lowest possible dose to obtain a beneficial response, is the key to decreasing the CAI side-effects. The site-selective pharmacologic action of a topically-administered carbonic anhydrase inhibitor would be an important advance in ocular therapy. The use of such a drug delivery system could dramatically improve the therapeutic indices of this important class of ocular hypotensive agents.

Beta-Adrenergic Receptor Blockers: Timolol Maleate

Unlike other areas of the body in which alpha- and beta-adrenergic stimulation has opposite physiologic effects, there is a more complex relationship between these receptors and the production and outflow of aqueous humor. The betareceptor blocker, timolol maleate, is an important component of this sensitive balance. The mechanism of action of timolol is explained by the decrease in the rate of aqueous formation with no clinically significant increase in outflow facility.[22] This beta-blocker has been shown to decrease intraocular pressure in normal as well as glaucomatous patients[23,24] and seems to be additive with current glaucoma medications.[25]

The dose response for timolol peaks at the commercially available 0.25% to 0.50% solutions. The maximal decrease in pressure occurs approximately two hours after topical instillation, and 24-hour control is attained with twice-a-day instillation. An increase in the frequency or concentration of the drug has no further ocular hypotensive benefit and may expose the patient to more systemic side-effects. During the first few weeks of administration, some patients respond to the beta-blocker with a dramatic drop in intraocular pressure after which a slight decrease in effect is seen. However, after stabilization from this rise in pressure, there is still the beneficial 25% greater decrease from the pretreated intraocular pressure.[26]

Ocular side-effects have been minimal with the beta-blocker. There is no change in pupillary size or accommodation but some patients experience burning, tearing, and foreign body sensation.

When used in the prescribed dosage and frequency, timolol has an excellent therapeutic index for most patients. However, because the beta-blocker can inhibit other beta receptors in the body, there is the possibility of systemic side-effects. It should be used with caution in patients with asthma, chronic obstructive lung disease, congestive heart failure, and bradyarrhythmias such as bradycardia or heart block.[27]

Hyperosmotic Agents

Hyperosmotic agents produce their ocular hypotensive effect through a diffusion gradient system by rapidly increasing the plasma osmolality relative to the intraocular fluids. There is a compensatory movement of water from the vitreous and anterior chamber into the plasma in an effort to equilibrate this osmolality difference, causing a decrease in the vitreous volume, anterior chamber depth, and intraocular pressure. The best ocular hyperosmotic agents include those drugs with a small molecular weight that do not corss the blood/aqueous barrier, and are easily administered and absorbed into the extracellular space. Clinically there are several osmotic agents that possess these necessary attributes. Their clinical use in glaucoma therapy is generally limited to the immediate short-term treatment of an acute, dangerously high intraocular pressure.[28]

Oral glycerin is available in 50% and 75% solutions and is given as a dose of 1.5 mg to 2.0 mg/kg of body weight. The maximal fall in intraocular pressure occurs approximately one hour after administration with a four- to six-hour duration of action. It is usually administered with orange juice through a straw to increase palatability. Prior administration of an intramuscular phenothiazine seems to decrease the gastrointestinal side-effects associated with this osmotic. Glycerin is a mild diuretic and has a large carbohydrate load, thus it should be used with caution in patients with glucose intolerance. Mild headaches, backaches, and dizziness associated with its use are attributed to the relative dehydration of the cerebrospinal fluid. It is the most accessible and easily-administered osmotic agent available.

If a parenteral osmotic is necessary, mannitol is the agent most often used. Mannitol is a hyperosmotic agent administered parenterally in a 10% to 20% solution at 1.5 gm to 2.0 gm/kg of body weight over 30 minutes. The maximal effect occurs in one hour with a five- to six-hour duration of action. Because of vascular overload, it should be used with caution in patients with compromised cardiovascular status or electrolyte imbalance tendencies.

Another oral hyperosmotic agent, isosorbide, is now being used especially in glucose-intolerant patients.[29] This clinically available drug (Hydronol®) is administered in a 50% solution at 1 gm to 2 gm/kg of body weight. It does not administer the glucose load of glycerin and thus will not increase the serum glucose. Other osmotic agents that decrese the intraocular pressure but are infrequently used are sodium ascorbate and ethyl alcohol.

Miscellaneous Agents for Control of Glaucoma

The use of cycloplegic agents and topical steroids is the accepted medical treatment for inflammatory or neovascular-induced glaucoma. With these agents, the inflammatory response will be suppressed and the alternate uveal-scleral outflow of aqueous will be utilized fully.

Miscellaneous therapeutic agents such as cardiac glycosides, ethyl alcohol, vasopressin, marijuana, phenytoin, clonidine, and the fungal metabolite, cytochalasin B, have all been shown to decrease intraocular pressure one way or another, but their use is presently limited to investigational studies.

As we understand more about the complex system of aqueous dynamics, more therapeutic agents will become clinically available. An example of this is the new alpha-adrenergic blocker, thymoxamine. This competitive antagonist with norepinephrine produces miosis without affecting intraocular pressure or accommodation.[30] It could have several applications in the management of glaucoma, especially in those cases secondary to the pigment dispersion syndrme. One theory regarding this disease is that there is a rubbing of the peripheral iris on the anterior ciliary zonules, thus causing loss of pigment into the anterior chamber and trabecular meshwork.[31] Iris-zonular contact can be prevented with miosis by thymoximine without the associated side-effects of our present miotics.

Principles of Clinical Applications

Providing a beneficial therapeutic regimen that is amenable to patient compliance is the goal of all medical therapy. Many patients who are unresponsive to the ocular hyypotensive agents fall into a category of "noncompliance." When the doctor/patient relationship becomes established and the decision to treat glaucoma has been made, the ophthalmologist should educate his patient in the nature of the disease and emphasize the need for and the proper use of the medications.

Following the principles of streamlining medications to a twice-a-day regimen whenever possible and prescribing the least amount of agents in the lowest concentration, will help the patient accept his therapy. By warning the patient of potential adverse effects prior to the prescribing of the medication, the side-effects will be more easily and less anxiously accepted. The teaching of punctal occlusion of the nasolacrimal system and the waiting of 5 to 10 minutes between successive topical drops will increase the therapeutic index of the medications prescribed.

Summary

The knowledgeable physician working with a patient who understands his disease and medications is the key to the successful use of ocular hypotensive agents in the medical management of glaucoma.

References

1. Koelle GB: Neurohumoral transmission and neuroeffector junctional sites. In: Goodman LS, Gilman A (eds), The Pharmacological Basis of Therapeutics. 5th Edition, New York: MacMillan Co., 1975, pp 404-410, 416-431.
2. Kaufman PL: Pilocarpine uptake. Ann Ophthalmol 11:631-632, 1979.
3. Creal AE, Newell FW: Effects of pilocarpine on ocular tension dynamics. Am J Ophthalmol 57:34-40, 1964.
4. Lyons JS, Krohn DL: Pilocarpine uptake by pigmented uveal tissue. Am J Ophthalmol 75:885-888, 1973.
5. Zimmerman TJ: Pilocarpine. Pharmacology of ocular drugs. Ophthalmology 88:85-88, 1981.
6. Chiou CY, Trzeciakowski J: Recent advances in cholinergic drugs for glaucoma therapy. In: Kaufman HE, Zimmerman TJ (eds), Current Concepts in Ophthalmology. St. Louis: Mosby, 1979, 6:134-143.
7. Macoul KL, Pavan-Langston D: Pilocarpine Ocusert system for sustained control of ocular hypertension. Arch Ophthalmol 93:587-590, 1975.
8. Niemeyer G: Carbaminoyl choline in glaucoma simplex: Comparative tonographic study of the effects of pilocarpine and carbachol in chronic simple glaucoma. Ophthalmologica 156:161, 1968.
9. Leader BJ, Zimmerman TJ: Advances in the pharmacologic treatment of glaucoma. In: Koch, Parke, Paton (eds), Current Management in Ophthalmology. New York: Churchill Livingston, 1983.
10. Axelsson V: Glaucoma, miotic therapy and cataract, III. Visual loss to lens changes in glaucoma eyes treated with paroaxon, echothiophate or pilocarpine. Acta Ophthalmol 46:831-845, 1968.

11. Alpar JJ: Miotics and retinal detachment: A survey and case report. Ann Ophthalmol 11:395-401, 1979.
12. Chamberlain W: Anticholinesterase miotics in the management of accommodative esotropia. Trans Ann Ophthalmol Soc 72:229-241, 1974.
13. Creel AE, Newell FW, Novack M: Early and long-term effect of L-epinephrine. Am J Ophthalmol 59:833-839, 1965.
14. McReynolds WV, Havener WHI, Henderson JW: Hazards of use of sympathomimetic drugs in ophthalmology. Arch Ophthalmol 56:176, 1956.
15. Michels RG, Maumenee AE: Cystoid macular edema associated with topically applied epinephrine in aphakic eyes. Am J Ophthalmol 80:379, 1975.
16. Lanscle RK: Systemic reactions to topical epinephrine and phenylephrine. Am J Ophthalmol 61:95, 1966.
17. Mandell AI, Stentz F, Kitabachi AE: Dipivalyl epinephrine in glaucoma. Ophthalmology 85:268, 1978.
18. Kohn AN, Moss AD, Hargett NA: Clinical comparison of dipivalyl epinephrine and epinephrine in the treatment of glaucoma. Am J Ophthalmol 87:196, 1979.
19. Ellis PP: Carbonic anhydrase inhibitor: Pharmacologic effects and problems of long-term therapy. In: Leopold IH (ed), Symposium of Ocular Therapy, Vol 4. St. Louis: Mosby, 1969.
20. Maren TH: Use of inhibitors in physiologic studies of carbonic anhydrase. Am J Physiol 232(4):F291-7, 1977.
21. Stone RA, Zimmerman TJ, Shin D, et al: Low-dose methazolamide and intraocular pressure. Am J Ophthalmol 83:674-679, 1977.
22. Yablowski ME, Zimmerman TJ, Waltman SR, Becker B: A fluorophotometric study of the effect of topical timolol on aqueous humor dynamics. Exp Eye Res 17:135, 1978.
23. Boger WP III, Steinert R, Puliafito C, et al: A double masked clinical trial comparing timolol ophthalmic solutions and pilocarpine in the therapy of open-angle glaucoma. Am J Ophthalmol 86:8, 1978.
24. Katz IM, Hubbard WA, Getson AJ, Gould AL: Intraocular pressure decrease in normal volunteers following timolol ophthalmic solution. Invest Ophthalmol Vis Sci 15:489, 1976.
25. Sonty S, Schwartz B: The additive effect of timolol on open-angle glaucoma patients on maximal medical therapy. Surv Ophthalmol 23:381, 1979.
26. Zimmerman TJ and Canale P: Timolol - Further observations. Ophthalmology 86:166, 1979.
27. Zimmerman TJ, Leader BJ, Golob DS: Potential side-effects of timolol therapy in the treatment of glaucoma. Ann Ophthalmol 13:683, 1981.
28. Becker B: Use of hyperosmotic agents in the treatment of glaucoma. Symposium on glaucoma. Trans New Orleans Acad of Ophthalmol. St. Louis: Mosby, 1967.
29. Becker B, Kolker AE, Krupin T: Isosorbide, and oral hyperosmotic agent. Arch Ophthalmol 78:147, 1967.
30. Wand M, Grant WM: Thymoxamine hydrochloride: An alpha-adrenergic blocker. Surv Ophthalmol 25:75, 1980.
31. Campbell DG: Pigmentary dispersion and glaucoma: A new theory. Arch Ophthalmol 97:1667, 1979.

Chapter 9

Medical Retina and Photocoagulation of Retinal Disorders

Joseph B. Walsh, MD
Paul R. Rosenberg, MD

MEDICAL RETINA AND PHOTOCOAGULATION OF RETINAL DISORDERS

Introduction

With the introduction of fluorescein angiography as a clinical device and the adaptation of the laser to ophthalmology, a revolution occurred in the diagnosis and treatment of retinal and choroidal diseases. This chapter will highlight some of the disease entities where these new techniques have been most beneficial. Emphasis is placed on retinal vein obstruction, diabetic retinopathy, and macular degeneration associated with aging.

Fluorescein Angiography

The blood-retinal barrier serves to protect the retina from a variety of blood components. This is analogous to that of the blood-brain barrier. This barrier exists at two points: the epithelial cell of the retinal capillary and the retinal pigment epithelial cell.[1] Although previous investigators used fluorescein and other dyes to investigate the retinal and choroidal circulation,[2-4] it was Norvotny and Alvis who defined the technique of present-day fluorescein angiography.[5]

This technique consists of a rapid (0.5 second interval) series of photographs of the retina following an intravenous injection of sodium fluorescein (10 cc of 5% or 5 cc of 20% NaF) (Figure 9-1). Using a fundus camera with appropriate filters and film, the fluorescence generated will outline the retina, the optic nerve head and, to a lesser extent, the choroidal circulation.

The onset of the retinal arterial phase usually occurs 7 to 20 seconds after dye injection (Figure 9-2A-E). The choroidal phase occurs within 1 second of the retinal arterial phase. From the onset of dye in the retinal artery to laminar flow in the major veins is usually 2 to 3 seconds. In another 3 to 4 seconds, the intensity of dye is equal in the arteries and veins; this marks the onset of the venous phase. Fading of the dye occurs in around 30 minutes but, because of recirculation, it can remain for hours. Because of the various cardiovascular and pulmonary functions, the exact timing of the various events may vary in the same patient from one study to another. When interpreting a fluorescein angiogram, it is most helpful for the reader to have examined the patient.

There is significant incidence of side-effects associated with fluorescein angiography.[6,7] Extravasation of the dye may cause local pain, redness, and edema. This responds to local injection of saline and cold compresses. In

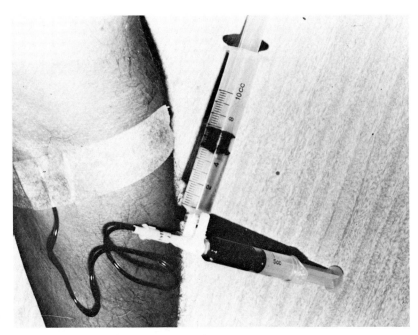

Figure 9-1. A technique for intravenous injection of sodium fluorescein. A 19-gauge butterfly is secured within an anticubital vein. A three-way stop-cock is employed with 5 cc of NaF in one syringe and 5 cc of NaCl in the other.

rare cases, necrosis of the skin may occur, necessitating plastic repair. Systemically, the most common side-effects include nausea and light-headedness, which occur in upwards of 10% of the patients. This is often transient and may be modified by supportive, quiet surroundings. The next most common symptom is emesis. Any of these conditions just listed may also be associated with a vasovagal response. Placing the patient in Trendelenburg's position will usually restore vascular stability. True allergies, such as represented by urticaria, bronchospasm, or anaphylaxis, are rare but require prompt supportive action including epinephrine, steroids, and appropriate life-support systems. It is obvious that, in the age group most commonly undergoing fluorescein angiography, cardiovascular conditions may be aggravated by any of the above complications and, in turn, lead to cardiac arrhythmias and coronary or cerebrovascular insufficiency. In any situation when fluorescein angiography is performed, cardiopulmonary resuscitation must be available quickly and performed efficiently.

There has been much discussion about the terminology used in describing fluorescein angiograms.[8] Basically there is a normal pattern which depends upon the individual patient. The blood-retinal barrier is normally intact. The only leakage noted is at the edge of the optic nerve head where, during the course of the angiogram, the disc may show increased fluorescence in a centripetal fashion due to leakage from the peripapillary choroid. Variations from normal may include more fluorescence (hyper) or less fluorescence (hypo). Hypofluorescence may be due to decreased vascular

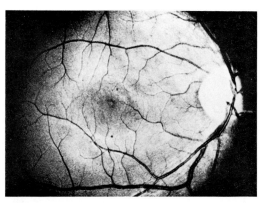

Figure 9-2A

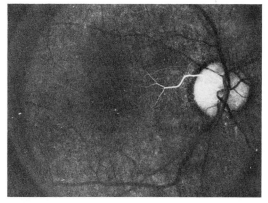

Figure 9-2B

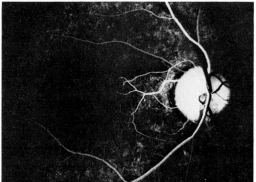

Figure 9-2C

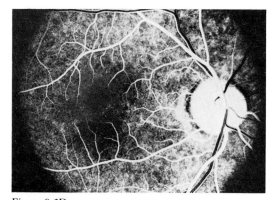

Figure 9-2D

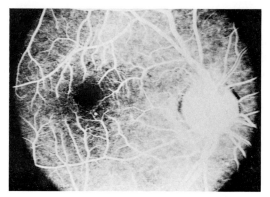

Figure 9-2E

Figure 9-2. Normal fluorescein angiogram demonstrating various phases. A. Red-free photograph of the posterior pole OD. B. Choroidal phase, 11.6 seconds. Note dye is present in the choriocapillaris, optic nerve and cilioretinal artery. C. Retinal arterial phase, 13.2 seconds. D. Arteriovenous phase, 14.1 seconds. Lamellar filling of the major veins entering the disc. E. Venous phase, 18.1 seconds. Note the retinal capillary detail and that the background fluorescence is peaked.

perfusion or blockage due to either blood, pigment, or retinal exudate. Hyperfluorescence may occur due to pooling of fluorescein beneath a detachment of the pigment epithelium, increased choroidal fluorescence due to decreased pigment of the pigment epithelium, or leakage due to breakdown of the blood-retinal barrier at the level of the retinal pigment epithelium and/or the retinal vascular endothelial cell.

Because both the choroidal and the retinal circulations are being studied simultaneously, stereoscopic analysis may be necessary in separating pathologies.

Retinal Artery Occlusions

Symptoms. The sudden and profound loss of vision as the presenting symptom of central retinal artery obstruction (CRAO) makes this one of the most frightening ophthalmologic entities, to both patient and physician.[9] Obviously the extent of the visual loss involved depends upon the retinal vessel(s) occluded. In some cases, the patient may report some transient obscurations of vision in the involved eye preceding the catastrophic event.

Associated Systemic Conditions. The over-65 age group is by far the most common group in which retinal artery occlusions occur and in this group, atherosclerosis of the carotid or, less commonly, the ophthalmic artery is the source of embolic material to the retinal arterial tree. This group has an association with other cardiovascular diseases such as coronary artery and cerebrovascular insufficiency.[9,10] Other factors contributing may include hypertension, diabetes, and hyperlipidemia. In some cases, atheromas of the central retinal artery at the level of the lamina cribrosa cause occlusion. In groups of younger patients a wide variety of diseases must be considered, among them cardiac valvular disease (including mitral valve prolapse and acute and subacute endocarditis), collagen vascular diseases, atrial myxoma, syphilis, and toxoplasmosis. In a patient where there is no obvious cause (such as listed above), a history of intravenous drug abuse, birth control pills, and/or an obstetric problem (amnionic fluid emboli) should be sought. Also to be considered are the hemoglobinopathies and cranial arteritis, as well as a history of possible emboli from diagnostic examinations, such as hysterosalpingography, or therapeutic, such as retrobulbar or parasinus injections.[11] Related to ocular surgery, intraocular pressure may be raised above that of the central retinal artery, producing arterial occlusion, by using preoperative devices to lower intraocular pressure by globe compression or by scleral indentation with retinal detachment surgery. Here the central retinal artery must be monitored periodically by ophthalmoscopy. Trauma may cause retinal arterial obstruction from retrobulbar hemorrhage or fat emboli from long bones. Preretinal arterial loops can occasionally kink and obstruct.[12]

Clinical Diagnosis. The findings depend upon the duration of the obstruction and the area of retina involved. In acute CRAO's, the vision is usually hand motion in the temporal periphery. Vision of no light perception indicates concomitant insufficiency of the choroidal system.[13] The pupil is dilated to about 7 mm and responds minimally to light and near. The retina and the retinal artery may be normal or a sluggish segmented dark blood column may be noted. The veins are usually moderately dilated. Within one to two hours, a whitening of the superficial retina occurs, most easily seen in the macula because of the volume of ganglion cells in this area and by contrast with the fovea, which has no ganglion cells. Variable amounts of retina may be normal, depending on the presence and extent of nonobstructed cilioretinal arteries. At this time, the retinal artery may still have the signs of sluggish flow or may be of normal appearance. The disc may appear blurred at the edges due to the adjacent intracellular retinal edema. Hemorrhages are rare. Over the next 48 to 72 hours, the intracellular edema fades and the retina appears normal. After several months, the picture is one of optic pallor, loss of the nerve fiber layer, and narrowing of the retinal vessels with or without halo sheathing. The retina has the appearance of a somewhat dull light reflex and foveal reflex. The pupil's response is that of an afferent pupillary defect. In some cases, patchy areas of choroidal hyper- and hypopigmentation may be noted, suggesting that choroidal vascular insufficiency was a concomitant, though unrecognized, event. Branch retinal artery occlusions have a similar course, limited to the section of the retina supplied by the involved artery.

Diagnostic Aids. The diagnosis is made by the history and clinical findings. Several additional modalities may be employed but are often unnecessary. Fluorescein angiography in the acute stage may be completely normal or show delay of retinal arterial filling and even late leakage from the prevenule capillaries. Rarely does the retinal artery fail to fill. Electroretinography acutely shows reduction of the b-wave. After reestablishment of retinal blood flow, the b-wave recovers although the photopic component may fail to recover as well as the scotopic.[14]

Natural Course History. The visual acuity loss in arterial obstructions of the retina is usually complete in the area involved. There is experimental and clinical support, suggesting that ischemia to the retina for 90 minutes or longer results in irreversible changes to the superficial retina.[15] It has been suggested that recovery of vision is related to an ischemia of less than 90 minutes or to a patent cilioretinal artery. In the latter case, the degree of final vision depends on the extent and area of retina supplied by the cilioretinal artery. In one series of 107 cases of central retinal artery occlusion, 26% had some sparing of vision due to a patent cilioretinal artery,[16] and 10% had a final visual acuity of 20/20 to 20/80. There continues to be a question of the benefit from treatment of central artery obstructions in relation to the final visual acuity. In one study of CRAO, which excluded those patients having a fovea-sparing patent cilioretinal artery, treatment was followed by 12 out of 34 cases showing a sustained improvement of vision to 20/100 or better, with 7 cases achieving a final visual acuity of 20/40.[17]

Treatment. Because of the usually dim prognosis linked with CRAO, it does not seem intemperate to initiate therapy in selected patients. Various regimens are listed below:

- Ocular massage and/or anterior segment paracentesis
- Diamox orally
- 95% oxygen/5% CO_2 delivered by face mask for five to ten minutes each hour
- Retrobulbar injection including anesthesia, vasodilators
- Systemic vasodilators
- Systemic steroids, especially in the presence of cranial arteritis
- Canthotomy or evacuation of clot if retrobulbar hemorrhage is present
- Cannulization of the supraorbital artery and retrograde injection of drugs, e.g., anticoagulants and vasodilators.[18]

As can be seen by the list above, no specific regimen has yet been proven to be the best. However, in patients having had symptoms for less than 24 hours, treatment should be considered and immediately instituted once the diagnosis is made. Treatment modalities 1, 2 and 3 (listed above) pose little risk to the patient and may assist in the visual recovery. Retrobulbar injections increase orbital pressure and systemic vasodilators may reduce systemic blood pressure and, therefore, ocular perfusion. Cannulization of the supraorbital artery is a procedure that requires surgery. If the obstruction is documented as having been present longer than 24 hours, treatment will depend on the individual case. The visual return may occur up to several weeks after the treatment is initiated. Ocular massage and the oxygen/carbon dioxide should be continued for at least 48 hours, and the Diamox for several weeks. It is of utmost importance to have a thorough systemic evaluation of the patient so that associated diseases may be diagnosed and treated. Rarely, rubeosis iridis may be seen in the involved eye. This may be due to the central retinal artery obstruction itself or to anterior segment ischemia from concomitant carotid disease.[19]

In branch artery obstruction, the choice of therapy depends on the duration of the obstruction as well as the area involved. If macular function or a hemisphere of retina is involved, treatment may be instituted as outlined above. Again, a thorough search for the associated conditions must be made and treatment for them performed.

Central Retinal Vein Occlusion

Central retinal vein occlusion has been described for well over 100 years. Recent efforts at classification have attempted to unify our thoughts on this subject. Hayreh[20] has proposed that we treat this condition as two separate entities: venous stasis retinopathy (VSR) and hemorrhagic retinopathy (HR). VSR was originally used by Kearns and Hollenhorst[21] to describe the retinal picture in chronic ischemic oculopathy. VSR is a term used by Hayreh to represent a condition in which there may be minimal or no visual symptoms. There is marked engorgement of the retinal veins with flame shaped, peripapillary hemorrhages and scattered midperipheral dot and blot hemorrhages (Figure 9-3). The disc is typically hyperemic, and macular edema is commonly present.

Angiographic features of VSR include engorged retinal veins and capillaries, with staining of venous walls (Figure 9-4). Cystoid macular edema may be present. The optic disc shows hyperfluorescence. The most critical finding is the presence of good retinal capillary perfusion. It is believed that VSR is due to stasis and occlusion of the central retinal veins but *without* any significant hypoxia. Affected individuals may be young, in which case inflammatory phlebitis is suspected to be present, or in older people in which arteriolar sclerosis of the adventitial sheath of the major vessels may be the etiologic event. The ocular complications of VSR include macular edema, pigmentary maculopathy, and/or macular gliosis. Late findings in this condition include opticociliary shunt vessels, and microaneurysms, but not neovascularization.

The second major class of vein occlusion has been called hemorrhagic or ischemic retinopathy. Middle-aged to elderly individuals are frequently involved, although this condition is much less common than VSR. There is usually a marked deterioration of vision, often of sudden onset.

There is marked dilation and tortuosity of the retinal veins (Figure 9-5). There is often diffuse retinal hemorrhage with minimal involvement of the periphery. Cotton-wool spots are typically present in contradistinction to VSR. There is frequently narrowing of the retinal arterioles.

The most salient angiographic feature of this condition is the presence of capillary non-perfusion due to the large component of arterial hypoxia (Figure 9-6). Late findings include neovascularization of the anterior or less commonly the posterior segment as well as permanent changes in the macula and opticociliary shunt vessels.

Both HR and VSR are frequently seen in association with other systemic problems. These include a high incidence of hypertension, as well as diabetes, hypercholesterolemia, hypercoagulability states, and hypertryglyceridemia.

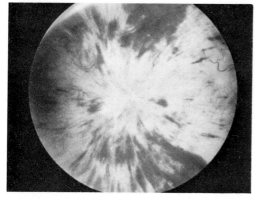

Figure 9-3. Venous Stasis Retinopathy (VSR)—retinal vascular tortuosity with flame shaped hemorrhages and swelling of the optic nerve are prominent features.

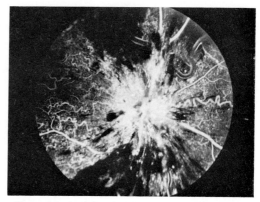

Figure 9-4. Angiography of the patient in Fig. 9-3 reveals unimpaired retinal capillary perfusion with blocking defects noted due to extravasation of blood. There is minimal edema.

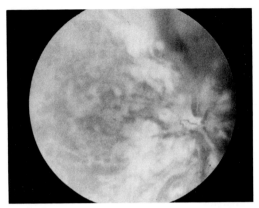

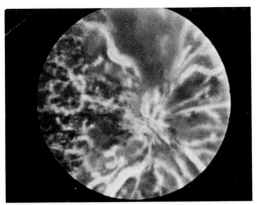

Figure 9-5. Hemorrhagic retinopathy is noted as evidenced by turgid retinal veins and numerous cotton-wool spots.

Figure 9-6. The angiogram of the patient in Fig. 9-5 shows the widespread obliteration of the retinal capillary bed with staining of the venule walls.

The differential diagnosis of vein occlusions should include central retinal artery occlusion, chronic ischemic oculopathy especially when due to carotid occlusive disease, diabetic retinopathy, papilledema, and Eales' disease.

Magargal[22] and co-workers confirmed that the risk of neovascular glaucoma after central vein occlusion was about 20%. However, those patients with VSR had essentially no risk of developing this complication. Patients with HR had about a 60% chance of developing neovascular glaucoma. The major reason for visual loss in both cases seemed to be prolonged macular edema when neovascular glaucoma does not develop.

There have been numerous treatment proposals for central vein occlusion. Among these are anticoagulants, dextran, fibrinolytic agents, vasodilators, and corticosteroids. There is no conclusive evidence to show that any of these modalities help at all.

Panretinal photocoagulation has been shown to be effective in prevention of neovascular glaucoma in eyes with HR and significant ischemia, both as a prophylactic measure or after the onset of rubeosis.[22] If the angle shows permanent damage, then photocoagulation therapy may be too late. Given the low morbidity rate of PRP, and the devastating effects of neovascular glaucoma, prophylactic PRP in patients with HR would seem pragmatic. As to the use of photocoagulation in cases of chronic macular edema, no conclusive evidence is available to determine the efficacy of treatment.

Branch Vein Obstruction

Branch retinal vein obstruction is, after diabetic retinopathy, the most common retinal vascular diagnosis made on a retinal service. Presenting symptoms include blurriness of vision, a sense of change in the quality of vision including metamorphopsia, visual field alteration usually segmental in nature, or a significant loss of vision.[23-25] It is not uncommon to make the diagnosis of a branch vein obstruction on an asymptomatic patient. Clinical findings include a wedge-shaped section of retina with the apex towards the disc wherein is found dot-and-blot hemorrhages, intraretinal edema (including subsensory retina), edema residue and cotton-wool spots. In the vast majority of the cases the obstruction occurs at an arteriovenous junction and the apex of the involved retinal segment points to the involved A-V crossing. In cases where the obstruction is not an A-V crossing, inflammatory diseases such as sarcoidosis or toxoplasmosis or other causes, e.g., trauma, should be considered. The obstructed vein in the acute stages appears dark, dilated and tortuous, and distal to the A-V crossing, and the proximate segment can be somewhat narrow. In the subacute or chronic phase, venous macroaneurysms[26] can be noted, as well as preretinal macular gliosis, pigmentary changes in the macula and venous sheathing both of the veins as well as secondary arteriosclerosis.[27] Venous-venous collaterals may be noted from the obstructed to the non-obstructed segment around the side of the obstruction, across the median raphe and from the obstructed vein to the non-obstructed veins or venules entering the disc. Neovascularization may be noted at the site of the obstruction or at the junction of the perfused and nonperfused retina as well as on the disc. Disc neovascularization may occur in quadrants not contiguous with the vein obstruction. In addition, retinal detachments may be noted either of a non-rhegmatogenous (effusion or traction) or rhegmatogenous.

Branch retinal vein obstructions commonly occur in patients with systemic diseases. The most common association is systemic hypertension and this may be found in 37-75% of the cases of retinal branch vein obstruction.[23,24] Diabetes may be found in anywhere from 2-30% of these patients and other atherosclerotic vascular diseases may be found in up to 4% of the patients. The relationship between chronic open-angle glaucoma and branch vein obstruction is somewhat controversial and elevated IOP has been reported in the literature to be 1% (i.e., no different than that of the general population) or in other studies up to 7-10%. There are many other associations with branch vein obstruction such as birth control pills, polycythemia, hemoglobinopathy, etc. In many of these cases, however, there is some dispute as to whether or not there is a cause and effect relationship between the systemic disease and the occurrence of the branch vein obstruction. The population in which branch vein obstructions are most commonly seen are over 60 years of age, and systemic abnormalities have an increased frequency.

The natural course history of branch vein obstructions is that approximately 50% of the patients have 20/40 vision or better at 6 months or more after their incident. About a quarter of the patients have visual acuity of 20/50-20/100 and about 22% have visual acuity of 20/100 or less. The major complications of vein obstruction involve the macula and include cystoid macular edema, preretinal macular gliosis, pigmentary mottling, macular cysts/holes or ischemia. The non-macula causes of decreased vision involve neovascularization either of the disc or elsewhere and result in vitreous hemorrhage, retinal detachment and, in rare cases, rubeosis iridis. Several characteristics of branch vein obstruction are able to be analyzed and give an estimate of the ultimate visual acuity. Foremost of these is the location of the obstruction. The more distal from the macula the less will be the alteration of the macular function. If a non-obstructed macular vein lies between the site of the obstruction and the macula so that the capillary network around the macula is normal, then the prognosis for good central vision is excellent. The establishment of good venous-venous collaterals will also allow the system to compensate and again a good prognosis is assured. If there is capillary nonperfusion involving the macular region, central vision will be poorer than with good perfusion.[28] If there is nonperfusion outside the macular region greater than 50-10 disc diameters in area, there is a reasonable incidence of neovascularization of the retina or disc.[29] It is interesting that although the incidence of neovascularization in vein obstruction is anywhere from 10-25%,[30] vitreous hemorrhage is not common. About 94% of the branch vein obstructions occur in the temporal retina. When the superotemporal branch vein is involved, the prognosis is better than the inferotemporal branch vein, perhaps because gravity aids edema clearing in the latter instance.

There has been much discussion on the medical treatment of branch vein obstructions but, except for controlling the systemic factors such as hypertension, diabetes, clotting disorders or hyperlipedema, there is no specific medical treatment. Systemic steroids have been mentioned to decrease macular edema in branch vein obstruction but indeed there are no sound supporting studies. Photocoagulation has been used for both macular edema and retinal neovascularization. With retinal disc neovascularization, quadrantic ablative therapy is used in the area of capillary nonperfusion. There is almost a 100% regression of neovascularization following this treatment. If significant hemorrhage is present the krypton laser is preferred over the argon-green. It has been reported that with chronic cystoid macular edema in branch vein obstruction, that is macular edema lasting 6 months or longer, 90% of these patients ultimately have 20/50 or poorer visual acuity.[31] Because of this, it has been suggested that focal photocoagulation be applied to the areas of capillary leakage in chronic cases. There have been some scattered reports in the literature[32-34]; but in the most recent study, which is the only controlled study yet available, by Shilling and Jones,[35] which involved two groups of patients, no statistical difference was noted in the final visual acuity between the treated and untreated cases. In this study 27 patients diagnosed within 3 months of the onset of the vein obstruction were randomized into treatment and non-treatment groups. They had 20/60 or poorer visual acuity. A second group of 63 patients, who had been followed for at least a year, with chronic cystoid macular edema, were also treated, and all had 20/60 or poorer visual acuity. At the end of one year follow-up posttreatment there was no statistical difference in the visual acuity between the treated and untreated groups. This study does not necessarily rule out the possibility that, in chronic macular edema in branch vein obstruction, photocoagulation would be of benefit, but does question the validity of the scattered reports that are present in the literature. There is a study sponsored by the National Eye Institute on the natural course history of branch vein obstructions as well as the alteration of this natural course history by treatment with photocoagulation. We await the results of that study. In those cases where traction retinal detachments occur, interventive therapy including vitrectomy and scleral buckling can be considered.

In summary, branch vein obstruction is one of the most common diseases that is seen in the retinal vascular service and has a relatively benign natural course history. By analyzing the characteristics of the branch vein obstruction one can determine to some extent the ultimate visual prognosis. In those cases with a poor prognosis, interventive therapy can be considered with the caution outlined in this chapter.

Diabetic Retinopathy

Incidence. Diabetes mellitus is becoming increasingly common in the USA. In 1978, it was estimated that 3-5% of the population in this country were diabetic. It is thought that, by the year 2000, this number will have risen to 10%. The incidence of diabetic retinopathy relates to the population under study. The Framingham study found that the incidence in the general population depended on the age of the group studied (Table 9-1).[36] In diabetics, the incidence of diabetic retinopathy seems to depend on the duration of diabetes as well as the age at onset. Several studies highlight these factors (Tables 9-2 and 9-3). Most studies have used ophthalmoscopic criteria such as retinal microaneurysms, exudate and hemorrhage. In one study several interesting trends were noted. One was that the incidence of diabetic retinopathy increased at age 15, suggesting a direct relationship to puberty.[37] These authors also felt that retinal fluorescein angiography was 1.4×'s more sensitive than retinal color photography in detecting diabetic retinopathy. Using vitreous fluorophotometry, it has been shown that there is a detectable breakdown of the blood-retinal barrier in all diabetics even with no clinical or fluorescein angiographic detectable retinopathy.[38] This latter finding supports the sensitivity of vitreous fluorophotometry in detecting leakage from retinal vessels or perhaps from the retinal pigment epithelium. These changes are not apparent clinically.

Clinical Findings. There are no pathognomonic findings ophthalmoscopically but rather a combination of findings plus systemic endocrine dysfunction. In general, diabetic retinopathy may be characterized as a bilateral, symmetrical, progressive disease affecting the posterior pole. It must be borne in mind, however, that it is most important to ascertain the status of the midperipheral capillary perfusion.[39] Specifically, the retinopathy may be divided into retinal vascular abnormalities and those nonvascular changes secondary to the primary vascular changes. The most common vascular findings are retinal microaneurysms and venous changes, such as segmental dilatation, beading, loops and reduplication. Capillary bed changes include a combination of dilatation, nonperfusion and remodelling. These are not typically noted clinically but are more a fluorescein finding. In areas of nonperfusion, a remaining tortuous capillary

TABLE 9-1
Diabetic Retinopathy
Incidence

General Population—Framingham Study*

Age group	% Diabetic retinopathy
52-64	2.1
65-74	2.9
75-85	7.0

Diabetic patients—Ophthalmoscopy

Duration of diabetes—yrs	Percentage of retinopathy by age at onset of diabetes		
	0-29	30-59	60+
0-4	4	22	34
10-14	45	53	44
20-24	74	68	—
30+	73	90	—

Fundus Photography/Fluorescein Angiography in 122 Juvenile Diabetics**

Duration of diabetes—yrs	Percentage of retinopathy
0-4	0
5-9	27
10+	71

* modified from The Framingham Eye Study. Surv Ophthalmol 24:355-620, 1980.
** Frank RN et al. Retinopathy in juvenile-onset diabetes of short duration. Ophthalmology 87:1-9, 1980.

TABLE 9-2.
Classification of Idiopathic Preretinal Macular Gliosis
Wise's Disease (IPRMG)

MILD
   no obvious membrane or glinting reflex
   no vascular changes
MODERATE
   obvious membranes
   traction lines (striae)
   vascular tortuosity
   no obscuration of retinal vessels
SEVERE
   obscuration of retinal vessels
   marked vascular tortuosity
   heterotropia of macula

TABLE 9-3.*
Visual Acuity at Initial Diagnosis
20/30 or better — 66%
20/50 or better — 84%
20/100 or worse — 11%
20/200 or worse — 4%

*adapted from Reference 60

channel may connect an artery to a vein. These arteriovenous connections are not shunt vessels but are low-flow much as are venous retinal collateral vessels. Arterial changes may be noted, as diabetes is one of the conditions that accelerate arteriolar sclerosis. The vascular change that is most striking is that of retinal neovascularization. These vessels arise from retinal vessels on the disc or retina. New vessels may also arise from cilioretinal vessels. Although these vessels begin within the retina (IRMA = intraretinal microvascular abnormalities), it is difficult to diagnose them with certainty until the vessels break through the internal limiting retina and occupy the retrovitreal space. The relationship between the retinal neovascularization and the vitreous is most important because of the complications of vitreous hemorrhage and retinal detachments related to neovascularization.[40] The non-vascular changes noted in diabetes reflect the vascular changes. Intra-retinal hemorrhages and edema residues (sometimes called "hard" exu-dates) reflect leakage of blood elements through the retinal vessels. Edema may accumulate in the macular area. Cotton-wool spots reflect retinal hypoxia due to arteriolar insufficiency, resulting in axoplasmic stagnation and nerve fiber layer infarct. It is important that, although flame-shaped intraretinal hemorrhages and cotton-wool spots are part of diabetic reti-nopathy, if they become the dominant picture, the presence of concomitant systemic hypertension should be considered. Also, in diabetics with diffuse and severe retinal edema, renal insufficiency should be suspected. Disc changes may also be present. As previously mentioned, this is a frequent site for retinal neovascularization. In addition, disc swelling may be seen in juvenile diabetics without functional alterations. However, in young and, more commonly, older diabetics, disc swelling may indicate ischemic optic neuropathy.[41]

Treatment. The treatment of diabetic retinopathy depends on the stage at which the retinopathy presents for evaluation and therapeutic consideration. It has seemed reasonable that control of blood sugar is of value in modifying the development and course of retinopathy in diabetics. In addition to that of the blood sugar, other factors such as systemic hypertension and renal insufficiency should be carefully monitored and controlled in diabetics. In recent years, development of methods of very strict blood glucose control have been achieved but, in spite of the tightest control, the course of diabetic retinopathy, once established, has not been altered in a positive fashion.[42] Perhaps as this strict control is maintained in patients before retinopathy is established, benefit in delaying the onset and modifying the severity of the course of diabetic retinopathy will be demonstrated. Obviously this type of study will take ten to thirty years to yield meaningful data. In the introduction to this section, the incidence of diabetic retinopathy in diabetics is mentioned. Of those people who develop diabetic retinopathy, 90% develop background diabetic retinopathy and 10% proliferative retinopathy.

Background (Non-Proliferative) Retinopathy. This includes the vast majority of the patients with diabetic retinopathy. Background diabetic retinopathy is most easily diagnosed by ophthalmoscopy. In any diabetic where macular function is not normal, fluorescein angiography is helpful in determining whether or not macular edema is present. Significant edema may be present with a few other signs of background retinopathy, such as microaneurysms, venous changes, retinal hemorrhages, and edema residues. Once macular edema is present, the course of the visual function is variable. Fluctuations are common in central vision, but over five years there is significant deterioration (2 or more lines in Snellen acuity) in 60% of the cases. In 1971, Spalter suggested that photocoagulation might improve the visual function in patients with diabetic maculopathy over the natural course history.[43] Many studies have followed, but the use of photocoagulation in diabetic maculopathy is still in question. In several studies a strong tendency toward treatment was suggested[44,45] and in others, this trend was not noted.[46,47] It has been suggested that the results of photocoagulation in diabetic retinopathy could be predicted on the type of maculopathy present.[48] In this study, maculopathy was divided into three categories:

(A) Focal diabetic maculopathy. Mild edema present with focal areas of retinal leakage not involving more than several parafoveal quadrants.

(B) Diffuse diabetic maculopathy. Leakage involved 360 degrees around the fovea with the typical picture of cystoid macular edema in the late phase.

(C) Ischemic diabetic maculopathy where the edema may be minimal or marked but the fluorescein picture is characterized by significant perifoveal capillary non-perfusion.

In group A, focal photocoagulation was applied to the discrete areas of leakage, producing a moderate coagulum. This group had stabilized or improved vision in all 24 eyes treated.

In group B, a grid pattern or "panretinal photocoagulation" of the macula was applied (avoiding the avascular zone), using moderate burns. This grid pattern was necessary because of the diffuse nature of the pathology on fluorescein angiography. In this group, the majority had stable vision at eight months.

In group C, a pattern similar to that used in group B was used because of the diffuse pathology. About 40% had poorer vision at a two-year follow-up. Of note in this group is the fact that some of the patients were also treated with panretinal photocoagulation outside the posterior pole and others were not. In the non-panretinal photocoagulation group, retinal neo-vascularization developed not uncommonly. This is not surprising, considering that these cases represent ischemic diabetic retinopathy.

This study suggests that carefully controlled studies might have a role in predicting which eyes with diabetic maculopathy might profit from photocoagulation. Perhaps those with focal leakage and good visual acuity (20/50 or better) would do better than the natural course history (Figure 9-7A-C). This is not yet proven. All studies indicate that photocoagulation has no effect on the maculopathy itself in patients who have ischemic maculopathy.

Proliferative Diabetic Retinopathy. Although much less common than background retinopathy in diabetics, proliferative retinopathy is feared because of its potential sudden and profound effect on ocular function. As opposed to diabetic maculopathy, where the use of photocoagulation may be questioned, in diabetic retinitis proliferation no such question exists. The Diabetic Retinopathy Research Study Group (DRS) showed the marked advantage of photocoagulation, using either xenon-arc or argon blue-green.[49] In this study, panretinal photocoagulation was

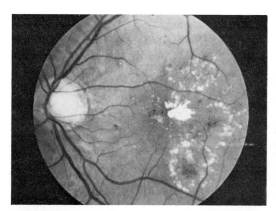

Figure 9-7A

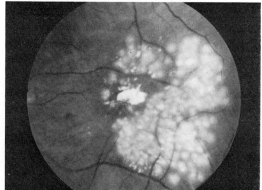

Figure 9-7B

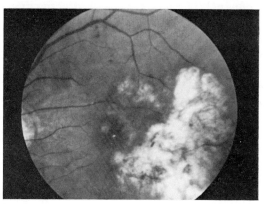

Figure 9-7C

Figure 9-7. Diabetic maculopathy and response to laser treatment. Patient is a 58-year-old white male diabetic with 20/50 VA OS. A. Fundus photograph. Macular edema is present, being most pronounced temporal to the fovea with confluent edema residues. Fluorescein angiography revealed good central perfusion with temporal leakage. B. Fundus photograph, immediately post-photocoagulation. The argon lsaer was used, directed to the areas of leakage. C. Fundus photograph, eight months later. Marked decrease in the retinal edema has occurred and the vision has improved to 20/25.

applied in a scatter fashion from the vessel arcade surrounding the posterior pole to the peripheral retina. New vessels on the disc (NVD) were not treated directly but new vessels elsewhere (NVE) in the retina could be treated directly at the time of the PRP or as necessary if regression was not deemed sufficient. The xenon-arc photocoagulator, while giving equally good results in relation to the argon laser, had a higher rate of complication related to peripheral field loss and, therefore, argon laser would seem to be preferred. In this study, the argon blue-green laser was used, but there is no benefit from the blue wavelength, so argon green or krypton red would seem to be more beneficial. In the DRS study group, several features of the retinopathy leading to visual loss could be isolated.[50] These so-called high-risk characteristics included: 1) new vessels present, 2) NVD, 3) NVD greater than ½ disc diameter, and 4) vitreous hemorrhage. In addition, extensive capillary non-perfusion on fluorescein angiography can be considered a risk factor whether retinal neovascularization is present or not. Shimizu, et al, have demonstrated the importance of the midperipheral retina in regard to determination of capillary perfusion or lack thereof.[39]

Once it is established that panretinal photocoagulation is needed, the treatment should be carried out with dispatch. Clear ocular media and a widely dilated pupil help to ease panretinal photocoagulation but are not common in diabetics. Usually 2000 to 3000 burns of 200 or 500 μ, using the three-mirror lens and the argon laser, are necessary to cause stabilization and/or regression of disc neovascularization (Figure 9-8A-E). If, however, after adequate treatment, satisfactory regression has not been achieved, further treatment may be applied. This may consist of filling in the PRP and focal treatment of the NVE (Figure 9-9A-C). In the latter case, care must be taken to achieve complete closure. Focal treatment must be carefully followed for the first 24 to 48 hours and re-treated if not obliterated. Lack of complete obliteration of NVE can lead to rapid growth of the NVE. Also, with focal treatment, destruction of part of the network can lead to the arterial input arising from the choroid for the remaining portion of the network. These chorioretinal neovascular membranes are most difficult to eliminate. For successful PRP, however, regression of disc neovascularization and of NVE does not have to be complete for the conversion of a florid retinopathy to one that is stable. The panfunduscopic Rodenstock lens allows a wider field of treatment than that of the three-mirror lens. This leads to more rapid PRP and better orientation of the macular region.

In cases where ocular media prohibit photocoagulation, several approaches are available. If no anterior segment neovascularization is present and ultrasound shows an attached retina, observation until the vitreous hemorrhage clears is warranted. Then treatment may be carried out as indicated above. If anterior segment neovascularization is present, panretinal cryopexy may be carried out to achieve effects similar to PRP.[51] Another option is to do a vitrectomy and apply endophotocoagulation at the time of surgery or, within the first several postoperative days, perform PRP. If the retina is detached in the posterior pole due to traction and the other characteristics of high risk in diabetic proliferative retinopathy, panretinal photocoagulation may be performed, avoiding the blue wavelengths and

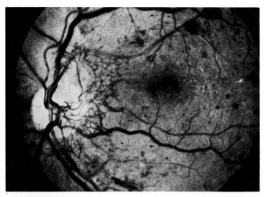

Figure 9-8A

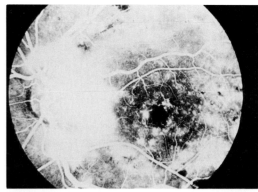

Figure 9-8B

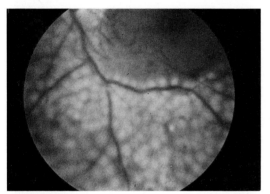

Figure 9-8C

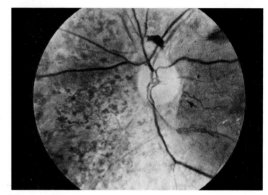

Figure 9-8D

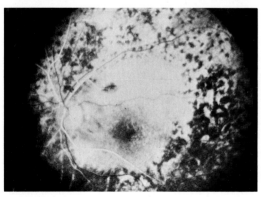

Figure 9-8E

Figure 9-8. Panretinal photocoagulation for disc neovascularization (NVD). 43-year-old white male on insulin for 20 years. VA 20/20 OS. A. Posterior pole fundus photograph. NVD is noted with background diabetic retinopathy. B. Fluorescein angiogram, venous phase. Diffuse leakage from the disc neovascularization. Although capillary perfusion is good in the posterior pole, the midperipheral retina shows massive non-perfusion. C. Fundus photograph, immediately post-photocoagulation. The lower half of the retina shows the response to laser photocoagulation. The macular area is not treated. The upper half of the retina was treated in a similar fashion one week later. D. Fundus photograph, three months post-photocoagulation. VA 20/20. Note the regression of the NVD but residual fibrosis. E. Wide-angle fluorescein angiography at the same time as Figure 9-8d. The regressed disc neovascularization, the shrunken veins, and the pigmentary changes are all in response to the panretinal photocoagulation.

the detached retina. After this procedure, subsequent vitrectomy may be done for retinal reattachment with decreased risk of anterior segment neovascularization. Some surgeons feel, however, that vitrectomy should be done for retinal reattachment and the PRP done intraoperatively.[52-54] Also, by releasing vitreous traction on retinal neovascularization, the risk of vitreous hemorrhage is diminished and even regression of the neo-

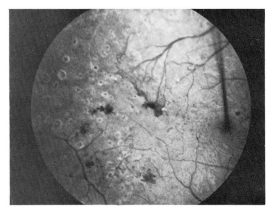

Figure 9-9A.

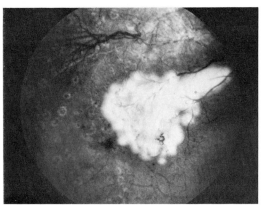

Figure 9-9B.

Figure 9-9. Focal treatment of retinal neovascularization not on the disc (NVE). 28-year-old white female diabetic whose left eye is NLP secondary to neovascular glaucoma. OD 20/20 with growing NVE responsible for several small vitreous hemorrhages. Panretinal photocoagulation with subsequent fill-in has caused no regression. A. Fundus photograph of the posterior pole. Frond of NVE from the superior temporal vein is noted above and temporal to the fovea. B. Fundus photograph, immediately post-focal photocoagulation. Heavy photocoagulation using the argon green laser was applied. Note the fragmentation of the NVE. Two additional treatments were needed the next day to secure permanent closure. C. Fundus photograph, eight months post-laser. Obliteration of the NVE remains but retinal striae involving the fovea have reduced the VA to 20/25 with minimal metamorphopsia.

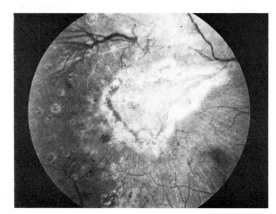

Figure 9-9C.

vascularization may be noted. In the phakic diabetic, the risk of anterior segment neovascularization is less than in the aphakic, so preservation of the lens during vitrectomy in diabetics is of concern.

Complications of panretinal photocoagulation include delayed dark/light retina adaptation, decreased pupillary response to light and near, and loss of accommodation. In presbyopic patients, near vision must always be considered after PRP. In diabetics without neovascularization but with good retinal perfusion on fluorescein angiography, PRP is not indicated. Also, post-PRP macular edema may cause decreased central vision of several Snellen lines or more. In about half of the cases, this edema spontaneously remits; in the other half, focal laser therapy may be considered, as outlined in the section on diabetic maculopathy.

When anterior segment neovascularization is present, panretinal photocoagulation is successful in causing regression of the anterior segment neovascularization in about 80-95% of the cases when media allows adequate treatment of the retina. Postoperative intraocular pressure depends on the state of the angle, however.[55-57] Direct laser treatment of the new vessels in the angle as they come over the scleral spur may be used to prevent further compromise of the angle while awaiting response from the panretinal photocoagulation.[58,59] If the media does not allow treatment of the retina, panretinal cryotherapy may be used to cause regression. Once the angle is devoid of new vessels, filtering surgery may be considered if the intraocular pressure cannot be kept under suitable control.

Although much progress has been made in the management of diabetic retinopathy in the past twenty years, visual rehabilitation must be available at any center where diabetic retinopathy is being managed because of the number of patients who, in spite of modern-day techniques, do not maintain useful vision.

Idiopathic Preretinal Macular Gliosis (Wise's Disease)

Idiopathic preretinal macular gliosis (IPRMG) may be defined as a preretinal membrane growing on the surface of the retina in an eye otherwise free from predisposing pathology, e.g., surgery or venous obstruction.[60] Terms used historically include idiopathic preretinal macular fibrosis, surface-wrinkling retinopathy, cellophane retinopathy, silk-screen retinopathy, macular pucker, primary retinal folds, silent retinal vein occlusion (central), shrinkage of the internal limiting membrane, and vitreoretinal interface maculopathy. This is a distinct entity first described completely by Wise in 1972.[61] Not included are membranes related to venous obstruction, diabetic retinopathy, post-trauma, post-intraocular surgery (especially retinal detachment surgery), inflammation, post-photocoagulation, macular degeneration associated with aging, heredoretinal degenerations (especially rod/cone dystrophies), and congenital preretinal membranes.

Incidence. In the Retina Service at Montefiore Medical Center, it has been estimated that idiopathic preretinal macular gliosis is found in approximately ten percent of patients over 50 years of age.[60] In a large autopsy study, it can be calculated that approximately 2% of the eyes sectioned had IPRMG.[62]

Symptoms. IPRMG is usually asymptomatic and is found on routine examination. When symptoms are present, the most common complaint is mild distortion or blurriness of vision. Forty percent have Amsler grid distortion on examination. The course of awareness of these symptoms is usually insidious. Occasionally a patient may present with a history of an "acute" symptomatology.

The clinical findings may be categorized into three classes: mild (Figure 9-10), moderate (Figure 9-11A-C), and severe. The characteristics of each are seen in Table 9-2. In some cases there can be focal thinning of the membrane, giving the appearance of a macular hole.[63] These "pseudoholes" have no effect on visual acuity. In 2-3% of the cases, lamellar or true retinal holes may be found. It is of interest that in two-thirds of the patients

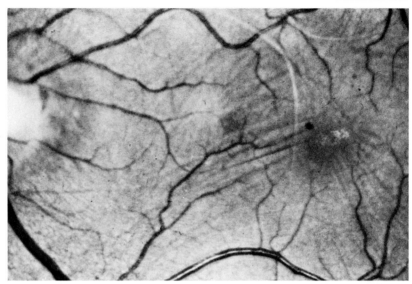

Figure 9-10. Fundus photograph OS of an asymptomatic 65-year-old white female. The preretinal membrane is noted crossing the superior temporal artery. Retinal striae (traction lines) are present throughout the macula.

with IPRMG, the posterior vitreous was detached at the time of diagnosis. In one-third, the posterior vitreous was attached.

The clinical appearance makes the diagnosis. Fluorescein angiography may show distortion of the retinal vasculature and occasional late leakage. One study noted fluorescein leakage in 34% of all cases with IPRMG.[60] Intraretinal edema was diagnosed clinically in 15% of these patients.

When Wise first described this condition, the term "fibrosis" was used. Pathology, however, has shown that the primary cells are glial.[64] These are probably from Müller's cells, responding to a break in the internal limiting membrane. These breaks are caused by the alteration of the vitreoretinal interface. Other cells have also been shown to be involved in severe cases, including fibrocytes and macrophages.[65] These may be derived from retinal pigment epithelial cells or even hyalocytes.

Prognosis. At presentation, the visual acuity is usually 20/30 or better (Table 9-3).[66-68] The natural course history shows that the visual acuity is stable in over 85% of the cases. In one series only 1% had decreased visual acuity related to the membrane alone.[60] Fourteen percent of the patients with decreased vision had associated lamellar macular holes/cysts.

Treatment. Because of the initial good visual acuity and high percentage of stable vision, the only treatment in most cases is observation. Two other treatment modalities have been suggested. The first was photocoagulation. In a small series of cases there seemed to be some positive benefit.[69] However, the argon blue-green laser was used. In further evaluating these cases (and in several other cases from the same group of

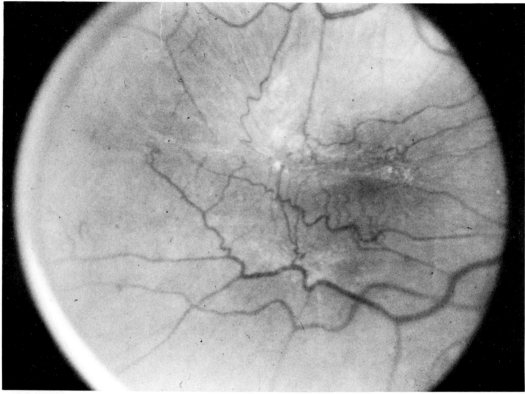

Figure 9-11A

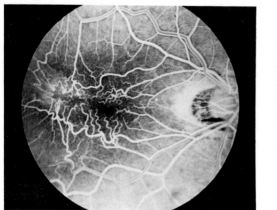

Figure 9-11B

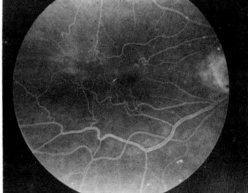

Figure 9-11C

Figure 9-11A. Fundus photograph of a 72-year-old white female with 20/40 VA OD. Note the membrane, as well as the distortion in the retinal vascular and foveal avascular zones. B. Fluorescein angiogram, arteriovenous phase. Distortion of the vessels is highlighted. C. Fluorescein angiogram, late stages. There is mild intraretinal leakage, most marked superior and temporal to the fovea.

investigators, not included in the original study), a negative effect was noted from photocoagulation. This is not surprising because of the well-known membrane-producing effect of this laser. Perhaps the use of an argon green or krypton red laser would be of benefit when there is mild membrane formation, and visual distortion is related to macular edema. The second modality is vitrectomy. When visual acuity is decreased to 20/70 or less, vitrectomy might be considered. In relieving the retinal traction, visual acuity may be improved.[70]

Isolated Acquired Retinal Arterial Macroaneurysm

Isolated acquired arterial macroaneurysms (IAM) present most commonly on routine examination. They may be associated with visual acuity loss from macular edema, usually gradual in nature, or, less commonly, sudden visual loss due to vitreous hemorrhage. IAM's are usually found in patients over 60 years of age and have a predilection for hypertensive females.[71] The patient should also be examined for cardiovascular disease, which can affect the carotid artery, the peripheral vasculature or the coronary system.

The clinical diagnosis is often apparent on ophthalmoscopy where saccular dilatation of a retinal artery is noted. This dilatation is usually 250-500 μ in size and often has a reddish-yellow appearance. It is not uncommon for it to be located near a bifurcation.[72] Adjacent capillary-bed dilatation, intraretinal edema and hemorrhage may be noted.[73] The distal portion of the artery may exhibit halo sheathing. Several aneurysms may be present on the same artery or noted in other quadrants of the retina, or in the opposite eye. Occasionally, transmitted pulsations of the artery may be noted.[74] Hemorrhage may also be located beneath the retinal pigment epithelium or in the vitreous. In the latter case, the diagnosis may await clearing of the vitreous hemorrhage. Fluorescein angiography may show prompt filling of the aneurysm, although there may be a segmental nature to this filling due to clot and scar formation with the aneurysm.[73] The surrounding capillary bed shows a widened capillary-free zone and an irregular formation that leaks fluorescein in the late stages. The artery distal to the aneurysm may show normal or delayed filling. It is unusual to see complete obstruction of this arterial segment. Other diagnostic tests are not helpful except in the case of vitreous hemorrhage where ultrasonography may suggest the diagnosis.

Because of the varied appearance of IAM, the differential diagnoses include diabetic retinopathy, macular degeneration, and vein obstruction. IAM also must be differentiated from hereditary retinal vascular disease. The natural course of these aneurysms is to fibrose over a period of several months to years. With the fibrosis, the surrounding capillary-bed abnormalities return to normal and there is absorption of the retinal hemorrhage and edema. This fibrotic process occurs more rapidly in those patients with

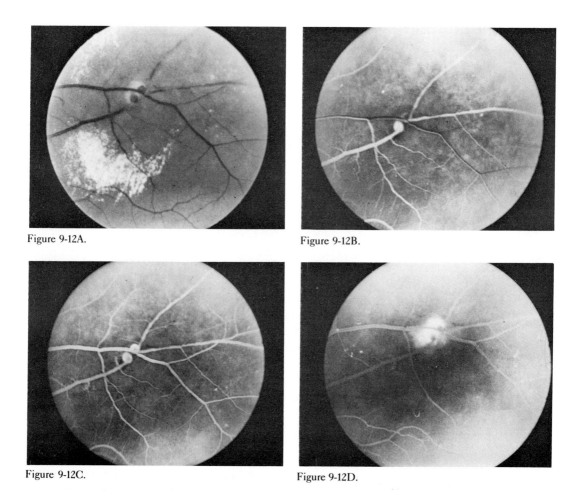

Figure 9-12A.

Figure 9-12B.

Figure 9-12C.

Figure 9-12D.

Figure 9-12. 56-year-old white female who, on a routine examination, was found to have a retinal lesion OS. Her past medical history included five years of systemic hypertension. Visual acuity 20/20 OD and 20/20 OS. A. Fundus photograph OS. The superior temporal artery has a double arterial macroaneurysm just proximal to a bifurcation. A surrounding halo of fibrosis and a wider ring of edema residues in a circinate pattern are noted. (b-d are fluorescein angiograms of Figure 9-1a) B. Arteriovenous phase. The proximal aneurysm is filled but only a rim of fluorescence is noted in the other one. The distal arterioles are irregular in caliber. C. Venous phase. Both aneurysms are filled with a relative hypofluorescent center. D. Late phase. Leakage is present both through the walls of the aneurysms and from the abnormal adjacent capillary bed.

marked hemorrhage. In looking at the effect on visual acuity, it is those cases with persistent macular edema that have residual visual acuity defects.[75] In these cases, photocoagulation may be considered, depending upon the extent and duration of the macular edema. Several techniques have been employed to help improve central vision. One technique is to treat the aneurysm directly with mild to moderate photocoagulation. The purpose of this treatment is to expedite involution of the aneurysm without causing obstruction of the distal arterial segment. Another method of therapy is to use photocoagulation to form a "diffusion" barrier between the leaking aneurysm and the macular region. Both of these techniques may be employed simultaneously.

Parafoveal Telangiectasia

Parafoveal retinal capillary telangiectasia is an entity which has appeared in the literature under many different terms. Localized Leber's, Leber's miliary aneurysms, and macular Coats' disease are some of these terms.[76-78] Affected patients usually present with decreased visual acuity and/or metamorphopsia. However, there are many reported cases in which the patients are asymptomatic. This condition is usually found in middle-aged people and there is currently no other association with systemic illness. It is known that patients afflicted with this condition will occasionally form subretinal neovascular membranes and/or have changes at the level of the retinal pigment epithelium.[79] There is one case reported with hereditary optic atrophy but no other ocular linkage has been reported.[79]

Although this condition has been linked under one common umbrella term, there are probably several categories of patients which fit the clinical and angiographic picture. Gass and Oyakawa[79] collected a large series of patients with this diagnosis and divided them into four categories. Group One consisted of males with uniocular involvement. They frequently had edema residues located in the temporal parafoveal region. Group Two consisted of mostly males with bilateral involvement. Their clinical and angiographic picture was characterized by symmetric temporal involvement of the retinal capillary bed. There was minimal evidence of edema residues. These patients had a high risk of subretinal neovascularization. Group Three consisted of bilateral involvement with an equal sex predilection. There was minimal evidence of edema residues, but involvement of the entire perifoveal capillary bed was noted. Group Four actually consisted of only one case with optic pallor and occlusive capillary disease.

There is one pathological case report of a patient with this clinical entity.[80] Green, et al,[80] have shown that this entity may not truly be a diffuse saccular aneurysmal dilatation of the retinal capillaries, but a disturbance primarily of the endothelial cells with secondary degeneration of pericytes. In addition, these vascular changes were not restricted to the clinically affected parafoveal region.

The differential diagnosis of this entity consists of small branch vein occlusions, diabetes mellitus, prior exposure to x-ray irradiation, and carotid artery obstruction. Patients with this condition may have minimal or no apparent findings on clinical exam. Angiography will often demonstrate the appearance of a dilated superficial or deep capillary plexus with late leakage (Figure 9-13A & B).

The prognosis of these patients is usually good. Patients with persistent edema residues and cystoid macular edema have occasionally been treated with laser, with variable improvement. Several patients have been noted to develop subretinal neovascular membranes, retinal pigment epithelial metaplasia or other signs of disturbance at the level of the retinal pigment epithelium. This has been felt to be due to chronic intraretinal edema with secondary pigment epithelial disturbance. In these patients the neovascular membranes should be managed in accordance with principles outlined for the treatment of neovascular membranes with macular degeneration.

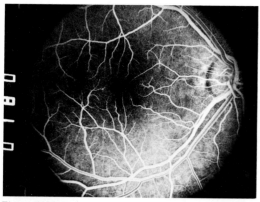 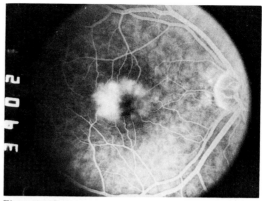

Figure 9-13A.   Figure 9-13B.

Figure 9-13 A and B. Although no abnormality of the retinal vasculature was seen on clinical examination of this patient, angiography revealed a dilated parafoveal capillary bed with diffuse leakage and cystoid edema temporal to the fovea.

Birdshot Retinochoroidopathy

Birdshot retinochoroidopathy, or vitiliginous chorioretinitis, is a recently described fundus disorder[81-85] characterized by multiple pigmented spots at the level of the retinal pigment epithelium, with an associated vitreous reaction. This disease occurs predominantly in middle-aged or older patients and ocular involvement is commonly bilateral and symmetrical. Affected patients often present with a history of floaters or photopsia, in a painless, non-inflamed eye. Night blindness occasionally occurs. Although vision may become progressively worse, about 50% of patients will stabilize and remain with a final visual acuity of 20/40 or better in at least one eye.[85] The anterior segment is uninvolved but clinical evidence of vitritis, depigmented spots, and cystoid macular edema is common in the posterior pole.

There are no known systemic diseases associated with this condition, but vitiligo has occasionally been reported.[82] A group of affected patients has been described who have a very high incidence of the HLA-A29 antigen.[84] A subgroup of this population showed a high incidence of in vitro response to testing with retinal S antigen.

The hallmark of the disease is the presence of depigmented areas in the retina without evidence of hyperpigmentation within or surrounding these areas. Most of these lesions are round or ovoid with regular "punched out" borders, and they appear to remain stationary. There is a diffuse and chronic vitreous inflammatory reaction, but no peripheral snowbanking. Cystoid macular edema has been noted in about 40% of patients.

Fluorescein angiography reveals diffuse staining of the walls of the retinal vasculature and subsequent leakage into the vitreous (Figure 9-14A). There is frequently a marked amount of leakage from a dilated perifoveal capillary bed (Figure 9-14B), which results in macular edema. The discrete areas of depigmentation appear as transmission defects without leakage of dye (Figure 9-15).

The majority of patients tested show abnormalities of the electroretinogram, often with diminished B wave amplitude.[84] Some of the

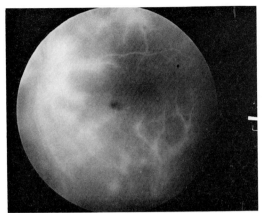 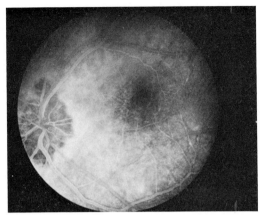

Figure 9-14A.   Figure 9-14B.

Figure 9-14A. Diffuse staining of the retinal vascular walls with leakage into the vitreous in a patient with active posterior pole inflammation. B. A dilated perifoveal capillary bed is often seen in conjunction with cystoid macular edema in this condition.

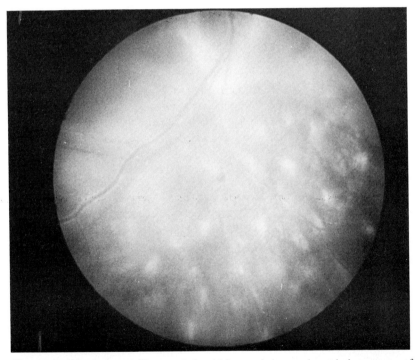

Figure 9-15. Discrete areas of increased choroidal transmission are the typical appearance of clinically detected atrophic spots.

patients show a diminished light peak to dark trough ratio in the electro-oculogram. This would seem to indicate a diffuse disturbance of the retinal pigment epithelium and photoreceptors.

The differential diagnosis includes sympathetic ophthalmia, pars planitis, Vogt-Koyanagi-Harada's disease, and Acute Posterior Multifocal Placoid Pigment Epitheliopathy. Other entities which might also be considered are geographic choroiditis, Behcet's disease, sarcoidosis, and histo-plasmosis. These conditions can often be ruled out by consideration of the history, ocular examination, and appropriate laboratory studies. Cortico-steroid therapy has been generally ineffective, although a few treated patients have shown some improvement.

Acquired Immune Deficiency Syndrome

Acquired immune deficiency syndrome (AIDS) is a serious disorder of the immune system affecting previously healthy individuals below the age of 60. Because this syndrome causes such a marked decrease in cellular immunity, patients typically present with systemic manifestations.[86] These include Kaposi's sarcoma, Burkitt's lymphoma and other oppor-tunistic infections including toxoplasmosis, Pneumocystis carinii, can-didiasis, and mycobacterial infections.

Certain individuals seem to be at a higher risk for development of this syndrome. These include homosexuals, hemophiliacs, Haitians, intra-venous drug abusers,[87] and possibly sexual partners and children of patients with this disorder. The cause of this condition is yet unknown, however the epidemiology seems to suggest that this condition is spread in a similar manner to the hepatitis B virus. Many ophthalmic manifestations have been seen in patients with this condition. The most common include cotton-wool spots (Figure 16A & B), hemorrhages and cytomegalovirus retinitis (Figure 17A & B). Other findings include cranial nerve palsies, conjunctival Kaposi's sarcoma, and orbital and conjunctival lymphoma.[88]

The diagnosis of AIDS is made by its systemic manifestations. These include cutaneous anergy, lymphopenia, depressed lymphocyte prolifera-tion to mitogens, and infections in which cell mediated immunity plays the major role in host defenses. The most consistent abnormality seen in these patients is the marked decrease of the helper-inducer phenotype and a relative increase in cells of the suppressor-cytotoxic phenotype as demon-

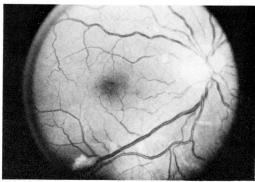

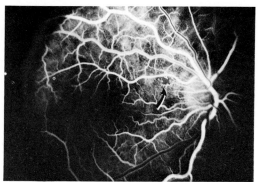

Figure 9-16A.   Figure 9-16B.

Figure 9-16A and B. Cotton-wool spots in a patient with AIDS. Areas of capillary non-perfusion are easily seen on angiography (16B).

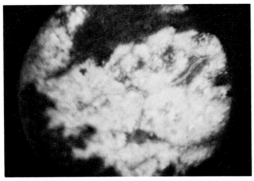

Figure 9-17A.

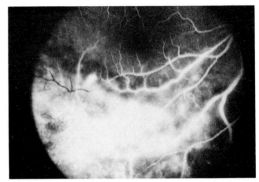

Figure 9-17B.

Figure 9-17A and B. Cytomegalovirus retinitis in a 34-year-old bisexual (17A). There is a cheesy white necrosis of the retinal tissue with areas of vascular infarction and diffuse leakage noted on angiography.

strated by monoclonal antibody analysis of T lymphocyte subpopulations. Those patients with evidence of immune deficiency, and unusual opportunistic infections or Kaposi's sarcoma are defined as AIDS.

Depending upon the criteria for diagnosis, probably between 40 to 70% of patients with this condition will not survive. There is no known treatment for this condition except specific therapy for opportunistic infections as well as localized tumors. There is experimental work with Interleukin 2 and Interferon which may prove useful in restoring and amplifying an individual's cell mediated immunity. There has been one reported case in which dapsone was useful in treating Kaposi's sarcoma in AIDS.

Presumed Ocular Histoplasmosis Syndrome (POHS)

POHS is a diagnosis which is based on clinical findings. The classic triad consists of peripheral atrophic choroidal spots, peripapillary choroidal changes and disciform detachments of the macula.

Patients usually come to the attention of the clinician when the disease affects the macula. They may complain of blurred vision, distortion, micropsia, and metamorphopsia. These classic symptoms of macular exudation and detachment may be due to choroidal neovascular membranes arising in the macula or spreading to the macula from a peripapillary location.[89]

Until the widespread use of histoplasmin skin testing, histoplasmosis was felt to be uncommon. We now believe that most cases of histoplasmosis are benign, self-limited infections occurring in childhood, and often are asymptomatic. It is likely, however, that this initial infection with the organism sets the stage for later ocular damage.

There are very strong endemic regions of histoplasmosis involvement. It is usually present in river basin areas. In the United States, the Ohio River Valley has a very high incidence of prior exposure to histoplasmosis, as determined by skin testing. There have been numerous reports of a decreased incidence of ocular involvement in blacks.[90] The disease may affect individuals in any age group and is typically bilateral.

Clinical diagnosis is based on previously mentioned ocular signs. Atrophic lesions are round to oval shaped and may have a greenish tint to the edge (Figure 9-18). The number of such spots may be a few to several dozen. Initially they may appear as raised lesions leading to the supposition that they may represent sites of Histoplasma induced granulomas.

The peripapillary changes seen in this condition have been described by Schlaegel in great detail.[91] The most common type is a confluent disturbance at the level of the retinal pigment epithelium. Hemorrhagic and nodular types of peripapillary involvement have been described. The sine qua non of ocular histoplasmosis remains macular choroidal neovascularization. In the early stages a focal yellow, white or gray area may be noted in the fovea. Histopathology[92] has shown a break in Bruch's membrane and the entrance of choroidal neovascular membranes into the subretinal space. Later evolution of the macular lesion reveals an end-stage disciform scar, heralded by recurrent hemorrhage and exudation in the macular region (Figure 9-19).[79] There is a belief that the presence of atrophic lesions in the macula predispose the eye to later development of choroidal neovascularization.[93] If the macula is uninvolved, the risk is low.

Although a high percentage of patients with ocular histoplasmosis have positive histoplasmin skin tests, this test is rarely used today due to the potential for exacerbation of a macular lesion. Complement fixation tests do not show a high degree of positive correlation with the ocular condition.[94] Fluorescein angiography has been very helpful in delineating the extent of pathology in the macular region and serves as a guidepost for therapy.

The differential diagnosis should include many of the other conditions associated with choroiditis, including toxoplasmosis, syphilis, toxocariasis, sarcoidosis, and tuberculosis. In patients presenting with peripapillary or macular neovascular membranes, angioid streaks, hyaline bodies of the optic nerve, and myopia should be considered.

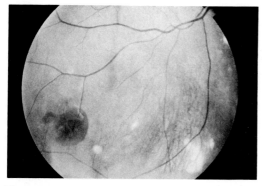

Figure 9-18. Several atrophic choroidal spots are noted, in addition to a small hemorrhagic retinal pigment epithelial detachment.

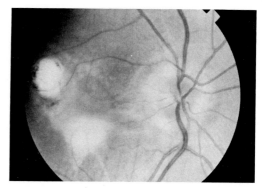

Figure 9-19. Peripapillary atrophy as well as a macular scar are present in this patient with POHS.

The natural course of this ocular condition is poor, and tends to vary with the extent of macular involvement.[95] Schlaegel, et al,[95] reported 59% of their untreated patients having visual acuity of 20/200 or worse.

Systemic antifungal agents have not been proven to be of significant value in the management of this condition. Corticosteroids may be of value in the early stages of macular involvement but this has not been proven conclusively. Recent experience with the use of laser therapy for control of choroidal neovascularization has proven encouraging. The ocular histoplasmosis study, using argon laser for treatment of neovascular membranes from 200 to 2500 microns away from the center of the foveal avascular zone, has shown that treatment was of benefit in an 18-month follow-up period.[96] Sabates, et al, studied patients with both argon and krypton red lasers, and concluded that patients treated with krypton laser have a better outcome.[97] However, further studies will be needed to validate this data.

Macular Degeneration Associated with Aging

Macular degeneration associated with aging is becoming increasingly more important and is being recognized as the most common cause of loss of visual acuity in the population over age 60 in the western hemisphere. In the Framingham eye study, which is a large prospective study, about a quarter of the patients examined were noted to have pigmentary mottling in the retina in all age groups, increasing to 40% when eyes over 75 years of age were examined.[98] Also, in about one-quarter of the eyes, retinal drusen were noted. Macular degeneration was rare under age 65, being 1.2%, but increasing in the group 75 years of age and older, being 19.7%. The male-to-female ratio was 4.2 to 6.7%. In another large study group done by the federal government, the incidence of macular degeneration in the age group of 45-64 years was 2.3%, increasing in the 65-75 years of age group to 9.6% for men and 6.9% for women.[99] This study is unusual in that a difference in the incidence of macular degeneration among races, comparing black to white, was not noted. It is also estimated that macular degeneration accounts for 17% of the new cases of blindness in the United States in the population over age 68.[100]

History. In 1927, Kuhnt and Junius described the clinical picture of macular degeneration with subretinal hemorrhage and scarring.[101] In 1929, Verhoeff and Holliday described the pathology of subretinal neovascularization in the macular region. They proposed that these new vessels were the cause of the condition known as "Kuhnt-Junius macular degeneration." Over the subsequent years there were many reports, both clinical and pathological, with the stress on the hemorrhage in the subretinal space producing the pathology. In 1963, Friedman, Smith and Kuwabara, using trypsin retinal digestion, showed that subretinal neovascularization was quite common in the periphery of the retina and was seen in almost 100% of the eyes older than 60 years of age. In 1967 and again in 1973, Gass suggested that subretinal neovascularization was the primary inciting pathology in disciform macular degeneration.[90] In 1973, Sarks in a monograph described subretinal neovascularization in the macular region of approximately 20% of aging eyes.[102] These studies, along with the increased use of fluorescein angiography, have helped to increase awareness of subretinal neovascularization as being a most important factor in the pathology in the disciform process. The basic abnormality in macular degeneration, however, is still not yet determined. One of the earliest histological changes related to aging in the retina is loss of the photoreceptors and their nuclei. These changes occur before any alterations in other than the retinal pigment epithelium and Bruch's membrane.[103] These changes at this time are not clinically detectable. Sarks noted, in a large series of clinical pathological correlations, a granular deposit between the pigment epithelium and Bruch's membrane.[102] These changes occur with variable changes in the overlying pigment epithelium. It has been suggested that the retinal pigment epithelial cell is the primary abnormality in macular degeneration.[104] The RPE cell may be unable to accommodate the debris from the shedding of the overlying rods and cones.[105] This may lead to sub-RPE deposits of material that may be similar to the basal laminar deposit of Sarks and/or retinal drusen. It is felt that these eyes are predisposed to the development of the changes under the category of macular degeneration. These include serous detachments of the retinal pigment epithelium and both atrophic and exudative macular degeneration.

Terminology. Macular degeneration associated with aging has also been called senile macular degeneration. It is felt that the term "senile" carries with it some loss of cognitive function and is therefore an inappropriate term. Macular degeneration of aging may be categorized as follows:
a. retinal drusen/pigmentary mottling
b. serous detachment of the retinal pigment epithelium
c. exudative, including subretinal neovascularization, hemorrhagic detachment of the retinal pigment epithelium, cicatricial stage
d. atrophic
This classification does not imply one stage leading to another, or cause and effect, but is a listing of the spectrum of changes noted. A combination of the above categories may be present together in the same eye.

Diagnosis. As previously noted, one-quarter of the population, especially in the older age group, have drusen and/or pigmentary mottling noted on ophthalmoscopic examination. Unless there is an unexplained alteration of central acuity or distortion on Amsler grid testing, fluorescein angiography rarely adds to the ophthalmoscopic examination. In those cases where visual acuity is altered quantitatively or qualitatively, fluorescein angiography can be justified in attempting to identify the reason for the altered acuity. In cases of serous detachment of the retinal pigment epithelium where there is good central visual acuity and no evidence of subretinal neovascularization clinically (as would be suggested with turbid subretinal fluid, hemorrhage or exudate), a fluorescein angiogram rarely adds to the diagnostic acumen of the ophthalmoscope and slit-lamp bio-microscopy. There is a group of patients with altered visual acuity who demonstrate drusen and multiple RPE defects on fluorescein angiography, as well as irregular late leakage due to a diffuse breakdown of the blood-retinal barrier at the level of the retinal pigment epithelial cell. This could be related to leakage through the pigment epithelial cells into the overlying sensory retina or, perhaps, inhibition by the retinal pigment epithelial cells of the dye. This condition is referred to as the "sick RPE syndrome." When patients appear with alteration of visual acuity and, on clinical examination, subretinal neovascularization is clinically suspected because of either a subretinal grayish area or frank hemorrhage beneath the pigment epithelium or breaking through the sensory retina, then fluorescein angiography is essential in localizing the extent of the subretinal neovascularization. It should be remembered that if the pigment epithelium is normal over the subretinal neovascularization, then the full extent of the pathology may not be noted on fluorescein angiography. In those cases where there is large subretinal and/or intraretinal hemorrhage, the fluorescein angiogram may also not yield the extent of the membrane, again because of masking of the underlying pathology. In these cases, follow-up examination is needed. When the cicatricial stage is present, fluorescein angiography serves no useful function. It should be noted that it was recently reported that a Marcus Gunn pupil may be detected in these cases without evidence of optic nerve disease.[106] Another diagnostic category could be considered, although it is relatively uncommon but has been increasingly recognized, and that is a tear of the retinal pigment epithelium.[107] These are associated with hemorrhagic or serous detachments of the pigment epithelium and may occur spontaneously or after photocoagulation, especially with the krypton red laser. Clinical examination usually reveals a dark area at one edge of a serous detachment of the pigment epithelium and, with slit-lamp biomicroscopy, one can almost see the pigment epithelium rippled and folded under. The overlying sensory retina is intact but an exposed choroid and Bruch's membrane are noted. As time goes on, this exposed area will become fibrotic and scarred and, in the late stages, will look much like a cicatricial stage with pigmentary changes. In the acute stage, on fluorescein angiography, the area lacking the retinal pigment epithelium usually fluoresces early with minimal, if any, leakage. The area of ripped pigment epithelium will remain hypofluorescent, and if there is a remaining serous detachment of the sensory retina, it will fill accordingly.

Natural Course History. The visual prognosis for patients with macular degeneration depends upon the type of pathology present. In cases where drusen and RPE defects are noted, visual acuity is usually excellent unless other pathology intervenes. Serous detachments of the pigment epithelium less than 1 disc diameter in area (even if they involve the foveal region) usually have a reasonably good prognosis, although subretinal neovascularization or atrophic macular degeneration may develop. Large serous detachments of the retinal pigment epithelium (i.e., 1 disc diameter or greater) have a poor prognosis for visual acuity. In 24 such cases followed from 14 months to 13 years, with a mean interval of follow-up of 4.5 years, Gass and Braunstein found that only three of these patients retained 20/40 vision or better at their last examination.[108] Fourteen of these developed subretinal neovascularization and four developed geographic atrophy of the pigment epithelium.

The presence of subretinal neovascularization in the macula is a poor prognostic sign for visual acuity. In a study of 96 eyes in 93 patients with a follow-up of 21 months, Bressler still found that, with both subfoveal and juxtafoveal subretinal neovascularization, 70% of the eyes ended up with 20/200 vision or worse.[109] In atrophic macular degeneration, which is perhaps three to five times more common than cicatricial, the visual acuity is usually lost slowly, but in 10% of the cases this leads to a significant visual handicap.

Therapy. In regard to macular degeneration, there are scientific studies related to photocoagulation. As for other treatment modalities, e.g., the use of vitamins (such as A, B or E) and trace metals (such as selinium), or protection of the retina from exposure to light (especially ultraviolet), there are no such studies. In the cases of drusen and pigmentary maculopathy, there has been no evidence that any current treatment modality has altered the outcome of these cases. In serous detachments of the pigment epithelium there have been several methods proposed for photocoagulation of these lesions. Using the argon laser and 200 μ spot size, moderate burns may be placed in a grid-like pattern over the lesion, avoiding the fovea and perifoveal regions, to cause collapse of the RPE detachment. It has also been suggested that the RPE detachment may be flattened by treating the edge of the lesion with similar treatment. The detachment usually flattens in two weeks but if not, treatment may be reapplied. There are many papers that discuss the benefit, or the lack thereof, from treatment of pigment epithelial detachments with photocoagulation. As noted in Table 9-4, there is not yet any evidence that photocoagulation significantly alters the natural course or history of serous detachments of the retinal pigment epithelium in a positive fashion.[108,110,111] In those detachments, when subretinal neovascularization is suspected, it is possible to flatten the RPE detachment by the method previously mentioned. Once the retinal pigment epithelial detachment is flattened, the identification and treatment of the subretinal neovascular membrane becomes feasible. It is possible that, because of the inherent qualities of the red light, krypton red laser could be more beneficial than the studies so far reported (which have used the argon blue-green and argon green).

It is in the case of subretinal neovascularization that photocoagulation has been proven of value in macular degeneration of aging. In the late 1960's and early 1970's, several studies of exudative macular degeneration treated with argon photocoagulation showed that this treatment could be of benefit in maintaining reasonably good central visual acuity (Figure 9-20A-D).[112-114] These studies were small and not randomized and the actual proof of the benefit of photocoagulation in such cases awaited the randomized trials done in both England and the United States.[115,116] Both of these studies used the argon blue-green laser in the treatment of patients 50 years or older, with evidence of subretinal neovascularization associated

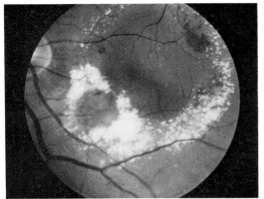

Figure 9-20A.

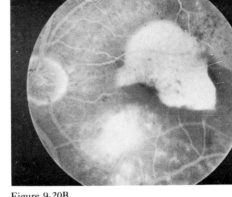

Figure 9-20B.

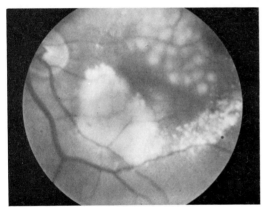

Figure 9-20C.

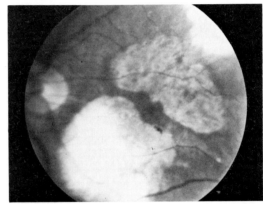

Figure 9-20D.

Figure 9-20A. Fundus photograph. A large area of intra-retinal and subretinal fluid, hemorrhage and exudate is present in the posterior pole. B. Fluorescein angiogram, late venous phase. An irregular detachment of the retinal pigment epithelium is present above the fovea and an area of irregular subretinal leakage is present below the fovea. C. Fundus photograph, immediately post-laser. The argon blue-green laser was used to apply heavy burns to the areas outlined above. D. Fundus photograph, 19 months later. VA has improved to 20/40 and the posterior pole is flat with much atrophy post-laser. E. Fluorescein angiogram, venous phase. Elimination of the subretinal neovascular membrane is confirmed.

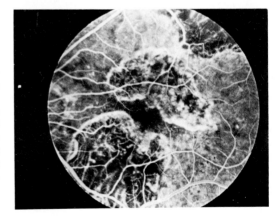

Figure 9-20E.

TABLE 9-4.*
SEROUS DETACHMENTS OF THE RETINAL PIGMENT EPITHELIUM

Study	Follow-Up Months	No. of Eyes	Treatment	Final Visual Acuity			
				Improved	Same	Worse	% 20/200 or Worse
Braunstein	54	24	no		5	19	42
& Gass		21	argon/ruby	6	6	9	38
Moorfields	18	24	no		14	10	20
		29	argon		6	14	33
Ho, et al	27	21	argon-green	7	1	13	62
Summary		48	no		40%	60%	33%
		62	yes	20%	20%	60%	31%

* adapted from references 108, 110, and 111.

Final visual acuity means percent of eyes showing a change of two or more lines in Snellen acuity posttreatment, as compared to pretreatment level.

with macular degeneration. In the American study the patients were limited to subretinal neovascular membranes that were from 200 to 2500 μ from the foveola, whereas the British group included subretinal neovascular membranes from 100 to 1500 μ from the foveola (Figure 9-21A-D). Analysis of both studies statistically determined that treatment was beneficial in the maintenance of central vision in those eyes that were treated versus those that were not treated. The American study had a higher incidence of significance than that of the British study (Table 9-5). There are significant problems using argon blue-green in the macular region due

TABLE 9-5.*
SUBRETINAL NEOVASCULARIZATION ASSOCIATED WITH MACULAR DEGENERATION OF AGING

Study	Follow-Up Months	No. of Eyes	Treatment	Final Visual Acuity—%			
				Improved	Same	Worse	20/200 or Worse
USA	3 or	98	no				50
	more	100	argon				18
England	18	51	no	2	25	73	51
		54	argon	9	73	51	28

* adapted from references 115 and 116.

Final visual acuity means percent of eyes showing a change of two or more lines in Snellen acuity posttreatment, as compared to pretreatment level.

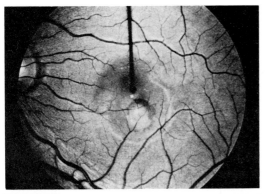

Figure 9-21A.

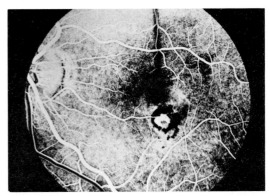

Figure 9-21B.

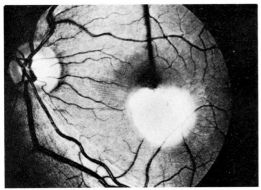

Figure 9-21C.

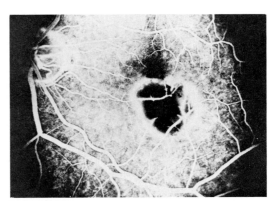

Figure 9-21D.

Figure 9-21. A 62-year-old white female complains of a blur OS. Examination revealed a VA OS 20/70. A. Fundus photograph. Inferior to the fovea is a subretinal neovascular membrane with some breakthrough hemorrhage. B. Fluorescein angiogram, arteriovenous phase. The membrane and corona of hemorrhage are well outlined. The membrane appears to be 350 μ from the foveola. C. Fundus photograph, immediately postoperative. The argon blue-green laser was used to cause a heavy coagulum to the area of the membrane with a most generous surrounding border. Note some retinal striae and retinal vessel occlusion. D. Postoperative fluorescein angiogram shows elimination of the subretinal neovascular net, a "dark" choroid and occluded retinal vessels.

to the absorption of that wavelength by the macular xanthophyll and the retinal blood vessels. These result in nerve fiber layer damage and can cause retinal vascular ischemia. To overcome these problems, the krypton red laser has been used in the obliteration of subretinal neovascular membranes in this region (Figure 9-22A-C). The benefits from use of krypton red are that the red wavelength: 1) is not absorbed by the macular xanthophyll, and 2) is less absorbed by the retinal blood vessels than argon blue-green or argon green. There are non-randomized studies that show that results with the krypton red are similar to those of the argon blue-green controlled studies, and in these krypton studies the treatment has been carried to within 50 μ of the foveal avascular zone.[117,118] This obviously allows treatment of many membranes that otherwise were excluded in the randomized trials of argon laser. Similar advantages have also been mentioned for the use of argon green photocoagulation within the avascular

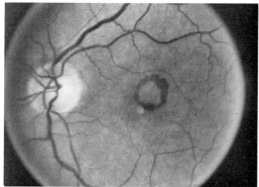

Figure 9-22A.

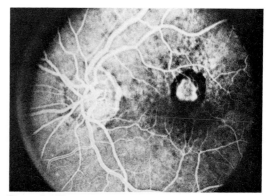

Figure 9-22B.

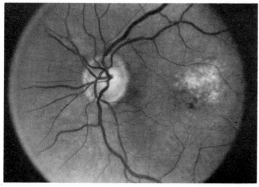

Figure 9-22. A 67-year-old white male presents with a blur OS for two weeks. Examination VA OD 5/400 (cicatricial disciform), OS 20/70. A. Fundus photograph. A subretinal neovascular network is superior to the fovea and ⅓ disc diameter in size. B. Fluorescein angiogram outlines the extent of the membrane with the rim of hemorrhage extending to the foveola. C. Fundus photograph, six months post krypton red laser. VA 20/40. Pigmentary changes extend through the foveola.

Figure 9-22C.

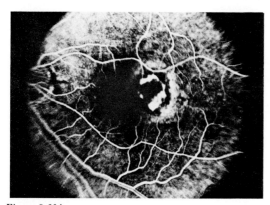

Figure 9-23A.

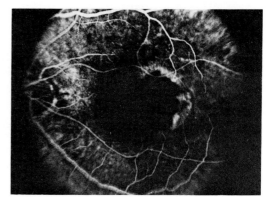

Figure 9-23B.

Figure 9-23. 42-year-old white female with 20/400 VA OS. (Courtesy of Drs. A. Ackerman and H. Topilow.) A. Fluorescein angiogram shows a large (1 disc diameter) subretinal membrane temporal to and extending to the foveola. B. Fluorescein angiogram, six months post argon green laser. The membrane has been obliterated and the VA improved to the 20/100 level.

227

zone (Figure 9-23A & B).[119] Regardless of which method of photocoagulation is used, several criteria are necessary for treatment. One is that a good fluorescein angiogram must be available to localize the area of subretinal neovascularization. The membrane must be completely eliminated when photocoagulation is applied and if hemorrhage is present (which may obscure some of the underlying neovascular membrane), a judgment must be made as to whether or not that area where the hemorrhage is present should also be included in the treatment. Postoperative examination is important to rule out residual subretinal neovascularization. Again the advantages of krypton red and argon green over argon blue-green are obvious. Because of the lack of absorption of the macular xanthophyll by the former two lasers, there will not be obscuration of the inner retina after photocoagulation, and fluorescein angiography of the treated pathology can be performed with much more clarity. There are as yet no firm conclusions about the treatment of subfoveal subretinal neovascularization, but the natural course history is such that a randomized trial is being undertaken by the National Eye Institute.

Summary In summary then, macular degeneration associated with aging is a significant problem affecting central vision in the population of the western hemisphere. Whether we will find that: 1) medical treatments such as use of antioxidants (e.g., vitamin E or selinium), or 2) protection of the retina from ultraviolet wavelengths, is going to prove beneficial is not yet known. At this time, photocoagulation with the argon green or krypton red laser or, if neither is available, the argon blue-green laser is of proven benefit in the treatment of subretinal neovascularization from 100 to 2500 μ outside the fovea. It is obvious, however, in both the natural course history studies and the randomized control studies, that a significant group of patients, even with the best present modalities of treatment, will end up with 20/200 vision or worse. It is, therefore, important that these patients have careful low vision evaluation and counseling by appropriate workers so that their quality of life may be maintained at the best level possible within reason.

Retinal Pigment Epithelial Hamartoma

Retinal pigment epithelial or combined hamartomas are uncommon tumors occurring in the first and second decades of life. They are most frequently located in the juxtapapillary region,[120] however a sizable number of eccentrically located tumors have been reported in all parts of the retina.[121] Clinically affected patients may be asymptomatic until late childhood when they may notice blurred vision, metamorphopsia, distortion, or a negative scotoma. A high percentage of affected individuals have strabismus or have been diagnosed as amblyopic. The lesion may be compatible with good visual acuity with many patients seeing 20/70 or better. Visual acuity may vary as contraction of glial tissue within the tumor causes increased traction upon the macula. There is no involvement of the

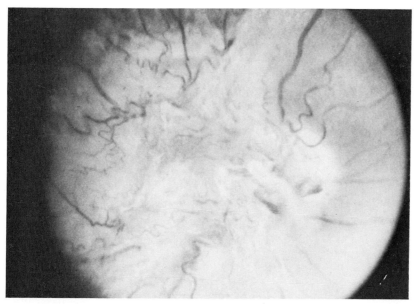

Figure 9-24. A juxtopapillary RPE hamartoma shows typical retinal vascular tortuosity with exuberant gliotic tissue.

anterior segment nor any associated systemic disease. There is one reported case showing late development of peripapillary subretinal neo-vascularization.[122]

Ophthalmoscopically the tumor presents as a dull gray or yellowish elevated retinal mass (Figure 9-24). There may be feathery fan-like projections from the tumor blending into the surrounding pigment epithelium. Dilated capillaries are commonly seen within or on the surface of the tumor and the retinal vasculature in the area of the lesion is usually dilated and tortuous. Although irregular hyperpigmentation of the surrounding retina may be present, atrophy of the retinal pigment epithelium is not a common finding. Ectopic maculae and pre-retinal striae have commonly been associated with this tumor. These structures may be obscured by the tumor. The vitreous is usually free of cells and the overlying retina is not detached.

Angiographic features of the tumor include marked hyperfluorescence from numerous small dilated capillaries within the tumor, which leak dye and cause staining of the tumor and associated glial tissue (Figure 9-25A & B). It is common to find zones of hyperfluorescence around the border of the tumor presumably due to pigment epithelial proliferation. The retinal vasculature not involved by the tumor is usually reported as normal.

RPE hamartomas are classically described as having no growth potential.[124] They have on occasion been misdiagnosed as juxtapapillary choroidal melanomas, especially in the small percentage of RPE hamartomas that were felt to exhibit growth. There are, however, several reported cases of tumors which have shown documented growth during puberty.[120,125] Ultrasonography of this tumor usually reveals a mildly elevated mass with high internal acoustical interfaces on A-scan.[125] In

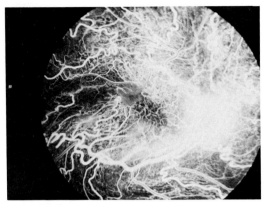

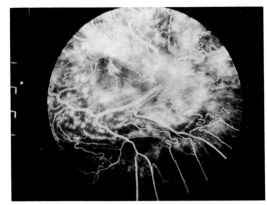

Figure 9-25A.   Figure 9-25B.

Figure 9-25A and B. The retinal vascular tortuosity (25A) and late tumor vascular leakage with staining of the gliotic mass is noted (25B).

general the natural course is good except when retinal striae involve the macula and cause distortion of vision. Although this tumor may simulate other ocular tumors such as melanoma or retinoblastoma, the clinical features usually enable accurate diagnosis.[126] As this is a benign condition there is no reason for intervention either with laser, radiation, or enucleation.

Summary

Disorders of the retina discussed in this chapter range from those related to systemic vascular disease, be it atherosclerotic or inflammatory, through those associated with a presumed systemic infection, to those associated with aging. Although our treatment for these disorders has improved with the maturation of fluorescein angiography and photocoagulation, management is far from perfect. Prevention remains the key to management and there is still much to be done.

References

1. Cunha-Vaz J, Shakib M, Ashton N: Studies on the permeability of the blood-retinal barrier. 1. On the existence, development, and site of a blood-retinal barrier. Brit J Ophthalmol 55:441-453, 1966.
2. Chao P, Flocks M: The retinal circulation time. Am J Ophthalmol 46:8-10 (July, Part 2, 1958.
3. Flocks M, Miller J, Chao P: Retinal circulation time with the aid of fundus cinephotography. Am J Ophthalmol 48:3-6 (July, Part 2), 1959.
4. MacLean AL, Maumenee AE: Hemangioma of the choroid. Am J Ophthalmol 50:3-11, 1960.
5. Norvotny HR, Alvis D: A method of photographing fluorescein in circulating blood in the human retina. Circulation 29:82-86, 1962.
6. Stein MR, Parker CW: Reactions following intravenous fluorescein. Am J Ophthalmol 72:861-868, 1971.

7. Pacurariu RI: Low incidence of side-effects following intravenous fluorescein angiography. Ann Ophthalmol 14:33-36, 1982.
8. Rabb MF, Burton TC, Schatz H, Yannuzzi LA: Fluorescein angiography of the fundus: A schematic approach to interpretation. Surv Ophthalmol 22:387-403, 1978.
9. Gold D: Retinal arterial occlusion. Ophthalmology 83:392-408, 1977.
10. Henkind P, Chambers JK: Arterial occlusive disease of the retina. Vol. V, Chapter 14, Duane TD (ed) *Clinical Ophthalmology.* Hagerstown: Harper & Row, pp 1-14, 1976.
11. Wilson RS, Havener WH and McGrew RN: Bilateral retinal artery and choriocapillaris occlusion following the injection of long-acting corticosteroid suspensions in combination with other drugs: I. Clin Stud Ophthalmol 85:967-974, 1978.
12. Limaye SR, Tang RA, Pilkerton AR: Cilioretinal circulation and branch retinal artery occlusion associated with preretinal arterial loops. Am J Ophthalmol 89:834-839, 1980.
13. Brown GC, Margargal LE: Central retinal artery obstruction and visual acuity. Ophthalmology 89:14-19, 1982.
14. Flower RW, Speros P, Kenyon KR: Electroretinographic changes and choroidal defects in a case of central retinal artery occlusion. Am J Ophthalmol 83:451-459, 1977.
15. Hayreh SS, Kolder HE, Weingeist TA: Central retinal artery occlusion and retinal tolerance time. Ophthalmology 87:75-78, 1980.
16. Brown GC, Shields JA: Cilioretinal arteries and retinal arterial occlusion. Arch Ophthalmol 97:84-92, 1979.
17. Augsburger JJ, Margargal LE: Visual prognosis following treatment of acute central retinal artery obstruction. Brit J Ophthalmol 12:913-917, 1980.
18. Yongue BR and Rosenbaum TJ: Treatment of acute central retinal artery occlusion. Mayo Clin Proc 53:408-410, 1978.
19. Hayreh SS, Podhajsky P: Ocular neovascularization with retinal vascular occlusion. II. Occurrence in central and branch retinal artery occlusion. Arch Ophthalmol 100:1585-1596, 1982.
20. Hayreh SS: Central Retinal Vein Occlusion: Differential Diagnosis and Management. Trans Am Acad Ophthalmology 83:379-391, 1977.
21. Kearns TP, Hollenhorst RW: Venous Stasis Retinopathy of Occlusive Disease of the Carotid Artery. Staff Meet Mayo Clinic 38(15):304-312, 1963.
22. Magargal LE, Brown GC, Augsburger JJ, Parrish RK: Neovascular Glaucoma Following Central Vein Obstruction. Ophthalmology 88:1095-1101, 1981.
23. Gutman FA, Zegarra H: The Natural Course of Retinal Branch Vein Occlusion, Trans Am Acad Ophthal Otolaryngol 78:178-192, 1974.
24. Michaels RG, Gass JDM: The Natural Course of Retinal Branch Vein Obstruction, Trans Am Acad Ophthal Otolaryngol 78:166-177, 1974.
25. Orth DH, Patz A: Retinal Branch Vein Obstruction: A Review, Surv Ophthalmol, 22:357-376, 1978.
26. Henkind P, Walsh JB: Retinal Vascular Anomalies: Pathogenesis, Appearance and History, Trans OSUK, 100:425-433, 1980.
27. Wise GN: Macular Changes After Venous Obstruction, 58:544-577, 1957.
28. Clemett RS, Kohner KM, Hamilton AM: The Visual Prognosis in Retinal Vein Occlusion, Trans OSUK, 93:523-535, 1973.
29. Shilling JS, Kohner EM: New Vessel Formation in Retinal Branch Vein Occlusion, Brit J Ophthalmol 60:810-815, 1976.
30. Hayreh SS, Rojas P, Podhajsky P, Montagque P, Woolson RF: Ocular Neovascularization with Retinal Vascular Occlusion III. Incidence of ocular neovascularization with Retinal Vein Occlusion, Ophthalmol, 90:488-506, 1983.
31. Gutman FA: Macular Edema in Branch Retinal Vein Occlusion: Prognosis and Management, Trans Am Acad Ophthal Otolaryngol, 83:488-493, 1977.
32. Blankenship GW, Okun E: Retinal Tributary Vein Occlusion. History and Management by Photocoagulation, Arch Ophthalmol, 89:363-368, 1973.
33. Wetzig P: The Treatment of Branch Vein Occlusion by Photocoagulation, Am J Ophthalmol, 87:65-73, 1979.

34. Gutman FA, Zegarra H, Rauer A, Zakov N: Photocoagulation in Branch Retinal Vein Occlusion, Ophthalmol, 13:1359-1363, 1981.
35. Shilling JS, Jones CA: Retinal Branch Vein Occlusion: A Study of Argon Laser Photocoagulation in the Treatment of Macular Edema, Brit J Ophthalmol, 68:196-198, 1984.
36. The Framingham Eye Study: Surv Ophthalmol 24:335-620, 1980.
37. Frank RN, Hoffman WH, Podgor MJ, Joondeph HC, Lewis RA, Margherio RR, Nachazel DP, Weiss H, Christopherson KW, Cronin M: Retinopathy in juvenile-onset diabetes of short duration. Ophthalmology 87:1-9, 1980.
38. Cunha-Vaz JG, Fonseca JR, Abreu JF, Ruas MA: A follow-up study by vitreous fluorophotometry of early retinal involvement in diabetes. Am J Ophthalmol 86:467-473, 1978.
39. Shimizu K, Yoshiharu K, Kanemitsu M: Midperipheral fundus involvement in diabetic retinopathy. Ophthalmology 88:601-612, 1981.
40. Takahashi M, Trempe CL, Maguire K, McMeel W: Vitreoretinal relationship in diabetic retinopathy: A biomicroscopic evaluation. Arch Ophthalmol 99:241-245, 1981.
41. Barr CC, Glaser JS, Blankenship GW: Acute disc swellling in juvenile diabetes: Clinic profile and natural course history of 12 cases. Arch Ophthalmol 98:2185-2192, 1980.
42. Puklin JE, Tamborlane WV, Felig P, Henel M, Sherwin RS: Influence of long-term insulin infusion pump treatment on type 1 diabetes in diabetic retinopathy. Ophthalmology 89:735-747, 1982.
43. Spalter HF: Photocoagulation of circinate maculopathy in diabetic retinopathy. Am J Ophthalmol 71:242-250;1971.
44. Patz A, Schatz H, Berkow JW, Gittelsohn AM, Ticho U: Macular edema—an overlooked complication of diabetic retinopathy. Trans Am Acad Ophthalmol Otolaryngol 77:34-41, 1973.
45. Rubinstein K, Myska V: Treatment of diabetic maculopathy. Brit J Ophthalmol 56:1-51, 1972.
46. Marcus DF, Aaberg JM: Argon laser photocoagulation: Treatment of diabetic cystoid macular edema. Ann Ophthalmol 9:365-372, 1977.
47. Blankenship GW: Diabetic macular edema and argon laser photocoagulation: A prospective randomized study. Ophthalmology 86:69-75, 1979.
48. Wiznia RA: Photocoagulation of nonproliferative exudative diabetic retinopathy. Am J Ophthalmol 88:22-27, 1979.
49. Whitelocke RAF, Kearns M, Blach RK, Hamilton AM: The diabetic maculopathies. Trans Ophthalmol Soc UK 99:314-320, 1979.
50. Diabetic Retinopathy Study Research Group: Photocoagulation treatment of proliferative diabetic retinopathy: The second report of Diabetic Retinopathy Study findings. Ophthalmology 85:82-106, 1978.
51. Diabetic Retinopathy Study Research Group: Four risk factors for severe visual loss in diabetic retinopathy: The third report from the Diabetic Retinopathy Study. Arch Ophthalmol 97:654-655, 1979.
52. May DR, Bergstrom TJ, Parmet AJ, Schwartz JG: Treatment of neovascular glaucoma with trans-scleral panretinal cryotherapy. Ophthalmology 87:1106-1111, 1980.
53. Michaels RG: Vitrectomy for complications of diabetic retinopathy. Arch Ophthalmol 96:237-246, 1978.
54. Miller SA, Butler JB, Myers FL, Bresnick GH: Pars plana vitrectomy: Treatment for tractional macular detachment secondary to proliferative diabetic retinopathy. Arch Ophthalmol 98:659-664, 1980.
55. Barrie T, Feretis E, Leaver P, McLeod D: Closed microsurgery for diabetic traction macular detachment. Brit J Ophthalmol 66:754-758, 1982.
56. Little HL, Rosenthal AR, Dellaporta A, Jacobson DR: The effect of photocoagulation on rubeosis iridis. Am J Ophthalmol 81:804-809, 1976.
57. Teich SA, Walsh JB: A grading system for iris neovascularization. Ophthalmology 88:1102-1106, 1981.

58. Pavan PR, Folk JC, Weingeist JA, Hermsen VM, Watzke RC, Montague PR: Diabetic rubeosis and panretinal photocoagulation: A prospective, controlled, masked trial using iris fluorescein angiography. Arch Ophthalmol 101:802-884, 1983.
59. Simmons RJ, Depperman SN, Dueker DK: The role of goniophotocoagulation in neovascularization of the anterior chamber angle. Ophthalmology 87:79-82, 1980.
60. Yagoda A, Walsh J, Henkind P: Idiopathic preretinal macular gliosis. Raab MF, (ed) International Ophthalmology Clinics. Boston: Little Brown & Co., Vol. 21:107-118, 1981.
61. Wise GN: Preretinal macular fibrosis. Trans Ophthalmol Soc UK 92:131-140, 1972.
62. Roth AM, Foos RY: Surface wrinkling retinopathy in eyes enucleated at autopsy. Trans Am Acad Ophthalmol Otolaryngol 75:1047-1058, 1979.
63. Allen Jr AW, Gass JDM: Contraction of a perifoveal membrane stimulating a macular hole. Am J Ophthalmol 82:684-691, 1976.
64. Bellhorn MB, Friedman AH, Wise GN, Henkind P: Ultrastructure of idiopathic preretinal macular fibrosis. Am J Ophthalmol 79:366-373, 1975.
65. Kampik A, Green R, Michaels RG, Nase PK: Ultrastructural features of progressive idiopathic epiretinal membrane removed by vitreous surgery. Am J Ophthalmol 99:797-809, 1980.
66. Wise GN: Clinical features of idiopathic preretinal macular fibrosis. The Schoenberg Lecture. Am J Ophthalmol 79:349-365, 1975.
67. Sidd RJ, Fine SL, Owens SL, Patz A: Idiopathic preretinal macular gliosis. Am J Ophthalmol 94:44-48, 1982.
68. Wiznia RA: Natural history of idiopathic macular fibrosis. Ann Ophthalmol 44:876-878, 1982.
69. Wise GN, Campbell CJ, Wendler P, Rittler MC: Photocoagulation of vascular lesions of the macula. Am J Ophthalmol 66:452-459, 1968.
70. Michaels RG: Vitreous surgery for macular pucker. Am J Ophthalmol 92:628-639, 1981.
71. Robertson DM: Macroaneurysms of retinal arteries. Ophthalmology 77:56-67, 1973.
72. Lewis RA, Norton EWD, Gass JDM: Acquired arterial macroaneurysms of the retina. Brit J Ophthalmol 60:21-30, 1976.
73. Gold DH, Walsh JB: Fluorescein angiographic patterns of retinal arterial aneurysms. DeLaey JJ, (ed) International Symposium on Fluorescein Angiography. Doc Ophthalmol Proc Series 9:541-547, 1976.
74. Shults WT, Swan KC: Pulsatile aneurysms of the retinal arterial tree. Am J Ophthalmol 77:304-309, 1974.
75. Cleary PE, Kohner EM, Hamilton AM, Bird AC: Retinal macroaneurysms. Brit J Ophthalmol 59:335-361, 1975.
76. Ehlers N, Jensen VA: ACTA Ophthalmologica 51:171-178, 1974.
77. Chopdar A: Brit J Ophthalmol 63:243-250, 1978.
78. Hutton WI, Snyder WB, Fuller D, Vaiser A: Arch Ophthalmol 96:1362-1367, 1978.
79. Gass JD, Oyakawa RT: Arch Ophthalmol 100:769-780, 1982.
80. Green WR, Quigley HA, De LaCruz Z, Cohen B: Parafoveal Retinal Telangiectasis Light and Electron Microscopy Studies. Trans Ophth Soc UK 100:162-180, 1980.
81. Ryan SJ, Maumenee AE: Birdshot Retinochoroidopathy. Amer J Ophthalmol 89:31, 1980.
82. Gass JDM: Vitiliginous Chorioretinitis, Arch Ophthalmol 99:1778, 1981.
83. Nussenblatt RB, Mittal KK: Birdshot retinochoroidopathy. Amer J Ophthalmol 94:147-158, 1982.
84. Kaplan HJ, Aaberg TM: Birdshot retinochoroidopathy. Amer J Ophthalmol 90:773, 1980.
85. Rosenberg PR, Noble KG, Walsh JB, Carr RE: Birdshot Retinochoroidopathy. Ophthalmology 91:304-306, 1984.
86. Drew WL, et al: Cytomegalovirus and Kaposi's Sarcoma in Young Homosexual Men, Lancet II 125-127 (July) 1982.
87. Rosenberg PR, et al: Acquired Immunodeficiency Syndrome-Ophthalmic Manifestations in Ambulatory Patients, Ophthalmol 90:874-878, 1983.
88. Holland GN, et al: Ocular Disorders Associated with a new Severe Acquired Cellular

Immune Deficiency Syndrome, Amer J Ophthalmol 93:393-402, 1982.

89. Gass JDM, Wilkinson CP: Follow-up Study of Presumed Ocular Histoplasmosis. Trans Am. Acad. Ophthalmol/Otolaryngol 76:672, 1972.

90. Gass JDM: Pathogenesis of Disciform Detachment of the Neuroepithelium. *Amer J Ophthalmol* 63:663, 1967.

91. Schlaegel TF Jr, Benney D: Changes Around the Optic Nervehead in Presumed Ocular Histoplasmosis. Amer J Ophthalmol 62:455, 1966.

92. Schlaegel TF (ed): Proceedings of the Ocular Histoplasmosis Symposium. Int Ophthalm. Clin 15.(No. 3):1, 1978.

93. Gass JDM: Pathogenesis of Disciform Detachment of the Neuroepithelium. V. Disciform macular degeneration secondary to Focal Choroiditis. Amer J Ophthalmol 63:661, 1967.

94. Schlaegel TF: Histoplasmic Choroiditis. Ann. Ophthalmol; 6:237, 1974.

95. Schlaegel TF Jr., Weber JC, Helveston E, Kenney D: Presumed Histoplasmic Choroiditis. Amer J Ophthalmol 63:919, 1967.

96. Macular Photocoagulation Study Group: Argon Laser Photocoagulation for Ocular Histoplasmosis. Arch Ophthalmol 101:1347-1357, 1981.

97. Sabates FN, King YL, Ziemianski MC: A Comparative Study of Argon and Krypton Laser Photocoagulation in the Treatment of Presumed Ocular Histoplasmosis Syndrome. Ophthalmol 89:729-734, 1982.

98. The Framingham Eye Study. Surv Ophthalmol 24:335-620;1980.

99. Klein BE, Klein R: Cataracts and macular degeneration in older America. Arch Ophthalmol 100:571-573;1982.

100. Walsh JB, Wright BE: Senile macular degeneration. Henkind P, Wright BE, (eds). Clinical Signs in Ophthalmology, St. Louis Mo: CV Mosby, 1983, Vol 3:1-10.

101. Henkind P: Ocular neovascularization. The Krill Memorial Lecture. Am J Ophthalmol 85:287-301;1983.

102. Sarks SH: Aging and degeneration in the macular region: A clinicopathological study. Brit J Ophthalmol 60:324-341;1976.

103. Gartner S, Henkind P: Aging and degeneration of the human macula. 1. Outer nuclear layer and photoreceptors. Brit J Ophthalmol 65:23-28;1981.

104. Green WR, Key SN: Senile macular degeneration: A histopathologic study. Trans Am Ophthalmol Soc LXXXV:180-250;1977.

105. Burns RP, Feeny-Burns L: Clinicomorphologic correlations of drusen of Bruch's membrane. Trans Am Ophthalmol Soc LXXXVIII:206-233;1980.

106. Newsome DA, Milton RC, Gass JDM: Afferent pupillary defect in macular degeneration. Am J Ophthalmol 92:396-402;1981.

107. Hoskin A, Bird AC, Sehmi K: Tears of detached retinal pigment epithelium. Brit J Ophthalmol 65:417-422;1981.

108. Braunstein RA, Gass JDM: Serous detachments of the retinal pigment epithelium in patients with senile macular degeneration. Am J Ophthalmol 88:652-660;1979.

109. Bressler SB, Bressler NM, Fine SL, Hillis A, Murphy RP, Olk RJ, Patz A: Natural course history of choroidal neovascular membranes within the foveal avascular zone in senile macular degeneration. Am J Ophthalmol 93:157-163;1982.

110. The Moorfields Study Group: Retinal pigment epithelial detachments in the elderly. Brit J Ophthalmol 66:1-16;1982.

111. Ho PC, Namperumalsamy P, Pruett RC: Photocoagulation of serous detachments of the pigment epithelium in patients with senile macular degeneration. Ann Ophthalmol 16:213-218;1984.

112. Zweng HC, Little HL, Peabody RR: Laser photocoagulation of macular lesions. Trans Am Acad Ophthalmol and Otolaryngol 72:377-388;1968.

113. Wise GN, Campbell CJ, Wendler PI, Rittler MC: Photocoagulation of vascular lesions of the macula. Am J Ophthalmol 66:452-459;1968.

114. Schatz H, Patz A: Exudative senile maculopathy. 1. Results of laser treatment. Arch Ophthalmol 90:183-196;1973.

115. Macular Photocoagulation Study Group: Argon laser photocoagulation for senile macular degeneration. Results of a randomized clinical trial. Arch Ophthalmol 100:912-918;1982.

116. The Moorfields Macular Study Group: Treatment of senile disciform macular degeneration: A single-blind randomized trial by argon laser photocoagulation. Brit J Ophthalmol 66:745-753;1982.

117. Yannuzzi LA: Krypton red laser photocoagulation for subretinal neovascularization. Retina 2:29-46;1982.

118. Yannuzzi LA: A perspective on macular degeneration. Bull NY Acad Med 59:803-817;1983.

119. Jalkh AE, Avila MP, Trempe CT, Schepens CL: Management of choroidal neovascularization within the avascular zone in macular degeneration. Am J Ophthalmol 95:818-825;1983.

120. Cardell BS, Starbuck MJ: Juxtapapillary hamartoma of retina. Brit J Ophthalmol 45:672-677;1961.

121. McLean EB: Hamartomas of the retinal pigment epithelium. Am J Ophthalmol 82:227-231;1976.

122. Yannuzzi LA, Gitter KA, Schatz H: In: The macula: A Comprehensive Test and Atlas. Baltimore MD, Williams & Wilkins Co., p. 298, 1979.

123. Gass JDM: An unusual hamartoma of the pigment epithelium and retina simulating choroidal melanoma and retinoblastoma. Trans Am Ophthalmol Soc 71:171-185;1973.

124. Laqua H, Wessing A: Congenital retino-pigment epithelial malformation, previously described as hamartoma. Am J Ophthalmol 87:34-42;1979.

125. Rosenberg PR and Walsh JB: Retinal Pigment Epithelial Hamartomas, Unusual Manifestations. Brit J Ophth: (in press) 1984.

126. Gass JDM: In: Differential Diagnosis of Intraocular Tumors, A Stereoscopic Presentation. St. Louis: CV Mosby Co., 1974, pp 222-224.

Section III

Neuro-Ophthalmologic Disorders

NEURO-OPHTHALMOLOGIC DISORDERS

Introduction

Neuro-ophthalmology has changed drastically in the past ten years. Medical imaging has been revolutionized with CT and NMR scanning. Wirtschafter and Gold guide the ophthalmologist through the rapidly changing world of diagnostic imaging and its applicability to ophthalmologic disorders. The chapter is long, but contains information not readily accessible to the ophthalmologist. This information enables us to utilize diagnostic imaging to our patient's advantage.

Optic neuropathies are a diverse group of afflictions involving the optic nerve. Tredici and McCrary present a concise and rational approach to the diagnosis and management of these disorders. This chapter really simplifies and facilitates understanding a very complicated subject.

The short chapter on pseudotumor cerebri emphasizes the importance of recognizing that visual loss is the only significant long-term complication of this disease and may occur any time after the diagnosis is made. Subsequently, these patients require periodic evaluation of their visual function for the remainder of their lives. This is the ophthalmologist's role. This chapter describes what the clinician needs to know to recognize, diagnose and manage these patients.

No discussion of neuro-ophthalmology is complete without mentioning syphilis—still the great imitator. The incidence of infectious syphilis is increasing at an alarming rate. These patients may present to the ophthalmologist with iritis, chorioretinitis, or swollen discs. Late syphilis may present as interstitial keratitis, iritis, chorioretinitis or optic atrophy. The key to diagnosing either late or infectious syphilis is suspicion and obtaining the appropriate serologic tests. This treatable cause of visual dysfunction is reviewed in this section.

(Editor)

Chapter 10

Medical Imaging in Ophthalmology: Interpretation and Misinterpretation

Jonathan D. Wirthschafter,
MD, MS, FACS
Lawrence H.A. Gold, MD

MEDICAL IMAGING IN OPHTHALMOLOGY: INTERPRETATION AND MISINTERPRETATION

The title of this chapter has been chosen to avoid instant obsolescence which may come about because of the introduction of a new imaging modality, (nuclear) magnetic resonance (MR) scanning that is becoming increasingly popular as this chapter is written less than one century since Wilhelm Roentgen discovered the short x-ray. The designation "medical imaging" has replaced "diagnostic radiology" and also encompasses ultrasonography, magnetic resonance scanning, and radionuclide scanning. Ophthalmologists will be pleased to learn that light is not yet included in "imaging."

The principles that govern the ordering, interpretation, and misinterpretation of images may be generalized and many of them apply whether or not potentially harmful ionizing radiation is used to obtain the image. Since many of the patients discussed in this chapter will require repeated scans, the ophthalmologist ordering the studies should remember that the recommended upper limit of total radiation to the lens of an infant should not exceed 450 rads while the dose to the lens of an adult should not exceed 700 rads. It is outside the scope of this chapter to discuss the technical aspects of radiation dosimetry, but a few facts may help gain some perspective protecting the eye. A single conventional skull x-ray will deliver about 3-5 rads to the entire head, thus a sinus series with 5 views might give a total exposure of 25 rads to the lens. Complex motion polytomography of the face results in doses of about 30 rads. A computed tomography (CT) scan delivers radiation primarily to the region studied in each slice, so that the radiation scattered from multiple thin sections does not more than double the dose to adjacent sections. Using the newest scanners typical doses to the lens are under 9 rads even when axial and direct subcoronal scans are used in combination. The radiation dose can be further controlled by proper orientation of the planes of section through the use of a localizer digital radiograph which itself adds less than 75 mrad to the dose. Figure 10-1 shows a digital skull radiograph with electronically generated lines in the coronal plane. An axial CT of the orbits would have lines parallel to Reid's base line, a line that extends from the inferior orbital rim to the upper margin of the external auditory meatus.

Comparison of Imaging Modalities

Plain Skull Films. Thus it is the role of the ophthalmologist to define the structures of interest and the kinds of processes that may occur in those structures. The examination can then be planned in collaboration with the neuro-radiologist. An examination is described as "plain" if no contrast material such as air or iodine containing media are used. The plain skull

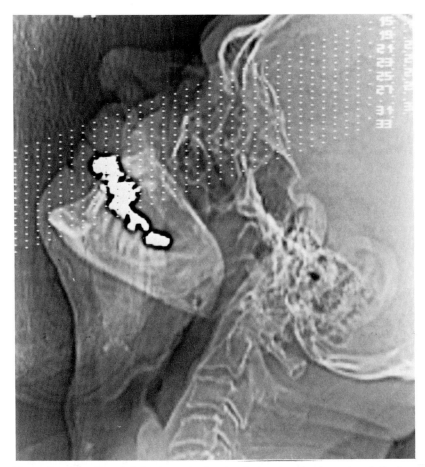

Figure 10-1. A localizer digital radiography showing the location of each numbered slice in a direct coronal scan. The relationships of the slices to the orbital structures can be seen. The angulation of the scan can be varied according to the location of metal dentures that create annoying lines and the flexibility of the patient's neck.

film used to be a required prerequisite to a CT, but such a tactic may waste both time and radiation exposure. "Routine" skull films in the management of head injuries would reveal only a small fraction of the total serious injuries, because skull fractures make up only a fraction of the brain injuries that occur in head trauma. If there is evidence of neurologic dysfunction, a CT scan would have a much higher yield.

In addition to the demonstration of fractures in trauma cases skull films may also show a radio-opaque foreign body, space intracranial air (this could be useful in a stab wound passing to the intracranial cavity via the superior aspect of the orbit), or blood or soft tissue in one of the paranasal sinuses. The presence of blood in the ethmoid sinuses may indicate that there could be a fracture that extends to the optic canal and that the optic nerve could be compromised by the manipulation of the fracture. In non-trauma cases, skull films may be useful in determining the integrity of the bony margins or the size of structures such as the optic canals or the sella turcica, the closure of the cranial sutures and other developmental and acquired abnormalities of the bones, and the presence of abnormal calcification of tissues.

Computed Tomography (CT). [1-5]The introduction of CT in 1972 has expanded the diagnosis of neurological and ophthalmological disorders because the vast majority of these conditions do not produce changes which can be imaged by plain films because they do not provide enough contrast to distinguish the regional variations in the attenuation of the x-rays by the tissues. Even without the addition of iodine-containing intravenous contrast material, the orbital contents are naturally contrasty ranging from about −100 H (Hounsfield units) for orbital fat to about +100 H for the arc of the cornea. This natural contrast is of practical significance because it may be possible to examine the orbit and the paranasal sinuses without the use of intravenous contrast materials when enhancement of intracranial structures is not required. The range of absorption coefficients is illustrated in Figure 10-2. Because of the overlap of absorption coefficients, measure-

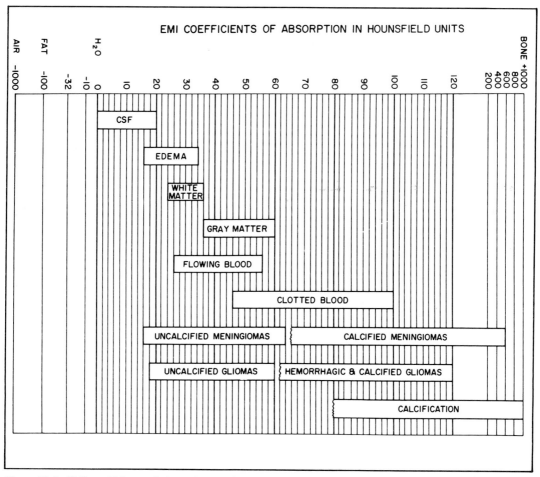

Figure 10-2. EMI coefficients of absorption in Hounsfield units. Reproduced with permission from Ramsay RG: Neuroradiology with computed tomography. Philadelphia, W.B. Saunders, 1981, p 128.

ment is rarely useful in the determination of the pathological process. Because of the overlap between brain edema and normal white matter, unenhanced scans of the head can be used instead of enhanced scans (the terms pre-infusion and post-infusion are also used) in the work-up of acute head trauma, to determine the ventricle size, and for the evaluation of dementia. Enhanced scans will be required to outline the parasellar regions, to define arteriovenous malformations, to locate and evaluate tumors, and to look for local enhancement or lucency in demyelinating disorders. Pre- and post-infusion scans may be required for several reasons including the differentiation of blood from calcium, isodense subdural hematomas from brain, and isodense regions of cerebral infarction from brain. A pre-infusion scan of the orbit should be converted to a post-infusion scan whenever a combined intraorbital-intracranial lesion is detected or if the lesion seems to extend into the temporal fossa. The allergic and renal complications which may follow the use of intravenous contrast media must also be considered before the test is ordered.

Angiographic Techniques. The essential equipment includes an image intensifier arranged so that both fluoroscopy and biplane arteriography can be performed. The ophthalmologist's decision to use angiographic imaging techniques will frequently involve other specialists such as the neurosurgeon. Two specific exceptions to this are dacryocystography and orbital venography. The former requires an ophthalmologist in attendance, if for no other reason than to prevent or treat corneal complications of injecting in the lacrimal puncta. The latter has been replaced by CT although it gave indirect information concerning vascular displacement by orbital masses or was a way of evaluating the blood flow or contents of the cavernous sinuses.

More frequently the ophthalmologist may wish to decide in consultation with the radiologist whether to perform a cerebral arteriogram that provides high resolution of the intra- and extracranial vessels with the risks associated with transfemoral catheterization, or to perform an intravenous digital subtraction angiogram which provides images of lower quality and is associated with the risks of injecting a much larger quantity of contrast material than is required for direct arteriography. In classical arteriography a high concentration of contrast material is required because the x-ray system provides high spatial resolution (image details) at the expense of low contrast resolution. Digital subtraction angiography uses electronic techniques to amplify the small amount of contrast material which appears diluted in the arteries following intravenous injection. This technique provides high contrast resolution but poor spatial resolution. At the time this is written, the author uses digital subtraction angiography when excluding operable occlusive disease of the carotid arteries and uses cerebral arteriography when it is likely to be a prelude to vascular surgical or neurosurgical procedures.

Radionuclide Scans. Radionuclide scans have ceased to have much application in ophthalmology. There are selected cases where imaging the passage or accumulation of a radioisotope can be of value.

Dacryocystography can be performed with sodium pertechnetate ^{99m}Tc and the movement of the dye through the lacrimal drainage system is followed with scintigraphy. The advantages of the technique are that the lens is subjected to much less radiation than with regular dacryocystography and that the tracer is placed in the lacrimal lake rather than injected into the puncta. The disadvantage of the technique is the inability to image the adjacent soft tissue and bony structures. This technique may thus be superseded by digital subtraction dacryocystography.

Radionuclide scanning may be useful in neuro-ophthalmology to locate a small arteriovenous malformation near the surface of the frontal lobe. Such lesions can be missed by CT because the lesions are averaged in with the adjacent brain and bone in what is known as a partial volume phenomenon. Dynamic radionuclide scanning can also be used to demonstrate cerebrospinal fluid leakage into the paranasal sinuses, nose or orbit, but CT metrizamide cisternography offers better spatial and contrast resolution.

Magnetic Resonance. Magnetic resonance[6,7] scanning is rapidly developing and will undoubtedly provide images that were not possible with CT. The method was first developed as a form of analytical chemistry and the term "nuclear" used because the nuclei of each species of atom has a spin that relates to the number of protons and neutrons that comprise the nucleus of the atom. For clinical use the term "nuclear" is being dropped because of the public fear and confusion that the technique is somehow related to x-rays. Actually the electromagnetic energy is in the 10 to 100,000 meter band of the radiofrequency spectrum and has less energy than x-rays, light, and microwaves.

Magnetic resonance scanning is performed by placing the patient in a powerful magnet to which are linked radio frequency (RF) transmitters and receivers and a computer to coordinate and time the RF stimulation and reception and to produce the image. Spatial localization is obtained because a smaller magnet called "the gradiant coil" produces a field at right angles to the main magnet. Nuclei closer to the magnet resonate differently than those at a greater distance. Radio frequency pulses are used to produce another and weak magnetic field that displaces the hydrogen (protons) in the tissue from their initial positions. After the pulse is removed the protons return to their original orientations, emitting a radio frequency that may resonate with that set in the radio antenna-tuner. The devices can be tuned for hydrogen nucleus (protons) or other specific atoms which are aligned by the magnet. The output reflects the location of the atoms, their rate of movement (for example in the blood flow), and the characteristics (for example, homo- or heterogeneity) of their molecular environment. The detailed description of these techniques is beyond the scope of this chapter. In clinical practice MR will be used to compliment CT in some cases while replacing it in others. At present MR is twice as expensive and twice as slow as CT. There are some instances where MR will be inferior to current imaging techniques because the signal from solids is very weak or because intrinsic motion of the organs degrades the image. Thus the outline of the optic canal or the location of a calcified lesion in the suprasellar cistern can be better demonstrated with a CT and bone windows. The details of lesions of the motile gastrointestinal tract may be best demonstrated with conventional radiographic techniques.[7] Nevertheless, it is clear that there are certain advantages over CT including the absence of ionizing radiation, inherent contrast between gray matter and white matter, identification of areas of abscess, infarction, or demyelination which might appear isodense with brain on conventional CT, and better detail of the posterior fossa including direct sagittal and direct coronal scanning. Recent papers have stressed that some intracerebral blood not detected by CT can be detected by MR. The age and distribution of blood in the vitreous cavity can also be better defined by MR than by CT (Figures 10-3 through 10-6).

Present disadvantages of MR include poorer spatial resolution, the high cost and special environment required by these magnetic devices, and the inability to scan patients who contain ferrous materials (prosthetic hips, heart valves, and surgical clips) which could be moved by the magnets. Dental appliances and stainless steel sutures are not a danger to the patient but they may distort the images. Recent studies have demonstrated that

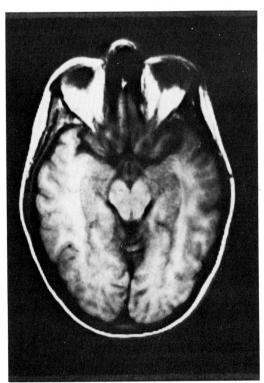

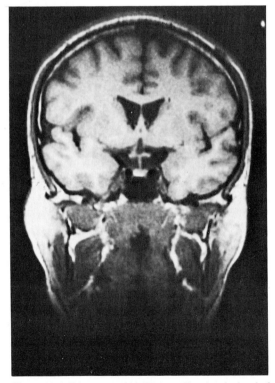

Figure 10-3. An axial magnetic resonance scan of head showing excellent definition of grey and white matter of brain and a slit-like third ventricle at a level above the optic chiasm. The details of the optic radiations are clearly demonstrated. The orbit fat is displayed as white while the skull and bony orbit appear black. (This and the three subsequent figures are copyright by and reproduced with the courtesy of General Electric Company Medical Systems Operations, Milwaukee, Wisconsin).

Figure 10-4. Direct coronal MR scan of head at the level of the pituitary fossa. The sphenoid bone appears black, the pituitary contents white. The pituitary stalk is seen below the third ventricle. The relationship of the temporal lobes lateral to the cavernous sinus is also demonstrated.

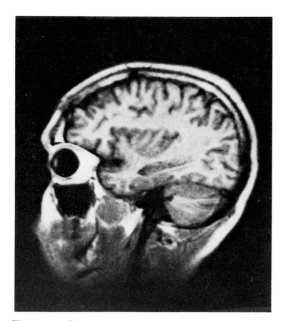

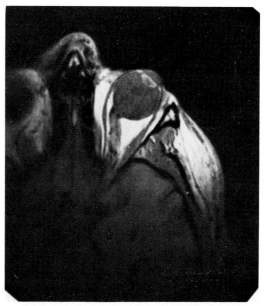

Figure 10-5. Direct parasagittal MR scan in the plane of the globe. The lens and extraocular muscles are seen. The relationship of the orbital fat to the floor of the orbit and the maxillary sinus is clearly demonstrated, as is the relationship of the frontal and temporal lobes of the brain to the superior and posterior orbital walls.

Figure 10-6. An MR scan of the orbit, produced with the use of special surface coils, shows even greater detail. The optic nerve and extraocular muscles are seen. A vessel (black) crosses the optic nerve. The bone of the frontal process of the zygomatic arch also appears black. The surface of the temporal lobe is seen with less detail posterior to the orbit, and the details of the temporalis muscle are seen lateral to the orbit.

MR may give information on the distribution, age, and organization of blood in the vitreous cavity. Other studies using special surface coil magnets have demonstrated orbital structures such as the vortex veins, the orbital septum, the details of the posterior orbit, and the intra-canalicular tumors of the optic nerve.

Positron Emission Tomography. Positron emission tomography (PET) is presently a research tool which will not be available at even all large institutions, because a cyclotron is required for the production of usable radioisotopes shortly before they are compounded into radio-pharmaceuticals and injected into the patient. Positron emitting sugars, for example, can be used to define the local metabolic activity of the brain during differing sensory stimulations. For example, the occipital lobes are more active when the patient is viewing an object, and the temporal lobes are more active when listening. Qualitative impressions of regional metabolism are now being replaced by quantitative studies of certain diseases and metabolic conditions such as increased intracranial pressure, cerebral edema, and anaerobic glycolysis in ischemic strokes. The clinical value of PET scans has yet to be demonstrated.[8]

Ultrasonography. Ultrasonography[9,10] has lost most of its applications in the evaluation of intracranial structures except for its use in probes used for intraoperative imaging. However ultrasonography remains of interest in measuring and imaging the eye and orbit. It is also used in the Doppler measurement of blood flow and to image irregularities of the extracranial arteries. Ophthalmologists may request cardiac echography for those conditions associated with mitral valve prolapse and emboli of cardiac origin. High frequency sound waves of 20 MHz and thus short wavelengths are used for ocular examination. The resolution is limited by one-half the pulse duration times the propagation velocity in the tissue. Thus the axial resolution is limited to about 0.11 mm. and lateral resolution to 0.2 mm. Due to absorption orbital examinations cannot be performed at as high frequencies as ocular examinations. When 10 MHz sound is used to examine the orbit, axial resolution is limited to 0.2 mm and lateral resolution to about 0.9 mm. Ultrasound can be refracted and this property can be used to measure the width of the optic nerve. Thus ultrasound images are generally more useful for intraocular than orbital diagnosis. A pulse-echo technique is used to measure the acoustic reflectivity and absorbtion of the tissue, thus providing different information than might be obtained with the other imaging modalities. The A-scan measures the reflection at points along a path while the B-scan is used to produce an image of one plane. As used diagnostically, ultrasound is not harmful to the eye, but there are high energy ultrasound systems that are cataractogenic.

Intraocular uses of ultrasonography include the detection of dislocated lenses, retinal detachment, vitreous hemorrhage, and intraocular foreign bodies and tumors. Extraocular uses of ultrasound may include presumptive preoperative tissue diagnosis, detection of the presence or absence of vascular flow within a lesion, determination of compressibility of a lesion, detection of increased optic nerve sheath width in increased intracranial pressure, and degrees of thickening of the extraocular muscles too small to be detected by CT.

Anatomical and Technical Considerations

Anatomical Considerations

The Axial Projection. Actually a family of projections in the general plane corresponding to the base of the skull, the axial projection takes its name from the prior definition by radiologists of axes connecting various bony landmarks. The orbit and optic nerve are generally imaged in the axial projection along the 0° axis parallel to Reid's base line as illustrated in Figure 10-7. Other variants of the axial projection vary from the axis parallel to the course of the optic canal (about − 30°) and the axial projection used in routine scanning of the brain (+15-20°) so as to include the posterior fossa structures and the frontal lobes in the lowest sections. It can be readily seen that the standard axial projection used for a scan of the brain will not have its axis projected through the optic canals, nor will it even be optimal for viewing the intracranial optic nerve or optic chiasm.

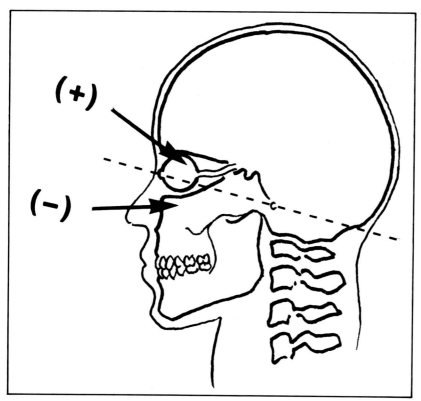

Figure 10-7. Diagram showing the direction of the x-ray beam in the axial plane. The dashed line through the orbit is parallel to Reid's base line. A section through the plane represented by the line is described as being at an angle of 0 degrees. Sections at negative angles of 30° can be in the long axis of the optic canal, the long axis of the intraorbital course of the optic nerve if the eyes are directed into upgaze, and, at a lower level, the long axis of the inferior rectus muscle. Sections at positive angles are normally used for brain scans and can show both the top of the orbit and the posterior fossa in the same image, but will fail to show important orbital details. When both brain and orbit are required, an initial scan at 0 degrees angulation is a good compromise. Reproduced from Wirtschafter JD, Taylor S: Computed Tomography: An Atlas for Ophthalmologists. American Academy of Ophthalmology, San Francisco, 1982.

The Coronal Projection. The coronal projection, at right angles to Reid's base line, requires the patient to severely hyperextend the neck into the gantry opening of the CT machine. In practice, subcoronal views are often obtained at less than a 90° angle. The interpretation of subcoronal views requires that you recognize that the orbit is sectioned obliquely. The angulation of coronal views must take into account the locations of dental fillings or other metallic foreign bodies which can cause significant artifacts. The coronal projection is useful for studying structures that are displaced vertically (for example, the inferior rectus muscle in an orbital floor fracture), especially when that structure is located near bony interfaces (such as the roof and floor of the orbit) that coincide with the axial plane. The coronal projection is also important in examining the suprasellar and parasellar region in neuro-ophthalmology.

The Sagittal Projection. At right angles to the axial and coronal projections, the sagittal projection is in the midline. Parasagittal projections may be to the right or left of the midline. Angulated parasagittal projections may be used to follow the orbital course of the optic nerve or the superior and inferior oblique muscles. Technical considerations have limited the usefulness of the sagittal and parasagittal projections in CT but new CT equipment and techniques are changing this. MR readily produces images in the sagittal projection.

Projections Used in Plain Skull Films. The projections used in plain skull films are illustrated in Figure 10-8. The lateral projection is the same as the midline sagittal projection and is used for the evaluation of facial trauma, localization of radio-opaque foreign bodies, and for determining the size and continuity of the sella turcica. The straight posteroanterior projection is about the same as the true coronal projection. The petrous pyramids are projected into the inferior orbits so that the view is useful for evaluating the upper orbit and the frontal bone.

Plain Skull Film Projections Not Used in CT. There are two projections regularly used for plain skull films that are not used for CT; these are the Caldwell's and the Waters' views. The inclined posteroanterior projection (Caldwell's view) is useful for viewing the superior orbital fissure and comparing the sizes of the two orbits. The Waters' view is useful for viewing the roof and floor of the orbit and demonstrating tumors of the lacrimal fossa and the frontal and maxillary sinuses. It is an oblique coronal

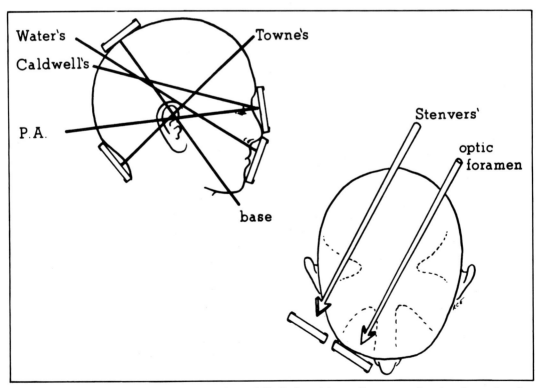

Figure 10-8. Radiological projections of skull: plane of film indicated by small cassettes; direction of central ray for each view is indicated by taglines and arrows.

projection of the orbit with the direction of the obliquity the opposite of that of the subcoronal view (Figure 10-8).

There are two special projections that may be useful in plain films. One is the optic foramen view with the axis of the projection rotated into that of the optic canal, normally 45° from the sagittal plane and 30° from Reid's base line. The examination of the optic canal will be discussed later. Stenver's view has been largely replaced by CT for the examination of the auditory canal.

Technical Considerations

Technical Aspects of Interpretation of Images. While this chapter cannot review the basic aspects of data acquisition for each of the imaging methods described above, it is possible to provide some information which will help in obtaining an interpretable image from the radiologist by manipulation of the console after the data has been gathered. The *spatial resolution* of an imaging system can be expressed in line pairs/cm and is currently about 10 line pairs/cm for CT scanners. The *contrast resolution* (the resolvable difference in contrast between two adjacent structures) of a system interacts with the spatial resolution in the identification of adjacent anatomic structures of specified size and contrast. For example, newer CT scanners usually provide sufficient spatial resolution to resolve the ophthalmic vein without the use of contrast enhancement.

A *pixel* is the smallest picture element seen on the cathode-ray tube (CRT). If the screen has 320 × 320 points in its matrix it will contain 102,400 pixels. Each pixel is the two-dimensional representation of the data from a three-dimensional volume element known as a *voxel*. The depth (out of the plane of the picture) of the voxel in the matrix corresponds to the *thickness of the slice* in the patient. The *level of the slice* refers to the midplane of the slice.

The signal computed for each voxel is stored as a number in the computer and represents the average signal obtained from all matter in that volume (plus any artifacts induced by matter in nearby voxels). For CT that number is the *attenuation coefficient* and can be printed as the *measure* for any pixel on the CRT screen. Since a given voxel could contain several tissues and forms of matter having high and low attenuation coefficients (for example, bone and air) an average value could result from each of the two materials that partially fill this volume. This is known as the *partial volume phenomenon* and is particularly troublesome in estimating the width of the intraorbital portion of the optic nerve because the nerve slips up and down through the plane of each slice and its density is averaged with that of the orbital fat.

The gray scale is the pictorial representation of the density or other data. There may be about 16 shades of gray shown on the screen. For CT the higher densities are usually shown as light (but this can be reversed when desired, for example, the suprasellar cisterns could be displayed as light and the optic nerves and chiasm as dark structures). Any density higher than the upper limit of the gray scale will thus appear light, and lower than the lower limit of the gray scale will appear black. These limits are known as the window, and the difference between its upper and lower limits are known as the *window width*, when the term should really be the window height. The average of the upper and lower density limits is *the window level*. It can be set for high density structures allowing all of the details of the brain and orbit soft tissue to be lost in black. No one print of a given scale can show both bony and soft tissue details well. An important application is that double prints are required of an axial CT of optic canals (with window level and width adjusted to show bony details), or the print can show low density structures causing all delicate bony detail to be lost.

Slice Thickness and Computer Reformation of Images. Reformation of an image can be used to improve the interpretation of information gathered during the direct scan. Thus reformation can produce an indirect coronal image from a direct axial scan in a patient who could not be positioned for a coronal scan. However the resolution is determined by the thickness of the slice which made up the original voxel. For the orbit this requires that the patient be able to hold still while multiple (about 25) thin (1.5 mm) contiguous axial slices are obtained. Conversely, the patient could be studied with about 15 (for each projection) direct axial and subcoronal slices of 5 mm thickness with 3 mm spacing so that the sections overlap one another by 2 mm. Either of these procedures will produce enough data to allow reformation of the images so that reformatted sagittal images can also be obtained. The radiation to the lens is about 50% greater when the coronal view is obtained directly than when it is obtained by reformation.

Regional Anatomy and Diagnosis

This section is organized so that for each region, first will be presented the anatomy (including aspects of the gross anatomy, imaging modality anatomy, developmental and aging changes, and normal variants), second will be presented the imaging indications and modalities, and last will be presented examples of pathology reflecting the imaging problems for each region except for the strictly intracranial regions. The examples are not intended to be encyclopedic but are chosen to help the reader in the selection and interpretation of images.

The Skull and Bony Orbit

Anatomy. *Anatomy of the Skull.* The skull can be divided into the skull vault and the skull base. The major anatomic features of the vault are its size and shape, its thickness and texture, and the sutures and fontanelles. Abnormalities of craniofacial proportion can be described as symmetric or asymmetric microcrania or macrocrania. Developmental defects in the skull can occur as developmental abnormalities, examples of which include meningoencephaloceles penetrating into the nasal aspects of the orbit and hypoplasia of the greater wing of the sphenoid giving rise to pulsating exophthalmos in neurofibromatosis. Hyperplasia of the skull can occur in acromegaly and in dystrophia myotonica.

The Anatomy of the Base of the Skull and Orbit. The embryological development of the sella turcica and the radiologic appearance of the cranial opening of the optic canal are interrelated and have been described by Kier.[11] The optic canal begins as a thin cartilaginous foramen, which later ossifies and lengthens into a bony canal in the lesser wing of the sphenoid bone. The inferior root of the lesser wing of the sphenoid is the optic strut that separates the optic canal from the superior orbital fissure. Loss of the optic strut is an important radiologic sign and usually results from an expanding mass in this region. However, in infants the roof of the optic canal may be much more prominent than the optic strut which forms the medial wall and floor of the canal. The result of this and other developmental features is that the normally prominent roof of the optic canal is misinterpreted on lateral films of infants as being all that is left after the floor and other presellar structures have been undercut by an expanding sellar mass. When it is fully developed the cranial opening of the optic canal comprises a vertical ellipse, while the orbital opening comprises a horizontal ellipse.

Anatomy of the Optic Canal. An optic foramen view projects an average of the profile transverse to the axis of the canal, (Table 10-1), thus thin-section tomography or CT will be required to more accurately define the dimensions of the optic canal (Figure 10-9). The overlap of the bony roof at the cranial opening of the canal is continued in a firm reflection of dura known as the falciform fold. The upper aspect of the optic nerves may be injured when pressed against the fold.

The Superior Orbital Fissure. Located in the sphenoid bone, the superior orbital fissure separates its greater and lesser wings. Because it is continuous with the cavernous sinus, the fissure transmits cranial nerves three, four, five (first division), and six, in addition to sympathetic nerves and the superior ophthalmic vein. The fissure is well seen on direct coronal CT and may also be visualized on axial CT (Figure 10-10). Through the fissure may pass important anastomotic circulation from the external carotid artery to the ophthalmic artery which may be supplied by branches of the middle meningeal artery. The fissure is best seen on plain films in the Caldwell projection. The fissure is asymmetric in about 9% of skull films. It may also be widened by tumors (Figure 10-11).

Differentiation of the Superior Orbital Fissure From the Optic Canal. The

TABLE 10-1. Measurements of the Optic Canal in Adults[12]	
Length of roof	8-10 mm
Length of floor and lateral wall	6-8 mm
Orbital opening height	6 mm
Orbital opening width	5 mm
Cranial opening height	4.5 mm
Cranial opening width	6 mm
Axis angle to midsagittal plane	38°
Asymmetry of axis angle	84% of skulls
Axis angle to Reid's base line	−38°

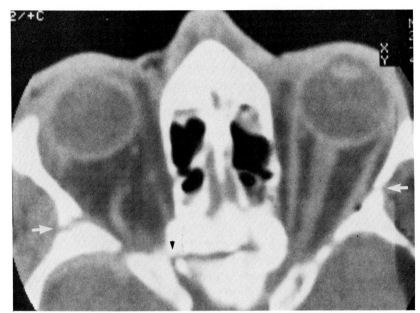

Figure 10-9. Axial CT demonstrating multiple facial fractures including bilateral LaForte 3 bilateral fractures of the lateral wings of the sphenoid bones (white arrows) and a fracture extending through the right optic canal into the body of the sphenoid bone (black arrow). In the setting of trauma, opacity in the ethmoid sinus may represent blood and can be associated with fractures that extend into the optic canal. Lower sections revealed blood in both maxillary antrums.

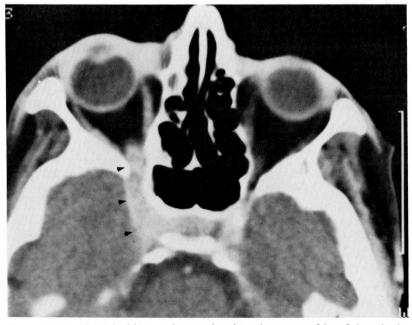

Figure 10-10. An enhanced axial scan at the same time shows the presence of the soft tissue density widening the cavernous sinus and extending into the superior orbital fissure (arrows). Compare with normal opposite side.

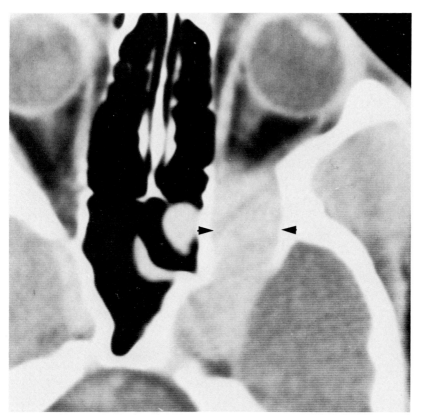

Figure 10-11. An angiofibroma of the nose is imaged in an axial CT with intravenous contrast enhancement as enlarging the superior orbital fissure (arrows) to approximately one-half the diameter of the globe. The tumor extends into the cavernous sinus. The patient first came to ophthalmological attention after a sudden loss of vision when a Foley catheter was inflated in his nose to control bleeding. Vision returned when the catheter was deflated.

superior orbital fissure curves from superolateral to inferomedial so that it is frequently confused with the optic canal on axial CT sections. It is important to recognize that the optic canal is less than 5 mm in height while the superior orbital fissure is 3 cm in height, and that much of the fissure lies inferior to the optic canal. The result of this is that the optic nerve will appear to lie anterior to a foramen that is really the superior orbital fissure. The ophthalmologist will need to review CT studies to be certain that the optic canal has been imaged. The minimum criteria for identifying that the optic canal are the presence of an anterior clinoid process lateral to the optic canal, and the superior orbital fissure lateral to the anterior clinoid process (Figure 10-13).

The Orbit. The orbit can be described as a hybrid between a four-sided pyramid and a pear so that the widest portions of the orbit are just posterior to the anterior rim. The orbital process of the frontal bone makes up most of the *roof of the orbit.* The irregular surface of this bone at the floor of the anterior cranial fossa may mimic bony destruction on axial CT (Figure 10-13). The gyrus rectus of each frontal lobe separates the superior orbits on

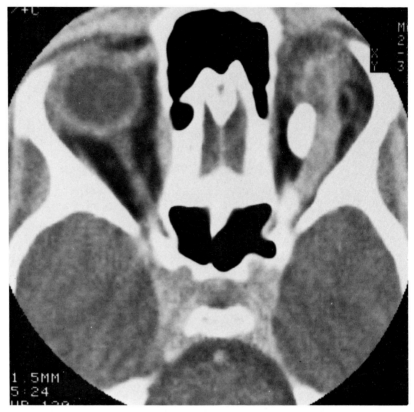

Figure 10-12. An enhanced axial CT showing two discontinuous regions of calcification of a rare osteogenic sarcoma. The more anterior region is in the plane of this coronal CT. The more posterior region lies just between the anterior openings of the optic canal (medially) and the superior orbital fissure (laterally).

scans at this level.

The Medial Walls of the Orbit. The medial walls of the orbit are formed by the thin laminae papyracea of the ethmoid bones that can be seen best with bone windows on axial CT. The lacrimal bones may have prominent anterior and posterior lacrimal crests that show well on posteroanterior (PA) skull films. Both the nasolacrimal ducts and the lacrimal fossa may be seen in axial CT scans.

The Lateral Wall of the Orbit. The lateral wall of the orbit is formed posteriorly by the greater wing of the sphenoid and anteriorly by the orbital process of the zygoma. The greater wing is less than a few millimeters in thickness posteriorly, where it separates the orbit from the middle cranial fossa, but it becomes thicker anteriorly where it can be seen as a triangle on axial CT. This thick portion of bone gives rise to the diagonal line (linea innominata) that passes through the orbit in PA skull films. Disappearance of this line is usually the result of destruction or thinning of the greater wing of the sphenoid. The junction of the zygoma and the greater wing of the sphenoid is also at the medial border of the temporal fossa.

The Floor of the Orbit. The floor of the orbit is made up of the maxillary bone with a lateral contribution from the zygoma, and medial contributions

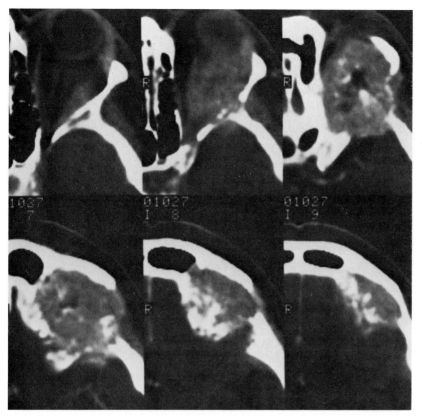

Figure 10-13. Carcinoma of the breast metastatic to the skull with involvement of the orbital roof is shown in portions of six CT images. From left to right and from top row to bottom row, six successive cuts starting below the roof of the orbit extend upward to the cranial vault. The tumor occupies the superior orbit and anterior cranial fossa with bony destruction. In the third scan of this series the tumor is extending through the roof of the orbit and the greater wing of the sphenoid bone as well as into the middle cranial fossa.

from the palatine bone and the bones of the medial wall. The posterior surface of the maxillary bone is the anterior boundary of the inferior orbital fissure through which the branches of the maxillary division of the trigeminal nerve will pass. One of these branches forms the infraorbital nerve and will pass through the infraorbital groove and foramen.

Imaging Indications and Modalities. Plain skull films continue to decrease in importance in imaging as the spatial resolution of CT improves. The obvious advantage of plain film is economic, and that they may be available without delay. The circumstances where plain films may be ordered first include:

- Isolated fractures of the midface and mandible including the orbital rim, maxillary sinus, and zygomatic bone.
- Gross abnormalities of the size or structure of the skull or orbit.

Conversely, CT will be required for the initial evaluation of all complex facial trauma even if it is not thought to involve an intracranial injury such as a brain contusion. This is because CT will not only identify soft tissue problems such as orbital floor fractures with muscle entrapment, but because the thin sections allow for identification of multiple displaced fragments of fractures. CT should always be obtained when plain films show blood in the ethmoid sinus as there is a high incidence of fractures extending into the optic canal, fractures that could lead to visual loss following early attempts at reduction (Figure 10-14). Coronal scans will be required to evaluate problems in the orbital roof or floor. If trauma or other conditions prevent positioning the patient for direct coronal scans, reformation will usually provide the desired information. Cerebrospinal fluid (CSF) leaks into the cribriform plate and paranasal sinuses may require metrizamide cisternography.

Plain films may also be required later in the work-up in the following circumstances:

- To evaluate the configuration and to measure the dimensions of the sella or the cranial foramina.
- To observe the vascular pattern of the skull for normal variations and changes induced by tumors.
- To locate normal and abnormal calcification.
- To distinguish between skull base abnormalities such as platybasia, basilar impression, and abnormal atlanto-occipital fusion.
- To follow primary or secondary disorders of the skull and the cranial sutures.

Even these conditions may require initial evaluation with CT to look for abnormalities in the brain or other soft tissues. In evaluating the optic canal, complex-motion polytomography can exceed the resolution of current CT scanners in determining the outline of the canal or to look for fractures of the roof. In most instances of pathology involving the optic canal, the CT is more rewarding because of tumor enhancement and other features.

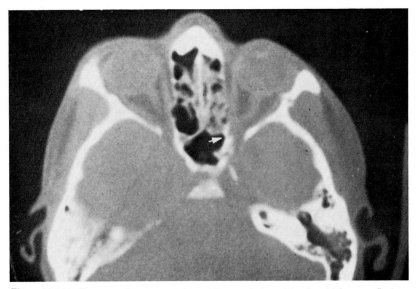

Figure 10-14A. Fracture of optic canal (arrow) in association with ethmoid fracture. Perhaps the radiologist's attention was not directed to this fracture because there were too many fractures to report. Vision was lost in the eye following surgery to reposition the nasal fractures.

Paranasal Sinuses

Anatomy. *The Paranasal Sinuses.* Associated with all but the lateral wall of the orbit, any of the paranasal sinuses can be a source of compression of the orbit via a mucocele, a mucopyocele, or a tumor. The frontal sinus pneumatizes and enlarges during and after the second decade of life after being a small extention of the frontoethmoid duct. A mucopyocele of the frontal sinus may take space in the orbit without actually penetrating the periorbita because this structure can be easily displaced except where it is tightly attached at the orbital rims and foramina. The mucosa of the sphenoid sinus may be in direct contact with the dura covering optic nerve in 20% of skulls. This contact occurs in the optic strut at the base of the anterior clinoid process of the sphenoid bone. Pneumatization of the anterior clinoid process gives rise to an artifactitious optic foramen on plain films. The mucosa of the ethmoid sinus has recently been demonstrated to cause an artifactual thickening of the intra-canalicular portion of the optic nerve when imaged in the axial plane by MR. The error is recognized when the coronal sections are obtained of the same structures.

The Floor and the Medial Wall of the Orbit. A direct blow to the globe may allow the medial walls of the orbit to fracture into the adjacent sinuses. Half of all floor fractures are associated with medial wall fractures. It was previously thought that restricted ocular movements following a floor fracture resulted from direct entrapment of the inferior rectus muscle, but CT examinations and cadaver studies now indicate that fibrous bands in the prolapsed orbital fat are the cause of the restriction, and that some of these may lengthen in time without surgical repair. Tumors in the *maxillary sinus* may extend to the orbit directly through the orbital floor while tumors of the nasopharynx may enter the orbit via the inferior orbital fissure (Figure 10-15).

Orbital Rim Fractures. Orbital rim fractures usually involve the contiguous paranasal sinuses. Inferior and lateral rim fractures involve the zygoma and result in a fracture at the zygomaticomaxillary suture, often leading to a palpable "step-off" along the rim. Superior rim fractures or puncture wounds of the superior orbit may or may not extend into the anterior cranial fossa with or without passing through the frontal sinuses. More medial fractures of the naso-orbital region can result in disinsertion of the medial canthal tendon and produce pseudo-hypertelorism. They can also extend into the cribriform plate and the ethmoid sinuses.

Craniofacial Disjunction. It has been postulated that there are four vertically oriented buttresses that translate masticatory forces through the maxillary bone to the base of the skull. These buttresses are resistant to vertical trauma but may fracture with a horizontal blow such as occurs in motor vehicle accidents, and thus may explain the relatively symmetrical bilateral orbital wall fractures known as Le Fort type II and Le Fort type III. The Le Fort type I fracture does not involve the orbit because it involves only the separation of the palate from the body of the maxilla. The Le Fort type II fracture is known as a pyramidal fracture because of its appearance *en face.* The nasal fractures extend into the frontal process of the maxillae, then to the lacrimal bones and the floor of the orbit and to the zygomaticofacial suture lines. The fracture may also extend posteriorly into

261

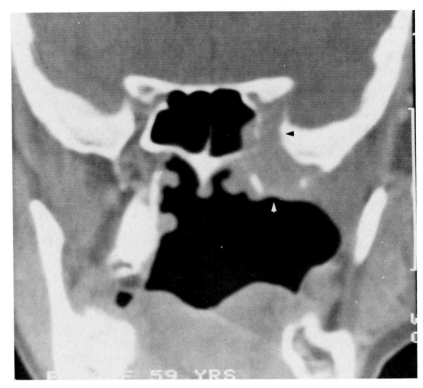

Figure 10-15. Extension of maxillary sinus carcinoma (white arrow) into the superior orbital fissure is demonstrated in a direct coronal CT. At age 58 a radical maxillectomy had been performed and this accounts for the absence of bone and the presence of air on the left side of the scan. Note that the tumor has also invaded the sphenoid sinus and destroyed the medial wall of the superior orbital fissure. The anterior clinoid process is intact. The coronal scan is particularly valuable in evaluating problems in the cavernous sinus and the superior orbital fissure because of the cross-sectional anatomy that is displayed.

the ethmoid and palatal bones. The Le Fort type III fracture completely detaches the middle third of the facial skeleton from the skull base because the fracture line extends completely across the orbit to the zygomaticofrontal suture (Figure 10-9).

Imaging. Plain films may be satisfactory for imaging isolated fractures of the zygomatic arch, maxillary sinus, and inferior orbital rims. They may also be useful for evaluating uncomplicated sinusitis. The remainder of the disorders may involve soft tissue components extending into one or more cavities. In such cases at least axial CT will be required and many cases would benefit from coronal CT as well.

Orbital Soft Tissues

Anatomy. Most of the pathological changes noted in disorders of the orbital soft tissues will be characterized by displacement, increased volume, or increased density of the normal structures. Thus a simple anatomic classification of the location of orbital masses is based on location inside or outside of the muscle cone (Figure 10-16).

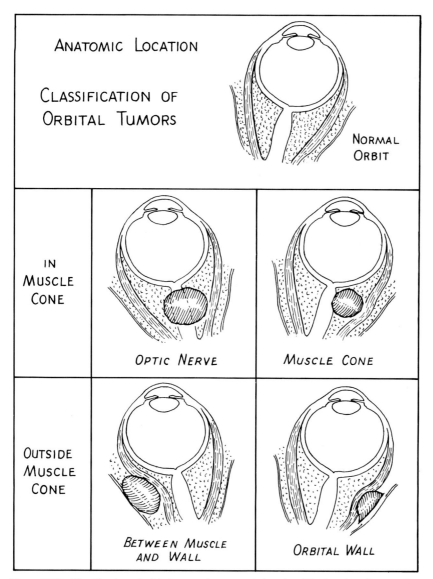

Figure 10-16. Classification of orbital tumors by anatomic location. The location of tumors in the orbit is an important aspect of acoustic evaluation. Tumors within the muscle cone are particularly susceptible to ultrasonic detection. Reproduced with permission from Coleman DJ, Lizzi FL and Jack RL: Ultrasonography of the Eye and Orbit, Philadelphia, Lea and Febiger, 1977.

The intraorbital portion of the optic nerve is approximately 20 percent longer than the distance from the back of the globe to the apex of the orbit. This gives rise to the vertically sinuous course of the optic nerve when the eyes are gazing straight ahead. Sagittal sections show that the central portion of the optic nerve dips toward the floor of the orbit so that the thickness of the nerve will vary on axial CT sections. The averaging of the optic nerve density with that of the orbital fat will cause the nerve to appear thin, especially in thick sections. The best way to straighten the nerve and obtain a uniform thickness is to have the patient look into extreme upgaze.

The Orbital Fat and the Fibrous Septa. These contribute most of the volume of the orbital contents other than the globe. The orderly arrangement of the septa has been explored in recent years and demonstrated to provide much of the basis for the support and movement of the globe in the orbit. The smallest of these septa divide the lobules of the orbital fat while the largest septa connect into the previously recognized orbital fascia. The central fat lobules are fine and loose and their septa insert into the retro-bulbar Tenon's capsule, the dura of the optic nerve, and the intermuscular membrane. The central fat occupies the region within the cone created by the four recti muscles, the intraconal space. The region peripheral to the four recti muscles and their aponeurotic extensions as the intermuscular membrane is known as the extraconal space and comprises four or more distinct lobules of fat.

The Orbital Septum. Constituting the anterior limit of the peripheral orbital fat, the orbital septum is contiguous with the periorbitum (periosteum) of the orbital rim. It acts as a diaphragm separating the orbital contents from the preseptal space. The tarsal plates form the central attachment of the orbital septum. In the upper lid a reflection of the orbital septum is fused with the aponeurosis of the levator palpebrae superioris and attached to the subcutaneous tissue and to the anterior aspect of the tarsal plate about 10 mm from the upper lid margin. The lower eyelid retractors are formed by a similar fusion of the orbital septum and the capsulpalpebral head of the inferior rectus muscle. The orbital septum transmits vessels, nerves, and the palpebral portion of the lacrimal gland. The orbital septum can be directly imaged with saggital MR scans.

Spaces. Two potential spaces in the orbit should be noted as their images change greatly in orbital inflammation: the episcleral space is located between the posterior aspect of the globe and Tenon's capsule, while the subperiorbital space may appear behind the orbital rim. The episcleral space may become radiographically more dense or ultrasonically "empty" when it becomes occupied by edemas and inflammatory reaction. The subperiosteal space may become elevated from the bone by the secretion, desquamation, and inflammation of an adjacent paranasal sinus containing a mucocele or mucopyocele. Subperiosteal abscess of the orbit can follow paranasal sinusitis without a mucopyocele.[13] Minimal elevation of the periorbitum can better be imaged with CT than with ultrasonography, a technique whose greatest usefulness is for conditions inside the globe or within the muscle cone.

The Extraocular Muscles. These muscles take their origins from the annulus of Zinn (the levator palpebrae superioris, superior, lateral, inferior, and medial recti), and contribute to the intermuscular membrane that defines the intraconal space. A three dimensional image of these muscles requires direct CT scans in two planes and it is best if one of the scan planes is parallel to the long axis of the muscle of special interest. Alternatively reformatted scans may be used. Ultrasonography can image the anterior portions of the four recti. The superior oblique muscle originates super-medial to the optic foramen and the annulus of Zinn and passes forward to the trochlea where it turns to attach behind the equator of the globe deep to superior rectus muscle. The portion of the muscle anterior to the equator is

usually recognized on axial CT scans. The muscle is sometimes congeni-
tally absent but making this distinction requires that the proximal portion
of the muscle is absent on direct coronal CT scans, as axial sections may
allow the superior oblique and medial recti to blend. The inferior oblique
muscle originates on the orbital floor and follows a course parallel to the
distal portion of the superior oblique muscle and tendon. MR scans can
image the oblique muscles.

The orbital vessels are best seen with intravenous contrast enhanced
CT, although the superior ophthalmic vein is sufficiently large and surrounded by sufficient fat that it can often be seen passing from its origin
near the nose within the supermedial extraconal fat, entering the muscle
cone in about the middle of the orbit, and exiting into the superior
cavernous sinus. The superior ophthalmic vein appears on higher axial
sections than the ophthalmic artery, which enters the orbit at the
inferomedial aspect of the optic foramen and curves superiorly above the
nerve (85% of the cases) to give rise to the central retinal and other arteries
(not identifiable) and to the ethmoidal and ciliary arteries which are identifiable. The inferior ophthalmic vein runs parallel to the inferior rectus
muscle and is not usually identifiable along its course or as it enters the
pterygoid plexus. While lymphatics are present in the lacrimal gland and
the tissues anterior to the orbital septum there is no lymphatic system in the
other orbital soft tissues.

The lacrimal system is represented by the lacrimal gland in the lacrimal
gland fossa superotemporally and the lacrimal sac inferonasally extending
into the nasolacrimal canal.

Imaging Indications and Modalities. Plain films have a minimal role
in the evaluation of orbital soft tissue disorders unless an exogenous foreign
body is present. All of the other problems in the *extraconal space* are best
evaluated by CT which can even detect degrees of calcification in tissue
that would be missed by plain films. Moreover, CT can determine if an
orbital soft tissue mass arises from or is invading the orbital margins and
adjacent cavities (Figure 10-17). CT can be used to determine the radiographic density and homogeneity of such masses. Quantitative echography
can provide some information concerning acoustical density and homogeneity but is of little value in determining the relationship of the soft tissue
mass to the orbital walls.

The extraocular muscles contributing to the muscle cone can be eco-
nomically studied with standardized A-scan and contact B-scan echography, especially if the findings include and are limited to bilateral involvement of multiple muscles characteristic of Graves' disease. All other
patients with disorders seeming to involve one muscle or to include
involvement of other structures (especially the optic nerve as manifested by
increased thickness or visual loss) should be studied primarily with CT or
MR. MR scans with surface coils can give better definition than CT in most
posterior coronal sections of the orbit. Ultrasound might then be used to
provide additional management information based on vascularity, compressibility, and change in size with corticosteroid therapy. CT has also
been used to explore the intraorbital anatomical causes for congenital and
acquired dysfunctions of the extraocular muscles.

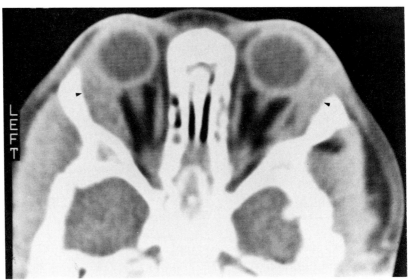

Figure 10-17. Acute myelogenous leukemia (arrows) metastatic to both orbits is seen in this intravenous contrast enhanced axial CT. On the right side the tumor is clearly extraconal as it is seen lateral to the lateral rectus muscle.

Intraconal abnormalities that involve the optic nerve require CT in the axial plane to follow the nerve into the intracranial cavity. Of course, other direct or reformatted views may also be required (Figure 10-18A & B). One of the most serious misinterpretations that may occur is interpreting the normally broad origin of the levator palpebrae superioris and superior rectus muscles as a thickened optic nerve presenting as an orbital apex tumor. This problem is exacerbated when the proximal portions of these muscles are thickened in Graves' disease. It is said that standardized A-scan ultrasonography can detect minimal thickening of the optic nerve sheaths not

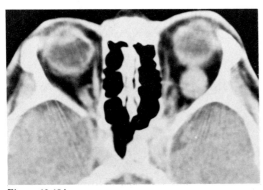

Figure 10-18A

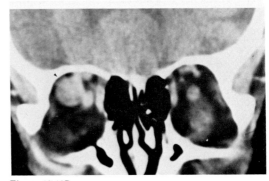

Figure 10-18B

Figure 10-18A. A neurofibroma presumably involving a branch of the trigeminal nerve is seen in the posterior lateral portion of the orbit. In this view it is very uncertain whether the mass is intra- or extraconal. Figure 10-18B. The direct coronal CT scan demonstrates the mass (arrow) displacing the optic nerve medially. The superior rectus levator palpebrae superioris complex and lateral rectus muscles are also seen. In this view it becomes much more likely that the mass arose in an extraconal location.

detectable by CT. Certainly A-scan and B-scan can detect markedly widened optic nerve sheaths associated with increased intracranial pressure, orbital congestion, or inflammation. Widened optic nerve sheaths are seen in a number of conditions including tumors (Figure 10-19A & B).

Both CT and ultrasonography can detect changes in vicinity of the sclera. Edema of the immediately retrobulbar portion of Tenon's capsule is easily detected with ultrasonography. One difference between Graves' disease and inflammatory orbital pseudotumor is that the tendonous portions of the extraocular muscles are much less thickened in the former than in the latter. Orbits or globes that may contain magnetic foreign bodies should not be imaged with MR because movement of the object could cause further injury.

The Globe

Anatomy. The diameter of the globe (about 24 mm) is correctly measured by CT scans in the axial section with the largest diameter.

Quantitative A-scan ultrasonography with the appropriate corrections for the differing acoustical properties of the components of the globe will give a more accurate measure. The anteroposterior dimension of the globe is between 50-55% of the anteroposterior dimension of the orbit. An increase in the portion of the cross-sectional area of the orbit occupied by the globe suggests an enlarged globe (infantile glaucoma or axial myopia) or

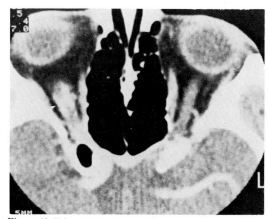

Figure 10-19A

Figure 10-19A. Vascular hamartoma of the optic nerve sheath mimicking an optic nerve sheath meningioma is seen on a CT scan with intravenous contrast enhancement. Figure 10-19B. Oblique sagittal reconstruction in the plane of the optic nerve (arrows) is shown in the upper part of the picture. The sagittal reconstruction aids in conceptualizing the relationship of the nerve sheath tumor to the inferior rectus muscle in the posterior portion of the orbit. Reconstructed or reformatted images do not provide the same quality of detail as a direct (non-reformatted) image. Some CT scanners now provide for direct oblique sagittal views through the orbit, and MR scanners are particularly useful for sagittal views.

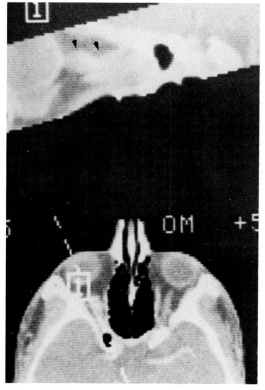

Figure 10-19B

a developmental abnormality with a small orbit. Conversely, a decrease in the ratio of globe/orbit area can result from forward displacement of the globe (proptosis) or a small globe. On CT scans, the normal structures seen include the cornea, the lens, and the retinochoroidalscleral (RCS) arc, and a vascular mound at the optic nervehead. This mound is more prominent when contrast media enhances the vessels at and around the junction of the optic nerve and globe. Calcific optic disc drusen may be seen at this location.

The cornea appears thicker by CT than its actual measurements and this thickness becomes even more exaggerated in the periphery. Contrast media further enhances the region of the cornea. The lens often appears to be more rectangular than biconvex and its thickness is more correctly displayed than its full diameter. The vitreous body is of low density unless there are abnormal cellular contents. The retinocorneoscleral arc should be about the same density as the cornea, however it measures less dense than the cornea due to the partial volume effect of the adjacent orbital fat which is included in the voxal. Conversely, air trapped underneath the eyelid adjacent to the cornea may give rise to a few low density pixels indenting the corneal outline.

Imaging. The globe will appear round in mid-orbital sections, but will

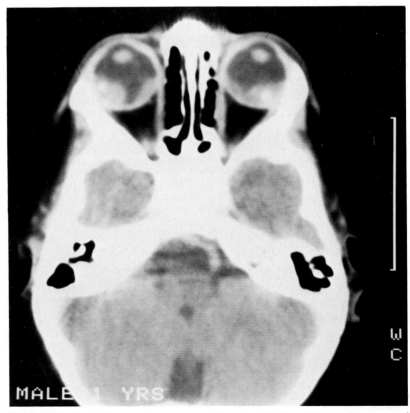

Figure 10-20. Retinoblastoma in a one-year-old male with bilateral intraocular tumor and multiple foci of calcification.

be elliptical or wedge-shaped near the boundaries of the orbits. The thickness and distance between the sections will control the number of times the globe will have a round appearance. For example the globe may appear round on only one or perhaps two 10 mm thick non-overlapping sections but at five levels with 3 mm thick sections. A single coronal section can include both the posterior aspect of the globe and the optic nerve. The availability of MR scanning will permit imaging of soft-tissue anatomic details that could not be resolved with CT. Some intraocular tumors can be well-visualized by CT (Figures 10-20 and 10-21).

The Optic Chiasm, Sella Turcica, and Adjacent Structures

Anatomy. The optic chiasm occupies the suprasellar cistern and can take a banana shape on an axial CT scan. In a sagittal section it fills the anterior recesses of the third ventricle like a bit fills the mouth of a horse. Enlargement of the optic chiasm beyond its usual dimensions of 8 mm anteroposteriorly and 12 mm transversely may raise the possibility of an anterior visual pathway glioma. The optic nerves pass forward on an inclined plane toward the optic canals. Laterally the chiasm is related to the

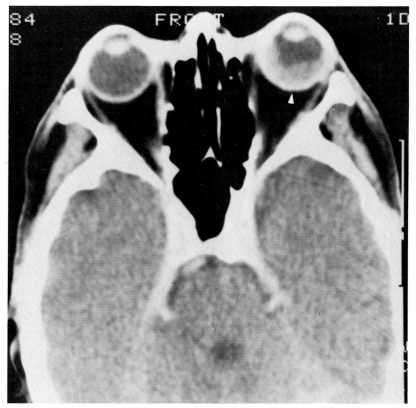

Figure 10-21. Diffuse posterior intraocular density (arrow), resulting from a primary melanoma of the skin metastatic to the globe, is demonstrated on an axial CT with enhancement.

269

suprasellar portions of the internal carotid arteries. Posteriorly the optic tracts embrace the lateral walls of the third ventricles and the hypothalamus.

The optic chiasm is usually located more than 1 cm superior to the top of the sella turcica so that tumors may reach at least this distance before they cause displacement of the optic nerves and chiasm or visual field defects. While the lateral walls of the sella can be visualized on axial scans, the location of the floor of the sella, and the height and configuration of the pituitary gland or other sellar contents requires coronal sections. The sellar contents normally enhance to about the same degree as the cavernous sinus on either side. The location of the diaphragm sella cannot usually be determined as CSF may be present below the diaphragm or above it in the suprasellar cistern. The pituitary stalk enhances with contrast media because of its many vessels.

The suprasellar cistern is bordered by the brain and has a star shape on axial CT sections. The appearance of the star is further accentuated by the circle of Willis which is contained within its borders. The six points of the star may not all be seen on any one section because of angulation or thickness of the slice. If the star is very large it may result from cerebral atrophy and if one portion is absent it may be filled with abnormal tissue. Since the suprasellar cistern is filled with CSF it is isodense with portions of the third ventricle from which it may not be further distinguished (Figure 10-22).

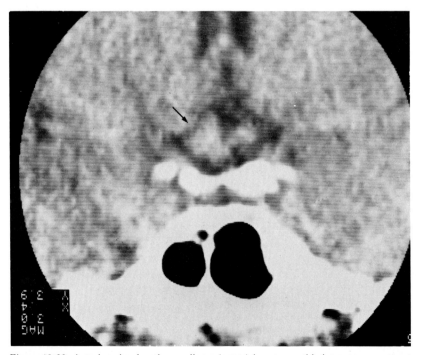

Figure 10-22. Anterior visual pathway glioma (arrow) is seen on this intravenous contrast enhanced coronal CT after an axial CT was initially interpreted as possibly being a pituitary tumor invading the suprasellar cistern. Courtesy of Saul Taylor, M.D.

The cavernous sinuses are located laterally to the sella turcica. They receive venous blood from the superior ophthalmic and other veins and normally drain posteriorly into the greater superficial petrosal sinuses. Each cavernous sinus contains an internal carotid artery and some fat which may take part in the inflammatory response of the Tolosa-Hunt syndrome. The abducens nerve runs the full posteroanterior length of the sinus having entered at Dorello's canal. The Gasserian ganglion and the branches of the trigeminal nerve enter the sinus from the CSF filled Meckel's cave which can be imaged at the posterolateral aspects of each sinus. The ophthalmic division of the trigeminal nerve and the abducens nerve are situated in the inferior portion of the cavernous sinus as they approach the superior orbital fissure. The oculomotor nerve enters the superior aspect of the cavernous sinus anterior to the midpoint of the diaphragm of the sella. The trochlear nerve enters more posteriorly and is positioned inferior to the oculomotor nerve. These relationships are important in deciding whether a process (such as an internal carotid artery aneurysm) is causing symptoms in or out of the cavernous sinus. The cavernous sinuses enhance with intravenous contrast and should have a symmetrically concave appearance on axial CT scans (Figures 10-10 and 10-15).

The retrosellar region is bounded posteriorly and laterally by the tentorium cerebelli whose margins enhance with contrast. The midbrain occupies most of the space between the clivus and the tentorium. The basilar artery may be located to either side of the midline, especially in older persons. The subarachnoid space in this area may be considered as the rostral extension of the prepontine or ambient cistern and is divided into the interpeduncular, perimesencephalic and cerello-pontine angle cisterns (Figure 10-23).

Imaging. The major consideration in imaging this region is the small size of the structures of interest and their complex three-dimensional relationships. Partial volume effects obliterate relationships adjacent to anatomic structures parallel to the plane of the scan. It follows that thin section CT scans will be required with images in more than one plane. Direct axial and direct coronal sections with 5 mm or thinner sections are preferred. If direct coronal views cannot be obtained, then thinner overlapping axial sections can be used to try to define the location of the floor and diaphragm of the sella and the cranial nerves within the cavernous sinus. MR scans are also of value in the parasellar region.

The Posterior Visual Pathway

Anatomy. The posterior visual pathway is comprised of the optic tracts, the lateral geniculate bodies, and the optic radiations in the temporal, parietal, and occipital lobes. On their way to the calcarine fissure of each occipital lobe, the optic radiation fibers course through the white matter that is located just lateral to the lateral ventricles. One anatomic point which may not be appreciated is the relatively caudal position of the occipital lobes within the skull so that persons unfamiliar with this may mistake the more rostral parietal lobe sections for occipital lobe sections (Figure 10-3). The calcarine fissures are not imaged on present CT scans, but their position can be inferred from the tips of the occipital horns.

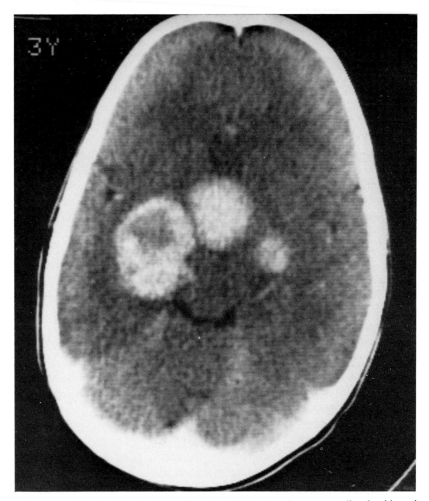

Figure 10-23. Anterior visual pathway glioma involving both optic tracts as well as the chiasmal region. The right optic tract (seen on the left) is the most greatly enlarged structure in this patient and has a central area of lucency, probably the result of necrosis.

Another anatomic consideration relates to the explanation of incongruous homonymous hemianopic visual field defects which may result from tumors which may simultaneously involve both the optic tract and the temporal lobe portion of the optic radiation (Meyer's loop).

Imaging. Large non-infiltrating lesions within the brain can be recognized on an enhanced CT with little difficulty because of differences in density or displacement of the ventricular system. We usually use an enhanced CT first because this brings out differences between white and gray matter and demonstrates some vascular abnormalities. Occasionally it is necessary to repeat the CT in the unenhanced state to distinguish calcification from an enhancing lesion. The greatest difficulty in unenhanced CT imaging occurs following an infarction where the area may show no change in density for 2 days and then become hypodense for as long as 14 days. Later the lesion may again become isodense for several months before assuming its final hypodense or frankly atrophic appearance. A phenomenon known as luxury perfusion can be seen in the enhanced scan during the second to sixth weeks after the infarct. The importance of this information is that the CT changes are evolutionary, and repeated examinations may be needed to distinguish infarcts from tumors or abscesses. Preliminary investigations with MR images indicate that they may supplement if not supplant CT in these examinations of the cerebral soft tissue. They seem particularly well suited for looking for demyelination in the periventricular regions.

Infratentorial Structures

Anatomy. The ambient cistern and its extensions have been described with the optic chiasm above. The oculomotor nerve passes through the interpeduncular cistern and passes over the dorsum sella to enter the superior portion of the cavernous sinus. The nerve can be compressed by lesions at the tentorial notch or by aneurysms of the circle of Willis. It can be involved within the cavernous sinus. The trochlear nerve has a parallel course after passing around the roof of the mesencephalon. The abducens nerve passes up the clivus but is not protected by dura until just before it enters Dorello's canal. As a result it is often affected by brain stem shifts resulting from increased intracranial pressure. Peyster and Hoover[2] state that CT scans will identify mass lesions in 40% of oculomotor palsies, 15% of trochlear palsies, 33% of abducens palsies, and 75% of multiple oculomotor nerve palsies. The cavernous sinus region is especially suspect if multiple oculomotor nerve palsies are combined with trigeminal nerve dysfunction (Figures 10-10 and 10-15). The normal anatomy of the other posterior fossa structures cannot be reviewed in detail here, but it is useful to review the anatomy of the various cranial foramen including the foramen magnum which is important in the Arnold-Chiari malformation.

Imaging. The imaging of the cavernous sinus with CT scans has been discussed above. The anatomy of the internal auditory canal and the inner ear can be demonstrated with CT scans having thin sections and bone window settings. Because the surrounding bone degrades the CT appearance of the brain stem it appears that posterior fossa scanning for intraxial neoplasms and other abnormalities will largely be accomplished with MR scans.

Avoiding Misinterpretations

In our experience the majority of misinterpretations and misdiagnoses result from failure of communication of the ophthalmologist and the radiologist as to the diagnostic considerations. The images obtained must be chosen to display certain tissues and tissue reactions at specified locations. The ophthalmologist should personally review the images to be certain that the images obtained are sufficient to answer the questions as to pathophysiology and location of the disease process.

Select the Best Imaging Modality. The selection of the imaging modality requires consideration of the structure and tissues to be imaged in addition to patient's general medical condition. Occasionally we see patients who have had CT scans when another modality would have better answered the anatomic and pathophysiologic questions.

Extracranial carotid occlusive disease investigated with CT instead of arteriography. One patient was a 49-year-old male who had a spinal fusion. One week postoperatively he noted blurred vision in both eyes. Venous stasis retinopathy was observed in both eyes (Figure 10-24A & B). An enhanced CT of the head and orbits was negative. Four months later rubeotic glaucoma was identified in the left eye and the patient treated with Coumadin, timolol, and topical steroids. Two months later the patient noted further visual loss in the right eye. When questioned the patient stated that he occasionally heard his own "heart beat." Carotid bruits could not be heard, but there was an intermittent bruit over the right temple. Figure 10-24C is from a digital subtraction angiogram that showed 90% stenosis at the aortic origin of the left common carotid artery and complete occlusion of the left internal carotid just beyond the bifurcation. The intracavernous portion of the right internal carotid artery was very stenotic. Comment: Enhanced CT scans will generally fill all of the major intracranial vessels so that flow problems can only be inferred from infarction or hemorrhage. CT can demonstrate large arterial aneurysms, calcified arteries, ectasia and displacement of the internal carotid arteries, however CT will not take the place of angiography in providing sequential studies of arterial blood flow through the head (Figure 10-24D).

Select the Optimum Plane. Important information may be lost when scanning parallel to an irregular surface such as the roof or floor of the

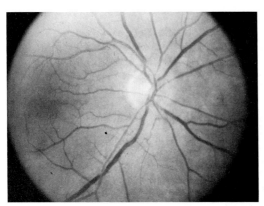 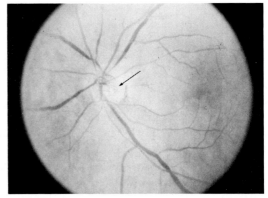

Figure 10-24A   Figure 10-24B

Figure 10-24A. Fundus photograph of right eye of a 49-year-old male who complained of poor vision in both eyes 1 week after a spinal fusion and 4 months prior to this photo. Blurred disk margins were noted and the clinical diagnosis was papilledema. An axial CT was negative. This photo shows mild arterial narrowing. Figure 10-24B. Fundus photograph of left eye showing neovascularization of the optic disk (arrow). At the time these photos were obtained the patient complained of an intermittent bruit in the right ear.

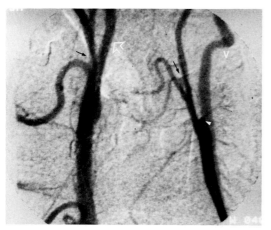

Figure 10-24C

Figure 10-24C. Digital subtraction angiogram showed complete occlusion of the left internal carotid artery (solid white arrow) just distal to the bifurcation. The right internal carotid artery (open white arrow) is patent at this level. External carotid arteries (black arrows), left vertebral artery (V). Figure 10-24D. Lateral arteriogram showing stenosis of the intracavernous portion (arrow) of the right internal carotid artery. Following a left temporal artery-middle cerebral artery bypass procedure, the patient had no worsening of the mild rubeotic glaucoma that was also present in the severely ischemic left eye.

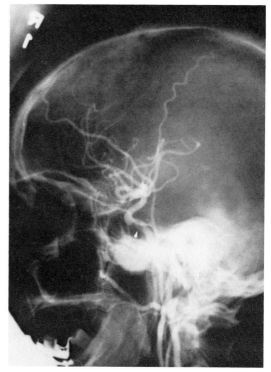

Figure 10-24D

orbit because each voxel may contain several tissues varying in density. The scanned or reformatted image should be perpendicular to the interfaces of interest. It is the average of these densities that may be recorded for a slice of a given thickness. Thus an axial scan is much less likely than coronal or sagittal scans to detect a small break in the optic canal or displacement of a thin plate of bone (Figure 10-14).

Perform Coronal Sections of the Orbit. In general, coronal scans of the orbit prove to be most helpful because they can section all of the extraocular muscles in one slice while it is unusual to see more than three extraocular muscles on any given axial section. In addition the cross-sectional area of the muscles is generally seen as compared to a longitudinal section. This is particularly helpful in appreciating possible compression at the apex of the orbit. On the other hand, orbital decompression for thyroid ophthalmopathy requires that it be known if both the medial and lateral recti are thickened (thus suggesting the need for a three-wall decompression) or if only the medial rectus is enlarged in which case only the medial and inferior walls of the orbit may be decompressed.

A patient with difficulty elevating the right eye had had an axial CT of the head and orbits, which was read as normal. A coronal CT demonstrated thickening of the levator palpebrae and superior recti. These two muscles are not differentiated on most CT scans.

Coronal CT scans may help in the diagnosis of inflammatory pseudotumor in that they may show an anterior ring of orbital density involving the tendonous insertions of the extraocular muscles and the tissues anterior to them (Figure 10-25). This predilection for anterior involvement is a characteristic of pseudotumor.

Perform Coronal Scans of Intracranial Structures. Coronal scans are essential to the evaluation of most problems involving the sella turcica or the cavernous sinuses, because the structures of interest lie in the axial plane. Thus superior displacement of the diaphragm of the sella of the

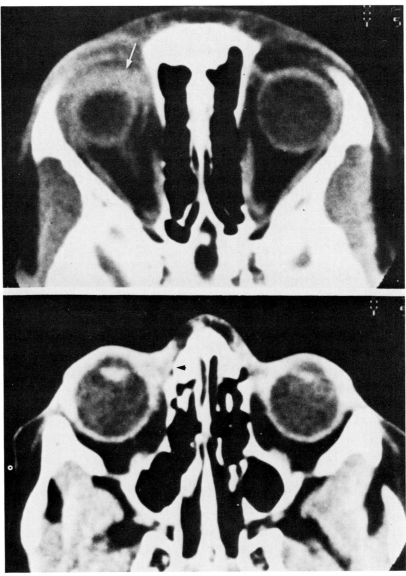

Figure 10-25. Top, inflammatory pseudotumor (arrow) of the anterior orbit is seen in this intravenous contrast enhanced axial CT section through the horizontal recti and the trochlear region. Coronal sections would be required to be certain that there was minimal involvement of the posterior portions of the extraocular muscles. Bottom, this section is at a lower plane passing through the maxillary sinuses posteriorly and through the lens anteriorly. The extraocular muscles are not specifically identified.

optic chiasm will best be seen with sections at right angles. The cranial nerves within the cavernous sinus can be appreciated as radiolucent areas with a cavernous sinus that has been enhanced with intravenous contrast media.

Select the Best Angulation. Select the best angulation within a plane so that the plane of the scan is parallel to the long axis of the structure of interest. For example, optic nerves can be misinterpreted as "thin" due to angle of axial CT scan (Figure 10-26A & B).

*Superior and Inferior rectus muscle enlargement in Graves' disease can be displayed by an axial scan (Figure 10-27A & B). An axial scan can display the widening of an enlarged inferior rectus muscle if the scan has sufficient negative angulation to be parallel to the plane of the muscle. Most axial scans are performed at angles that only display a small portion of this muscle or its insertion.

Perhaps the best clue to the presence of an optic canal fracture is the presence of blood in the ethmoid sinus on either plane films or thick section CT scans (Figure 10-9). The recognition of such fractures is important to avoid dangerous manipulation that may occur during repair of maxillofacial trauma. We have one case of a male who had multiple fractures in an auto accident and who lost vision in the left eye following surgery to reposition the facial and nasal bones. An axial section showed blood in the ethmoid but careful review of the thin axial sections shows a fracture of the ethmoid extending into the optic canal (Figure 10-14A).

Thickness and Overlap. Select the thickness and overlap of the sections so as to demonstrate the structures of interest while optimizing radiation dose and scan time.

Contrast Studies. Use special contrast studies to improve images or demonstrate pathophysiology.

Valsalva Maneuver. Perform a Valsalva maneuver to fill an orbital varix. We have seen a male with a 6-year history of intermittent painful swelling in the right orbit, where a routine CT scan had shown a small enhancing region in the posterior medial aspect of the orbit. Because the proptosis increased when the patient's head was recumbent, the scan was repeated following the Valsalva maneuver and the mass was greatly enlarged.[14]

Intrathecal Metrizamide. Performing an intrathecal metrizamide CT of the foramen magnum region will demonstrate an Arnold-Chiari malformation with hydromyelia in a patient with downbeat nystagmus.

A 50-year-old female presenting with difficulty seeing, particularly when walking or riding in an automobile, had downbeat nystagmus and abnormal vestibuloocular reflexes, with no long tract abnormalities. A routine CT showed a large cervical spinal cord "shadow" at the C1 level (Figure 10-28). The scan was repeated after intrathecal injection of contrast material. Positioning of the patient in a Trendelenburg position revealed large dysplastic cerebellar tonsils and flattening of the cervical cord at the C1 and C2 levels (Figure 10-29).

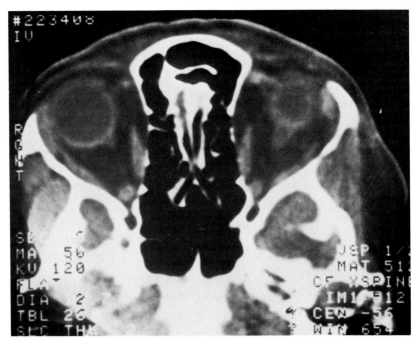

Figure 10-26A

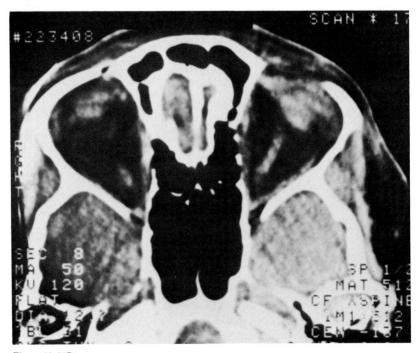

Figure 10-26B

Figure 10-26A. This case was misinterpreted as "thin or absent" optic nerves, because the angles of the axial CT scan were too positive. This section shows the base of the clivus and the trochlea in the same plane. The medial recti are seen in front of the inferior orbital fissures. Figure 10-26B. The next higher section skims the top of the optic nerves that appear thin due to the partial volume effect.

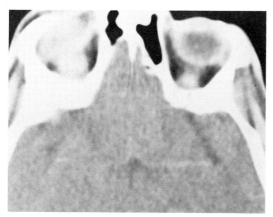 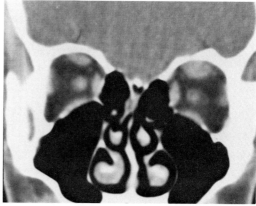

Figure 10-27A   Figure 10-27B

Figure 10-27A. Graves' disease with widening of the superior rectus/levator palpebrae superioris complex (on the left side of the illustration) is identified in this axial CT scan with intravenous contrast enhancement. The usual lucency of the orbital fat has disappeared. Figure 10-27B. Direct coronal CT obtained at the same time reveals that the optic nerve is normal and that it is the left superior rectus/levator palpebrae superioris muscle complex that is thickened. When only one extraocular muscle and one orbit is thickened, the diagnosis of Graves' disease is still possible. However, the diagnosis is on more certain ground when more muscles are involved.

Furthermore, six hours following the initial study, the entire cervical cord should be rescanned without further contrast enhancement to demonstrate the presence of any associated syringohydromyelia. The findings of Arnold-Chiari malformation, type 1, can also be identified using MR scanning and it is likely that asymptomatic Arnold-Chiari malformations will be frequently detected as an incidental finding with this new technique.[15]

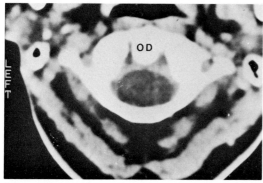 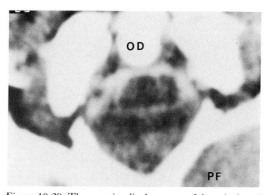

Figure 10-28. Slightly cervical spinal cord shadow at medullary-cervical junction as seen with conventional CT scan and intravenous contrast. The cerebellar contribution to the dimension of the shadow cannot be distinguished. The arch of the first cervical vertebrae is seen. The plane of the slice can be oriented at (1) in Figure D, Hostovsky. Odentoid process (OD).

Figure 10-29. The anterior displacement of the spinal cord is readily distinguished with the addition of intrathecal metrizamide in a repeat CT scan at a slightly higher level but with different angulation. The posterior portion of the slice is higher than the anterior portion, and passes through the foramen magnum, occipital bone, and floor of the posterior fossa (PF). The cerebellar tonsil limits the spread of the contrast agent posteriorly.

Intrathecal metrizamide scans should be used to determine the emptiness of an "empty sella," or to demonstrate the size of the anterior visual pathway structures in the suprasellar cisterns.

Adjacent Abnormalities. Image and interpret significant abnormalities in adjacent anatomic structures. Examples of possible findings include:

- ethmoitis extending into cranial cavity and orbit (Figure 10-30);
- petrous pyramid (meningioma) (Figure 10-31); and
- greater wing of the sphenoid invaded by meningioma and ignored as a cause of proptosis in a patient with a lymphoma (Figure 10-32).

Repeat Imaging. Repeat imaging at a later date to monitor change in size, contrast, or luxury perfusion of a lesion. This can be particularly useful in multiple sclerosis and cerebral infarctions when the pathological process or the blood may be isodense with brain. Presumably MR will make these differentiations possible in many cases at the time of the initial examination. However, it will be important to know the indications for re-examination as the disease process evolves.

Conclusion

This chapter has reviewed aspects of the various imaging techniques used in ophthalmologic diagnosis. While the role of the various techniques is constantly undergoing change, the duty of the ophthalmologist will remain relatively constant, that is, to request that the imaging techniques answer specific anatomic and pathophysiologic questions and to review the images obtained to ascertain that they are sufficient. In our experience the majority of misinterpretations and misdiagnoses result from failure of

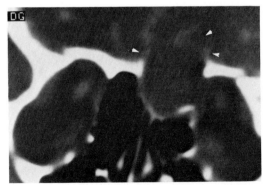

Figure 10-30. Ethmoiditis has created a mucopyocele that has extended into the orbit and the anterior cranial fossa (arrows). The coronal CT shown here determined these relationships much better than the axial scan. The patient was a 38-year-old male with a one-week history of intermittent blurry vision.

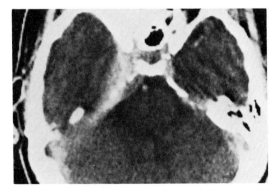

Figure 10-31. A meningioma involving the petrous pyramid has invaded the cavernous sinus and caused oculomotor and trigeminal nerve dysfunction.

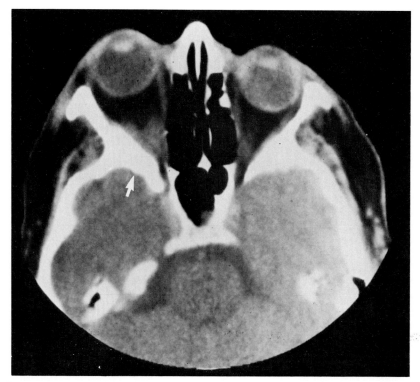

Figure 10-32. Misinterpreted enhanced axial CT of a 71-year-old woman with unilateral proptosis. Her current medical diagnoses were chronic lymphocytic lymphoma and diabetes mellitus. The density in the posterior orbit was thought to be due to the lymphoma for which she received radiation therapy. The proptosis was really due to a meningioma expanding the greater wing of the sphenoid bone (arrow). Courtesy of Lanning Kline, M.D.

communication between the clinician and the radiologist of the exact nature of the information that is required.

References

1. Moseley IF, Sanders MD: Computerized Tomography in Neuro-Ophthalmology. Philadelphia: Saunders, 1982.
2. Peyster RG, Hoover ED: Computerized Tomography in Orbital Diseases and Neuro-ophthalmology. Chicago: Year Book Medical Publisher, 1984.
3. Ramsey RG: Neuroradiology with computed tomography. Philadelphia: Saunders, 1981.
4. Jacobs L, Weisberg LA, Kinkel WR: Computerized Tomography of the Orbit and Sella Turcica. New York: Raven Press, 1980.
5. Hammerschlag SB, Hesselink JR, Weber AL: Computed Tomography of the Eye and Orbit. Norwalk, CT: Appleton-Century-Crofts, 1983.
6. Koutcher JA, Burt BT: Principles of imaging by nuclear magnetic resonance. J Nucl Med 25:371-382, 1984.
7. Young SW: Nuclear magnetic resonance imaging: Basic principles. New York: Raven Press, 1984.
8. Walker MD (ed): Research issues in positron emission tomography. Ann Neurol 15(Suppl):S1-S204, 1984.
9. Coleman DJ, Lizzi FL, Jack RL: Ultrasonography of the eye and orbit. Philadelphia: Lea & Febiger, 1977.

10. Ossoinig K: Echography of the eye, orbit, and periorbital region. *In:* Arger P (ed): Orbit Roentgenology. Wiley, 1977, pp 224-269.

11. Kier EL: Fetal skull. *In:* Newton TH, Potts DG (eds): Radiology of the Skull and Brain. St. Louis: Mosby, 1971, Vol. 1 pp 106-117.

12. Potter GD, Trokel SL: Optic Canal. *In:* Newton TH, Potts DG (eds): Radiology of the Skull and Brain. St. Louis: C.V. Mosby Co., 1971, Vol. 2, pp 487-507.

13. Harris GJ: Subperiosteal abscess of the orbit. Arch Ophthalmol 101:751-757, 1983.

14. Shields JA, Dolinskas C, Augsburger JJ, Shah HG, Shapiro ML: Demonstration of orbital varix with computed tomography and Valsalva maneuver. Am J Ophthalmol 97:108-109, 1984.

15. Hostovsky M, Tubman DE, Wirtschafter JD: Intrathecal metrizamide computed tomography: Diagnosis of downbeat nystagmus in Arnold-Chiari I malformation. Surv Ophthalmol 27:123-125, 1982.

Chapter 11

The Diagnosis and Management of Optic Neuropathies

Thomas D. Tredici, MD
John A. McCrary, MD

THE DIAGNOSIS AND MANAGEMENT OF OPTIC NEUROPATHIES

Introduction

The optic neuropathies are a diverse group of afflications which affect the optic nerve. As such, the optic neuropathies can be confusing to the general practitioner in ophthalmology. We will present here a reasonable approach to the diagnosis and management to these disorders.

Basically, an optic neuropathy is classified as having one or more of the following etiologies[1,2]:

- Inflammation or demyelination
- Ischemia
- Toxic or deficiency state
- Compression
- Hereditary

Most of these etiologies produce either an anterior optic neuropathy with papillitis (disc swelling) or a retrobulbar optic neuropathy (with normal discs) in the acute presentation. Slow compression and congenital causes are more likely to reveal optic atrophy at the time of initial presentation. Each etiology will later be discussed in detail.

When a patient presents with a possible optic neuropathy, the work-up of this patient would include the following:

- Detailed history emphasizing time course of visual loss (acute loss suggests a vascular insult whereas chronic loss suggests a toxic or compressive etiology), dietary habits, toxic substance exposure, and the possibility of involvement of other family members.
- Best corrected vision (distance and near) with and without pinhole.
- Color vision testing in each eye (D-15 or D-100 tests are best).
- Pupil exam for afferent pupillary defects in unilateral optic neuropathies.
- Peripheral visual fields (Goldmann, Aimark) and central fields (tangent screen and Amsler grid).
- Examination of fundus with special attention to the optic discs with Hruby lens and indirect ophthalmoscope. In addition, Hoyt, et al,[3] advocate the examination of the nerve-fiber layer of the retina with a direct ophthalmoscope using red-free illumination. Slit-like gaps in the nerve fiber pattern of the retina signify *permanent* axonal involvement.

In addition, the following tests are useful:

- 2 × disc photographs are useful for detailed study and for follow-up exams.

- Hematological studies (including sed rate, CBC, collagen vascular screen, B_{12} level, folate level, VDRL, FTA-ABS).
- CT scans with particular attention to the orbits and optic canals (axial and coronal cuts).[4]
- The photostress test of Glaser[5] may be useful in differentiating retinal pathology from optic nerve pathology. It is performed as follows:

A penlight is held for 10 seconds at 2-3 inches in front of an eye with the other eye occluded. Then the time required to read three lines larger print than was needed to record the best acuity is recorded. Both eyes are compared. Prolonged recovery indicates *macular* disease rather than *optic nerve* disease.

- Electrophysiology - Visual evoked response (VER) test may be helpful in following patients with an optic neuropathy.[6]
- Finally, hospitalization with more invasive procedures (lumbar puncture, angiography and even craniotomy) may be necessary if an optic neuropathy has a progressive decrease in vision and is of unknown etiology. Always remember that *chronic optic neuritis* is never an acceptable diagnosis, and a negative CT scan does not guarantee that a lesion does not exist.[7]

Inflammation and Demyelination — Optic Neuritis

Optic neuritis is basically a clinical diagnosis. Characteristically, these patients present with mild to severe visual loss. Usually, the loss is acute and unilateral. The disease most often affects patients in the 20-40 age range (predominantly women). They usually complain of pain in and around the affected eye, and they display defective color vision, a central scotoma and an afferent pupillary defect.

In addition, some of these patients may complain of Uhthoff's phenomenon, that is, deterioration of vision with increased exercise, stress, or heat. The cause of the symptom is unknown, but it has been suggested that it is caused by a reduction in the venous pH with elevation of lactic acid. Apparently, the denuded internodal nerve segments are quite vulnerable to this metabolic change.[8]

In general, these patients regain their vision quite rapidly (usually within one month) without treatment. Some evidence of optic nerve dysfunction often remains, however, albeit minimal (that is, afferent pupillary defect or mild disc pallor). Remember that chronic optic neuritis is not a reasonable diagnosis, and the possibility of a tumor should not be lightly dismissed in those cases that continue to lose vision (see section on compressive optic neuropathies).

Ophthalmoscopic signs of optic neuritis include peripapillary hemorrhages and retinal vein sheathing. In addition, vitreous inflammation may be present. Remember that the disc may be swollen (papillitis) or normal (retrobulbar optic neuritis). Bilateral involvement may be seen in children or in systemic inflammatory conditions.

If a patient presents with a first attack of optic neuritis, he or she can usually just be closely followed after obtaining skull films with optic canal views, chest x-ray, sed rate, CBC and serology. However, if the vision continues to deteriorate or if the problem is recurrent or bilateral, additional studies are warranted including: neurological consultation, CT scan of the optic nerves and orbit, and CSF examination (particularly for oligoclonal banding, presence of lymphocytes and level of myelin basic protein).[9]

The entire issue of progression to multiple sclerosis is best *not* discussed with a first attack unless the patient asks for this information. The frequency with which multiple sclerosis follows an attack of optic neuritis is controversial, but one study[10] suggests that 30-40% of these patients will eventually have the disease manifest itself. One cannot predict *which* patients will develop multiple sclerosis (an essentially untreatable condition), but women in the 20-40 age range with recurrent optic neuritis appear to be especially susceptible. Always remember that *one* attack of optic neuritis is never *multiple* sclerosis!

Although demyelination is a common cause of optic neuritis, inflammation of the optic nerve can be caused by a wide variety of inflammatory conditions including bacterial, viral, mycotic and parasitic infections along with many systemic inflammatory conditions. A list of some of these conditions[11] is found in Table 11-1. Obviously, each of the conditions found in Table 11-1 must be treated with regard to the specific etiology.

There is no specific treatment known to be effective for optic neuritis, unless a specific underlying etiology that is amenable to treatment can be found. Close follow-up of the patient is recommended; the prognosis is generally good. High dose oral steroids, (80-100 mg prednisone per day) may decrease the periocular pain and speed recovery, but they have *no* effect on the final visual outcome. Steroids are usually reserved for patients with severe involvement of one eye or in those with an attack in the second eye, when vision in the fellow eye is very poor.

Ischemia

The onset of visual loss in ischemic optic neuropathy (ION) is sudden (like optic neuritis), and the visual loss ranges from mild to severe. In addition, visual loss is also accompanied by acquired dyschromatopsia, and an afferent pupillary defect. However, unlike optic neuritis, this disease occurs in older individuals (50-75 years range), and the most common visual field defect is an *altitudinal* defect, not a central scotoma.[16] In fact, an altitudinal field defect alone is highly suggestive of this disorder.

It has been commonly observed that, although patients afflicted with ION are usually in good health, they have a high incidence of mild vascular disease. For example, as many as 44% of patients with ION have hypertension, and indeed, it has been suggested that ION may be an early complication of systemic hypertension.[17] It is well known that chronic hypertension causes specific pathologic changes in the walls of cerebral, coronary and retinal arteries. Although we do not know the specific pathogenesis of ION, it is reasonable to assume that these vascular changes lead to occlusion of some of the posterior ciliary vessels behind the globe with subsequent infarction of the optic nerve.

It has also been found that the most important intraocular factor related to the production of ION is elevated intraocular pressure,[18] and therefore this should be treated if it exists.

Most importantly, a small group of older patients with giant cell arteritis (a severe, life-threatening, systemic disorder) will first present with ION, and this possibility must *always* be excluded with an erythrocyte sedimentation rate so that appropriate therapy can be instituted (e.g., high-dose steroids and temporal artery biopsy).

Although an optic nerve affected by ION rarely has a recurrent attack (unlike optic neuritis), the subsequent risk of developing ION in the fellow eye after the first eye has been affected is about 40%.[16] The second attack may occur weeks to years after the first attack. Also, it is not unusual for the visual loss of ION to develop during sleep (like stroke) because of arterial hypotension.[17] In fact, nonsimultaneous ION is the most common cause of

---

Table 11-1.

Etiologies of Optic Nerve Inflammation

Collagen vascular disease[12]

Syphilis

Sarcoidosis

Tuberculosis

Nematode infections

Acute toxoplasmosis

Presumed ocular histoplasmosis[13]

Cysticercosis

AMPPE birdshot retinochoroidopathy

Herpes zoster[14]

Cat scratch fever

Crohn's disease

Ulcerative colitis

Whipple's disease

Measles, rubella, chicken pox, mumps, influenza

Sinus disease (rarely)[15]

Polio, coxsackievirus

Mononucleosis

Behcet's and Reiter's diseases

Post-vaccination optic neuritis

```
┌─────────────────────────────────────────────────────────────────┐
│                          Table 11-2.                              │
│                                                                   │
│                     Treatable Etiologies of                       │
│                    Ischemic Optic Neuropathy                      │
│  ───────────────────────────────────────────────────────────     │
│  Giant cell arteritis                                             │
│  Collagen vascular disorders                                      │
│  Cardiac disorders                                                │
│  Systemic hypertension                                            │
│  Diabetes mellitus (esp. juvenile onset)[19]                      │
│  Hematologic disorders and blood dyscrasias                       │
│  Carotid artery disease (auscultate the carotids, obtain carotid  │
│    Doppler studies and digital subtraction angiography)[20]       │
└─────────────────────────────────────────────────────────────────┘
```

pseudo Foster Kennedy syndrome. This can be differentiated from true Foster Kennedy syndrome by the clinical history alone. Bilateral simultaneous attacks are most suggestive of collagen vascular disease.[11] Because in ION there is infarction of the optic nerve, it is difficult to tell the patient about the level of his final visual acuity as his acuity may or may not improve.

Most patients with ION present with a swollen disc. The swelling is often sectoral, and corresponds to the visual field defect. The swollen disc may be pale or hyperemic. In addition, peripapillary flame-shaped hemorrhages or cotton-wool patches usually accompany arteriolar narrowing. In severe cases, an incomplete macular star will be detected as testimony to the severe exudation derived from the vessels of the disc. In a short period, the disc swelling may resolve leaving optic atrophy.[11]

As mentioned above, most cases of ION present with a swollen disc (papillitis). Although there have been several reports of ION *without* disc swelling following trauma or irradiation, we are not sure why the posterior (retrobulbar) form of ION is so rare (poor recognition).

The first step in the effective management of a patient with ION is a complete medical evaluation to treat any systemic vascular condition which may be present. Conditions which need to be excluded and should receive special emphasis and treatment are found in Table 11-2.

Two special forms of ION need to be mentioned. Hayreh[21] has directed our attention to the fact that ION may develop after a cataract extraction. This may be related to the acute intraocular pressure rise in the immediate postoperative period, and its probable effect on the circulation of a susceptible optic nerve. Hayreh warns us that if ION occurred in one eye after a cataract extraction, it will probably occur in the other eye following cataract surgery. Preventive measures are indicated when the second eye is operated. He recommends antiglaucoma medications (esp. Timoptic and Diamox) for one week after surgery.

Finally, a central retinal artery occlusion is the most advanced form of

ION. However, despite the usual poor prognosis of this disorder, several case reports exist[22] to demonstrate that immediate vigorous therapy (usually consisting of digital massage, 5% CO_2 breathing mixture and use of Timoptic and Diamox) of those eyes afflicted with CRAO from an emboli source may completely regain vision up to *6 hours* after the original insult. Obviously, all of these patients need a complete medical evaluation.

In summary, all patients with ION need a complete medical evaluation with treatment of any underlying vascular disorder. Arteritic ION is treated with high dose steroids (80-100 mg qd), but presently there is no effective treatment for nonarteritic ION.

Compression

Retrobulbar compression of the optic nerve without optic disc swelling may procede insidiously with few if any overt signs until optic atrophy occurs. As in the other optic neuropathies, the process is usually accompanied by dyschromatopsia, an afferent pupillary defect and a visual field defect. The hallmark of an optic neuropathy of compressive origin is a progressive, chronic loss of vision. When compression is suspected, neuroradiologic studies (particularly axial and coronal CT scan) should be performed. It cannot be overstated that a high index of suspicion is required in these cases. Several reports[23,24] demonstrate that lesions in the posterior part of the orbit are quite difficult to evaluate radiologically. A patient with severe, progressive visual loss with repeatedly negative neuroradiological studies may require an exploratory craniotomy, if no valid explanation for visual loss can be invoked.

As opposed to the diagnostic subtleties of retrobulbar compression, compression of the optic nerve with disc swelling may be accompanied by all of the signs of orbital disease including periorbital pain and proptosis. In addition to the usual signs and symptoms of optic neuropathy, these patients may develop an acquired, unilateral hypermetropic refraction change, and may display choroidal folds on ophthalmoscopy.[25] Both of these changes can be signs of a compressive mass.

Hodes and Weinberg[26] have demonstrated that the combined use of CT scan and A-scan echography provides the best approach to the evaluation of orbital disease. The management of the compressive optic neuropathies is diverse because treatment depends on etiology. For example, compression caused by dysthyroid disease in the orbit is best treated with higher dose steroids (80 mg/day) or orbital irradiation (2000 R over 10 days). Only if these conservative modalities fail is orbital decompression attempted.[27] On the other hand, a slowly growing optic nerve glioma in an eye with good visual acuity is presently followed in a conservative manner unless the tumor begins to threaten the optic chiasm or begins to grow rapidly.[28]

Some patients with compression of their optic nerves develop decreased vision, optic atrophy and optociliary disc vessels. This triad of findings should signify the presence of a spheno-orbital meningioma or optic nerve glioma until proven otherwise. Optociliary shunt vessels overlie the optic disc and shunt blood between the retinal and choroidal venous circulations. Disc collaterals can be congenital or acquired, and fluorescein angiography can effectively differentiate between these two categories.[29]

Prompt restoration of vision often occurs following decompression of these lesions. This is probably due to the reestablishment of axoplasmic and vascular flow, and possibly also to slow remyelinization of the optic nerve.[30]

Toxins and Deficiencies

In this section, we will first briefly discuss the toxins thought to produce optic neuropathies.. These toxins usually cause painless, *bilateral* symmetrical visual loss. (Some toxins like hexachlorophene need to be ingested over months to produce optic nerve damage, whereas ethylene glycol produces its damage quickly.) Patients who have toxic or deficiency neuropathy usually have cecocentral scotomas and bilateral acquired dyschromatopsias, and display light/near dissociation of their pupils.[11] The Farnsworth D-15 or D-100 test color vision tests are very effective in the early detection of these disorders before visual field or visual acuity changes are detected.[31] After visual system damage has been disclosed and the offending toxin has been recognized, its use must be stopped. Visual recovery depends upon whether irreversible optic nerve damage has already taken place.

A firm association between toxin and optic neuropathy is claimed for the following drugs.[32] The optic neuropathy resulting from these drugs, which are listed in Table 11-3, may or may not result in disc swelling.

The deficiency state optic neuropathies comprise a very large and confusing portion of the neuro-ophthalmologic literature. Well designed and well controlled animal and clinical experiments and data are lacking for these conditions. These optic neuropathies have been known since the 19th century, but are still poorly understood. For example, we know that cyanide is toxic to myelin,[40] and may play some role in some of these disorders, but experimental evidence indicates that cyanide is *not* an overt factor in the production of *human* disease.[41] Despite this evidence, you will find cyanide discussed as an etiology in most deficiency state optic neuropathies and even in some hereditary optic neuropathies.

The most common deficiency state optic neuropathy in the US is the so called "Tobacco-Alcohol Amblyopia." The name is inappropriate since the condition is clearly due to nutritional deficiency. The disease usually affects middle-aged males who may or may not smoke tobacco or consume alcohol, but have poor dietary habits. This disease causes decreased vision *bilaterally* with *cecocentral* field defects. (We don't know why the papillomacular bundle is particularly susceptible in this disorder.) These field defects may be subtle, and may only be detected by thorough tangent screen examination with red test objects. The optic nerves may only show mild temporal pallor. Temporal disc pallor is usually a late finding.

Although we don't know the exact pathogenesis of this disorder, it is felt thta it probably is *not* caused by a toxic substance (or inborn error of cyanide detoxification) but is a true nutritional deficiency disease.[42] At present, the most effective management of this condition consists of having the patient stop tobacco and alcohol intake, and reestablish a good diet with daily supplementation with vitamins (especially B-complex) and minerals. This regimen is usually beneficial to vision.

For completeness, it should be mentioned that an entity called "Tropical Amblyopia" exists. This optic neuropathy is found in Nigeria and is thought to be related to the heavy ingestion of cassava, a plant staple from which tapioca is made. Cyanide is suggested to be the toxin involved, but the etiology remains unproven.[43]

Finally, it should be mentioned that specific vitamin deficiencies are associated with optic neuropathies. The most well-known associations include[11]:

- Vitamin B-12 (cobalamin) - In fact, optic neuropathy may be the earliest manifestation of pernicious anemia[44].
- Vitamin B-1 (thiamine) - Beriberi in POW's is a well-known cause of optic neuropathy.
- Niacin (nicotinic acid) - Pellagra may be associated with optic nerve disease.
- Vitamin B-2 (riboflavin).

In these deficiency states, proper nutrition and supplementation is necessary for effective management of the optic nerve disease. Vision may or may not return after therapy.

Table 11-3.

Possible Causes of Toxic Optic Neuropathies

Carbon tetrachloride (cleaning fluid)

Chloramphenicol (oral ingestion)[33]

Ethambutol (up to 15 mg/kg/day found to be safe dosage)[34]

Ethchlorvynol (Placidyl)

Ethylene glycol (2-3 oz. is lethal)[35]

Hexachlorophene[36]

Hydroquinolines (Entero-Vioform)

Isoniazid (beware of synergism with ethambutol)[37]

Lead (penicillamine effective in therapy)[38]

Methanol[39]

Organophosphates

Toluene

Trichlorethylene (cleaning fluid)

Vincristine

Heredity

There are two general categories of hereditary optic neuropathies: those that occur *without* systemic or neurological disease, and those optic nerve disorders that occur in the presence of systemic disorders.

One of the more common forms of hereditary optic neuropathy is dominant optic atrophy. Kline and Glaser[45] describe the characteristics of this disorder as:

- develops during the first decade of life,
- the visual loss is often asymmetrical in nature,
- cecocentral scotomas are present,
- Tritan (blue/yellow) defects are common in this disorder in contrast to the more common protan/deutan (red/green) defects of other optic nerve diseases. (in fact, a tritan defect in the presence of optic atrophy should always raise the possibility of dominant optic atrophy),
- the visual loss is insidious, but not totally debilitating,
- the condition has an autosomal dominant mode of inheritance, and
- these patients exhibit temporal pallor rather than diffuse optic nerve pallor.

Johnson, et al,[46] feel that this optic neuropathy derives from a primary degeneration of the retinal ganglion cells.

As with all hereditary optic neuropathies, all family members should be examined, and genetic counseling given. Hoyt[47] reiterates that we should emphasize to parents that this disorder does not result in *severe* visual disability.

Leber's hereditary optic neuropathy is a disease that primarily afflicts adult males with a sudden decrease in their central vision accompanied by cecocentral scotomas. The genetic transmission pattern of this disorder suggests a sex-linked recessive mode of inheritance, but because some women have been affected by this disease, it has also been suggested that cytoplasmic inheritance is involved.[11] The true pattern of inheritance remains unknown.

The fundus changes of this disease are more striking and distinctive than those encountered in any other optic neuropathy. In fact, this disorder has been mistaken for papilledema or papillitis. Smith, et al,[48] list the fundus changes in the acute phase of Leber's optic neuropathy as:

- circumpapillary telangiectatic microangiopathy,
- swelling of the peripapillary nerve fiber layer, and
- no leakage from the disc on fluorescein angiography.

These changes gradually resolve as the optic nerve becomes atrophic.

The exact nature of this neurovascular disorder is unknown, and unfortunately there is no effective therapy. Some of these patients undergo complete or partial spontaneous recovery.[49] Certainly more research is needed on this visually destructive condition.

The largest category of hereditary optic neuropathies are those associated with overt systemic or neurologic disease. All of these patients need a thorough medical and neurological evaluation. The main groups of these optic neuropathies include:[11]

- autosomal recessive, progressive optic atrophy with juvenile diabetes mellitus, diabetes insipidus and hearing loss (DIDMOAD or Wolfram's syndrome),[50]
- optic neuropathy with the hereditary ataxias, specifically Friedreich's (spinal) ataxia and Marie-Brown's (cerebellar) ataxia,
- optic neuropathy with Charcot-Marie-Tooth disease (progressive peroneal muscular atrophy),[51] and
- optic neuropathy with degenerative and storage diseases such as the lipidoses and mucopolysaccharidoses.

Summary

The complexity and spectrum of the optic neuropathies is great, but we have attempted to discuss the optic neuropathies with regard to their major etiologies.

Remember that in evaluating a patient with an optic neuropathy, a detailed *clinical history* is the key asset in establishing the probable etiology of an optic nerve disease.

References

1. Smith JL: The Optic Nerve Workup. Trans Am Acad Ophthalmol Otolaryngol 83:778, 1977.
2. Rosen JA: Pseudoisochromatic Visual Testing in the Diagnosis of Disseminated Sclerosis. Trans Am Neurol Assoc, 90:283, 1965.
3. Hoyt WF, Schlicke B, Eckelhoff RJ: Fundoscopic appearance of a nerve-fibre-bundle defect. Brit J Ophthal 56:577, 1972.
4. Osher RH, Tomsak RL: Computer Tonographic Features in Optic Neuritis. Am J Ophthalmol 89:699, 1980.
5. Glaser JS, Savino PJ, Sunens KD, et al: The Photostress Recovery Test in the Clinical Assessment of Visual Function. Am J Ophthalmol 83:255, 1977.
6. Ikeda H, Tremain KE, Sanders MD: Neurophysiological investigation in optic nerve disease: Combined assessment of the visual evoked response and electroretinogram. Brit J Ophthal 62:227, 1978.
7. Burde RM, Gittinger J, Keltner JL, Miller NR: Neuroophthalmologic Dilemma: Chronic Optic Neuritis? 23:173, 1978.
8. Selhorst JB, Saul RF, Waybright EA: Optic Nerve Conduction: Opposing Effects of Exercise and Hyperventilation. Trans Am Neurol Assoc 101, 1981.
9. Cohen SR, Herndon RM, McKhann GM: Radioimmunoassay of Myelin Basic Protein in Spinal Fluid. New England J Med 295 (No. 26): 1455, 1976.
10. Cohen MM, Lessell S, Wolf PA: A prospective study of the risk of developing multiple sclerosis in uncomplicated optic neuritis. Neurology 29: 208, 1979.
11. Miller NR: Walsh & Hoyt's. Clinical Neuro-Ophthalmology. Baltimore: Williams and Wilkins, (4th ed, Vol I): 212-329, 1982.
12. Fulford KWM, Catterall RD, Delhanty JJ, Doniach D, Krener M: A collagen disorder of the nervous system presenting as Multiple Sclerosis. Brain 95:373, 1972.
13. Husfed RC, Shock JP: Acute presumed histoplasmosis of the optic nerve head. Brit J Ophthal 59:409, 1975.
14. Ramsell TG: Complications of Herpes Zoster Ophthalmicus. Am J Ophthalmol 63:1967.
15. Tarkkanen J, Tarkkanen A: Otorhinolaryngological Pathology in Patients with Optic Neuritis. Acta Ophthalmol 49:649, 1971.
16. Boghen DR, Glaser JS: Ischemic Optic Neuropathy, The Clinical Profile and Natural History. Brain. 98:689, 1975.
17. Ellenberger C: Ischemic Optic Neuropathy as a Possible Early Complication of Vascular Hypertension. Am J Ophthalmology 88:1045, 1979.

18. Hayreh SS: Anterior Ischemic Optic Neuropathy. I. Terminology and Pathogenesis. Brit J Ophthal 58:955, 1974.

19. Hayreh SS, Zahoruk RM: Anterior Ischemic Optic Neuropathy. VI. In Juvenile Diabetes. Ophthalmologica (Basil) 13:182, 1981.

20. Waybright EA, Selhorst JB, Comes J: Anterior Ischemic Optic Neuropathy with Internal Carotid Artery Occlusion. 93:42, 1982.

21. Hayreh SS: Anterior Ischemic Optic Neuropathy. IV. Occurrence After Cataract Surgery. Arch Ophthalmol 98:1410, 1980.

22. Stone R, Zink H, Klingele T, Burde RM: Visual Recovery After Central Retinal Artery Occlusion: Two Cases. Am Ophthalmol 445, April 1977.

23. Susac JO, Smith JL, Walsh FB: The Impossible Meningioma. Arch Neurol 34:36, 1977.

24. Pruett RC, Wepsic JG: Delayed Diagnosis of Chiasmal Compression. Am J Ophthalmol 76:229, 1973.

25. Cangemi FE, Trempe CL, Walsh JB: Choroidal Folds. Am J Ophthalmol 86:380, 1978.

26. Hodes BL, Weinberg P: A Combined Approach for the Diagnosis of Orbital Disease (Computed Tonography and Standardized A-Scan Echography). Arch Ophthalmol 95:781, 1977.

27. Kennerdell JS, Rosenbaum AE, El-Hosky MH: Apical Optic Nerve Compression of Dysthyroid Optic Neuropathy on Computed Tonography. Arch Ophthalmol 99:807, 1981.

28. Wright JE, McDonald WI, Call NB: Management of Optic Nerve Gliomas. Brit J Ophthal 64:545, 1980.

29. Irvine AR, Shorb SR, Morris BW: Optociliary Veins. Trans Am Acad Oph Oto 83:541, 1977.

30. Kayan A, Earl CJ: Compressive Lesions of the Optic Nerves and Chiasm. Brain. 98:12, 1975.

31. Trusiewiez D: Farnsworth 100—Hue Test in Diagnosis of Ethambutol-Induced Damage to Optic Nerve. Ophthalmologica (Basel). 171:425, 1975.

32. Grant WM: Toxicology of the Eye. Springfield, Illinois: Charles C. Thomas, 1975.

33. Godel V, Nemet O, Lazan M: Chloramphenical Optic Neuropathy. Arch Ophthalmol 98:1417, 1980.

34. Carr RE, Henkind P: Ocular Manifestations of Ethambutol. Arch Ophthal 67:50, 1962.

35. Ahmed MM: Ocular effects of antifreeze poisoning. Brit J Ophthal 55:854, 1971.

36. Slamovits TL, Burde RM, Klingele TG: Bilateral Optic Atrophy caused by Chronic Ingestion and Topical application of Hexachlorophene. Am J Ophthalmol 89:676, 1980.

37. Kass I, Mandel W, Cohen H, Dressler SH: Isoniazid As a Cause of Optic Neuritis and Atrophy. J Amer Med Assoc 164:1740, 1957.

38. Baghdassarian SA: Optic Neuropathy due to lead poisoning. Arch Ophthal 80:721, 1968.

39. Benton CD, Calhoun FP: The Ocular Effects of Methyl Alcohol Poisoning: Report of a Catastrophe Involving Three Hundred and Twenty Persons. Trans Amer Acad Ophth Otol 875, (Nov-Dec) 1952.

40. Foulds WS, Chisholm IA, Pettigrew AR: The toxic optic neuropathies. Brit J Ophthal 58:386, 1974.

41. Lessel S: Experimental Cyanide Optic Neuropathy. Arch Ophthal 86:194. 1971.

42. Potts AM: Tobacco Amblyopia. Surv Ophthal 17:313, 1973.

43. Osuntakum BO, Osuntokum O: Tropical Amblyopia in Nigerians. Am J Ophthalmol 72:708, 1971.

44. Foulds WS, Chisholm IA, Steward JB, Wilson TM: The Optic Neuropathy of Pernicious Anemia. Arch Ophthalmol 82:427, 1969.

45. Kline LB, Glaser JS: Dominant Optic Atrophy. Arch Ophthalmol 97:680, 1979.

46. Johnston PB, Gaster RN, Smith VC, Tripathi RC: A Clinicopathologic Study of Autosomal Dominant Optic Atrophy. Am J Ophthalmol 88:868, 1979.

47. Hoyt ES: Autosomal Dominant Optic Atrophy. Ophthalmology 87:245, 1980.

48. Smith JL, Hoyt WF, Susac JO: Ocular Fundus in Acute Leber Optic Neuropathy. Arch Ophthalmol 90:349, 1973.
49. Constantine EF: Leber's disease with recovery. Arch Ophthalmol 53:608, 1955.
50. Lessel S, Rosman NP: Juvenile Diabetes Mellitus and Optic Atrophy. Arch Neurol 34:759, 1977.
51. Hoyt WF: Charcot-Marie-Tooth Disease with Primary Optic Atrophy. Arch Ophthalmol 64:925, 1960.

Chapter 12

Pseudotumor Cerebri and the Ophthalmologist

Thomas C. Spoor, MD, FACS

PSEUDOTUMOR CEREBRI AND THE OPHTHALMOLOGIST

Introduction

Patients with pseudotumor cerebri (benign intracranial hypertension) have increased intracranial pressure and papilledema. Except for a unilateral or bilateral sixth nerve paresis secondary to elevated intracranial pressure, there are no localizing neurologic or neuro-ophthalmic signs. Spinal fluid is normal except for an elevated opening pressure. Computed tomography reveals normal to small-sized ventricles and is otherwise normal.

Pseudotumor cerebri may have an identifiable etiology. Examples include: middle ear disease with subsequent intracranial venous sinus thrombosis, radial neck surgery, trauma, lupus erythematosis, hypoparathyroidism, carbon dioxide retention and certain drugs (Table 12-1).[1] Associated obesity and menstrual irregularities are common.[1] An often self-limiting form may develop during pregnancy and remit during the third trimester or after delivery.[2] The etiology for increased intracranial pressure in pseudotumor cerebri is unknown. Both cerebral edema and diminished cerebrospinal fluid absorption have been postulated.[1,3] More than 90% of patients present with a headache, which most always precedes visual symptoms. Visual symptoms occur in 35-70% of patients and include transient (seconds) loss or blurring of vision (obscurations), diplopia and convergence insufficiency.[1,3,4]

This syndrome is important to the ophthalmologist for three reasons: First, patients may present with visual complaints (obscurations, diplopia and convergence insufficiency) accompanied by headache. Second, the major complication of pseudotumor cerebri is visual loss, occurring in 4-26% of patients.[3,5,6] It is also important to recognize that pseudotumor cerebri may have a protracted course and is not always a benign, self-limiting disease. Corbett, et al,[6] reviewed long-term visual complications in patients with pseudotumor cerebri and found that visual loss was common (26%) and occurred months to years after the initial symptoms appeared.[6] Visual loss resulted from optic atrophy secondary to protracted elevation of intracranial pressure. In 80% of these patients, CSF pressure remained elevated regardless of treatment. Subsequently, these patients need long-term follow-up and repeated ophthalmologic evaluation, including reproducible visual fields, to detect and obviate visual loss.

Finally, the ophthalmologist may be asked to determine whether apparent disc swelling is real or represents pseudopapilledema secondary to buried drusen or hyperopia. This requires a cycloplegic refraction and a compulsive dilated fundus exam. The discs should be examined with a Hruby or contact lens. Ultrasonography, fluorescein angiography and disc photos may be helpful in demonstrating buried or subtle drusen. Differentiating pseudopapilledema from true papilledema is the ophthalmologist's job. If properly done, this may save your patient a good deal of expense, discomfort and anxiety. Serial fundus photos are an excellent method for documenting disc changes compatible with subtle papilledema.

The obese 35-year-old lady complaining of headaches, obscurations and diplopia is not a diagnostic dilemma. Exam may reveal a sixth nerve paresis and markedly swollen discs (Figure 12-1A & B). Computed tomography is normal, excepting small ventricles, as is the neurologic exam. Lumbar puncture documents a markedly elevated opening pressure, and spinal fluid is otherwise normal.

If this patient is not properly treated and followed, she may eventually develop a marked loss of vision and field. Figure 12-2A & B depicts the fundus from a patient with visual loss due to pseudotumor cerebri. Note the peripapillary pigmentary changes indicative of previous disc swelling, the secondary optic atrophy and optociliary shunt vessels. These changes

TABLE 12-1
Drugs and Toxins Associated with Pseudotumor Cerebri

Hypervitaminosis A
Hypovitaminosis D
Tetracycline
Nalidixic Acid
Nitrofurantoin
Indomethacin
Corticosteroids
    Prolonged use
    Rapid withdrawal
Heavy Metals
    Lead
    Arsenic

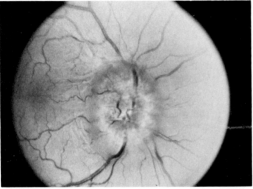 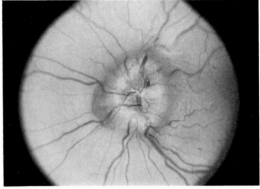

Figure 12-1. Patient with pseudotumor cerebri and obvious, bilateral disc swelling.

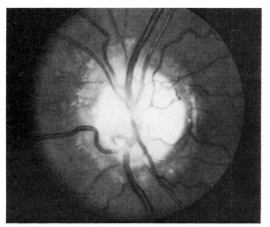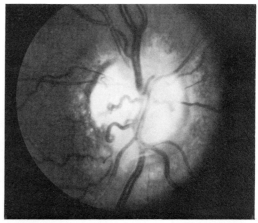

Figure 12-2. Chronic atrophic papilledema with secondary optic atrophy and optociliary shunt vessels. This patient had marked visual loss due to neglected pseudotumor cerebri.

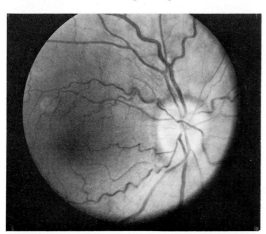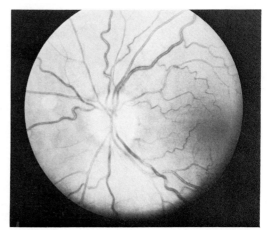

Figure 12-3. Subtle disc swelling in a patient with pseudotumor cerebri.

are bilateral and secondary to chronic papilledema from neglected pseudotumor cerebri. They should be easily differentiated from similar appearing discs due to uniocular abnormalities; for example, perioptic meningiomas, gliomas and central retinal vein occlusions.[7,8]

Visual loss is the only serious long-term complication of pseudotumor cerebri.[6] The degree of visual dysfunction, in my experience, is related to the degree of disc swelling; but this may not be a statistically valid observation.[5] However, patients with a mild disc swelling rarely have significant visual dysfunction. For example, the patient whose discs are shown in Figure 12-3A & B complained of severe headaches and dizziness. She had no visual complaints and a complete neuro-ophthalmologic exam was normal except for the swollen discs. Computed tomography was normal. An opening pressure of 350 mm H_2O was documented on lumbar puncture. Spinal fluid was otherwise normal.

Patients with pseudotumor cerebri are supposed to have obviously swollen discs. Many do, and present with headaches and papilledema, prompting neuroradiologic and neurologic evaluation. A minority of patients have subtle to mild disc swelling that is often overlooked. They complain of headaches and occasionally diplopia. Diplopia is due to a subtle abducens paresis. Such subtle to mild disc swelling is rather common with pseudotumor cerebri, and these patients have minimal visual symptoms.

Asymmetric disc swelling may also be a manifestation of pseudotumor cerebri. One disc may be markedly swollen, the other only mildly swollen. The patient in Figure 12-4A & B presented with headaches and obscurations in the right eye. The right disc was rather markedly swollen, the left minimally swollen. Opening pressure on lumbar puncture was 350 mm H$_2$O.

Management of pseudotumor cerebri should begin with a high index of suspicion, in order to make the diagnosis in the presence of subtle or asymmetric disc changes, followed by a careful history to detect an offending drug or medication (Table 12-1). Computed tomography should be promptly obtained to rule out a mass lesion as the cause of the headache and papilledema. If none is found, a neurologic examination to rule out focal deficits and a lumbar puncture to document elevated intracranial pressure with otherwise normal cerebrospinal fluid should be obtained.

Treatment consists of lowering intracranial pressure to alleviate symptoms and obviate visual loss. Hypertension is a statistically significant risk factor for visual loss.[6] Blood pressure should be checked and, if elevated, controlled. If the patient is obese, weight reduction should be encouraged.

There is little agreement concerning more specific treatment. Serial lumbar punctures, systemic steroids and acetazolamide all have their advocates.[9-11] Serial lumbar punctures may be technically difficult in an obese patient, and patient acceptance and compliance may be a problem. High dose systemic steroids, used to decrease cerebral edema and lower intracranial pressure, may not be tolerated by an already obese, hypertensive patient. They may also elevate intraocular pressure, adding an additional risk factor for visual loss.

I have found initial treatment with acetazolamide 500 mg. sequels

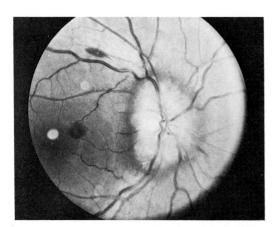 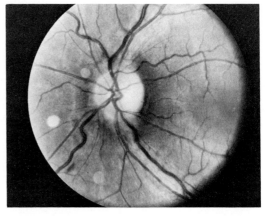

Figure 12-4. Markedly asymmetric disc swelling in a patient with pseudotumor cerebri.

(Diamox) twice a day to be well tolerated and effective in the majority of patients.[10,11] Acetazolamide is usually better tolerated and safer over the long term than systemic corticosteroids. It can easily be decreased and discontinued as signs and symptoms abate, and re-instituted periodically as required during long-term follow-up evaluations. Additionally, all ophthalmologists are familiar with its use and side-effects.

If visual function fails to improve or deteriorates during treatment with acetazolamide, management should be altered to obviate visual loss.[1]

Medical options include the use of systemic corticosteroids or osmotic agents. Surgical options include repeat lumbar puncture, lumbo-peritoneal shunting or optic nerve sheath decompression. These options all have their advocates and have been extensively reviewed elsewhere.[1,5,11]

Patients with pseudotumor cerebri should be routinely evaluated by an ophthalmologist for the rest of their lives. Evaluation should include reproducible visual field examinations to detect subtle changes in visual function. Deteriorating visual function should prompt more aggressive medical or surgical therapy.

Summary

The ophthalmologist needs to recognize, diagnose and follow the visual function in patients with pseudotumor cerebri. An identifiable etiology may be present and should be sought. The presentation may not be obvious. Patients may complain of headaches and have minimal or asymmetric disc swelling. The degree of visual dysfunction is directly related to the degree of disc swelling. Visual loss may occur in 25% of patients and is the only serious long-term complication. These patients' visual function should be evaluated regularly for the rest of their lives. Treatment consists of lowering intracranial pressure, medically or surgically, to obviate visual loss from chronic disc edema.

References
1. Keltner JL, Miller NR, Gittinger JW, Burde RM: Pseudotumor Cerebri Surv Ophthalmol, 23:315-322, 1979.
2. Greer J: Benign Intracranial Hypertension. III. Pregnancy. Neurology 13:670-672, 1963.
3. Johnston I, Paterson A: Benign Intracranial Hypertension. Brain 97:289-312, 1974.
4. Weisberg LA: Benign Intracranial Hypertension. Medicine 54:197-207, 1975.
5. Rush JA: Pseudotumor Cerebri—Clinical Profile and Visual Outcome in 63 Patients. Mayo Clin Proc 55:541-546, 1980.
6. Corbett JJ, Savino DJ, Thompson HS, et al: Visual Loss in Pseudotumor Cerebri. Arch Neurol 39:561-574, 1982.
7. Spencer WH, Hoyt WF: Chronic Disc Edema From Neoplastic Involvement of Perioptic Meninges. In: Smith ME (ed): Ocular Pathology. Boston: Little, Brown & Co., 1971, p. 171.
8. Perlmutter JC, Klingle TG, Hart WM, Burde RM: Disappearing Optociliary Shunt Vessels and Pseudotumor Cerebri. Am J Ophthalmol 89:703-707, 1980.
9. Ahlsrog JE, O'Neill BP: Pseudotumor Cerebri. Ann Internal Med 97:249-256, 1982.
10. Lubow M, Kuhr L: Pseudotumor Cerebri: Comments on Practical Management. In: Glaser JS (ed) Neuro-Ophthalmology, Vol IX, St. Louis: Mosby, 1977.
11. Katzman B, Lu LW, Tiwari RP, Bansal R: Pseudotumor Cerebri: An Observation and Review. Ann Ophthalmol 13:887-892, 1981.

Chapter 13

Ocular Syphilis

Paula J. Wynn, MD
Thomas C. Spoor, MD

OCULAR SYPHILIS

INTRODUCTION

Syphilis has been called the "great imitator" of diseases. This particularly applies when considering its ocular and neurological manifestations. Ocular involvement may be limited to the eyelids and conjunctiva, or involve the orbit, cornea, iris, ciliary body, retina, choroid, optic nerve, cerebrum and spinal cord. Unfortunately, the number of reported new cases continues to rise (Figure 13-1) and standard screening ability remains limited.

Syphilis is caused by *Treponema pallidum* and may be congenital or acquired. Both forms have ocular manifestations. Congenital syphilis is transmitted prenatally from an infected mother to her fetus. Acquired syphilis is transmitted by direct contact with an infective lesion of early syphilis. Diagnosis is based upon history, clinical appearance, and serologic testing.

Nontreponemal serologic tests are used for screening because of availability and lower cost. These include the Rapid Plasma Reagin (RPR) test and the Venereal Disease Research Laboratory (VDRL) test. The VDRL is reported as nonreactive, weakly reactive, or reactive. If any degree of reactivity is present, a quantitative titer is reported which may be useful in following disease activity. If the screening test is reactive, a specific treponemal antigen test is performed. The fluorescent treponemal antibody absorption (FTA-ABS) test is highly specific with a 1% false positive rate. It is reported as nonreactive, borderline, or reactive. Although a reactive FTA-ABS test indicates infection at some time, it does not necessarily mean active infection. A borderline FTA-ABS may be clinically significant. Seeley, Sarkan and Smith showed an increased incidence of syphilitic pupillary abnormalities and optic atrophy in a group of patients with borderline FTA-ABS reactivity.[2] Another specific test is the microhemagglutination for *Treponema pallidum* (MHA-TP). Recent studies have shown the MHA-TP equal to or more specific and sensitive than the FTA-ABS test, except in early syphilis.[3,4] Neither the FTA-ABS or MHA-TP revert to nonreactivity with treatment; but once reactive, remain reactive. They subsequently are not useful for posttreatment follow-up. Problems with serologic testing will be discussed later.

Clinically, syphilis is divided into primary, secondary, and tertiary stages. Primary syphilis is usually manifest by the appearance of a chancre at the site of inoculation. This appears an average of 21 days after contact, most often as a single papule which is painless, erodes and becomes indurated at the base. Frequently it involves the genitalia, mouth (Figure 13-2), and perianal areas, but may occur anywhere and is often unnoticed,

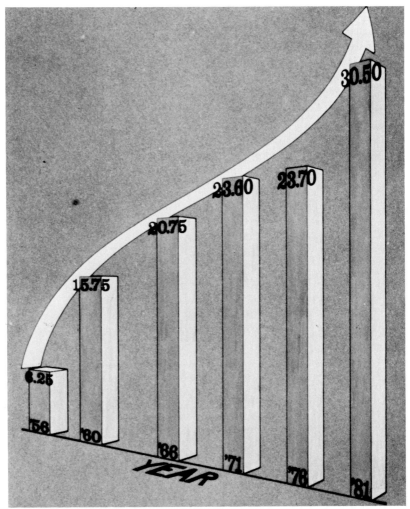

Figure 13-1. Increasing incidence of reported and new cases of infectious syphilis over the past thirty years.

especially in women and homosexual men. Chancres are usually accompanied by regional lymphadenopathy.

Ocular involvement in primary syphilis is limited to the appearance of a chancre of the eyelids or bulbar conjunctiva. This occurs so infrequently that it may be unrecognized or misdiagnosed. Chancres may heal without treatment within two to twelve weeks leaving a thin atrophic scar. The diagnosis of syphilis is confirmed by observing spirochetes on darkfield examination of scrapings from the lesion. When the chancre appears, only 25% of patients will have a reactive VDRL or RPR. After two weeks, 75% are reactive.[5] The FTA-ABS becomes reactive earlier than the MHA-TP, however all tests are usually reactive within a month of infection.

Secondary syphilis appears two to eight weeks after the chancre. This is the most florid stage of infection and manifestations are widespread and protean. The most common clinical manifestation is a rash which may be macular, maculopapular, or papular and is typically nonpruritic (Figure 13-3). It is most often bilaterally symmetrical involving the palms and soles. Other manifestations include mucous patches, general adenitis, condyloma lata, alopecia and mild constitutional symptoms with slight fever, malaise, anorexia, pharyngitis and arthralgias. The central nervous system may become involved, but is usually asymptomatic at this stage. Darkfield examination of moist, cutaneous lesions reveals spirochetes and most all serologic tests are reactive at this stage. The VDRL titer is usually 1:32 or higher. With treatment this will gradually revert to nonreactive, with 75% becoming nonreactive after two years.[5] The most common forms of ocular involvement in the secondary stage include iritis, chorioretinitis, optic neuritis, and interstitial keratitis. These and other ocular manifestations will be discussed later.

Latent syphilis is manifest by a reactive FTA-ABS (VDRL is nonreactive in 30% of cases).[6] Clinical manifestations are absent and cerebrospinal fluid (CSF) is normal, as is the chest x-ray. It is a serologic diagnosis, persisting from one to many years. The first four years are referred to as early latency and relapses are common in this stage. Thereafter it is referred to as late latency.

Late or tertiary syphilis is a slowly progressive disease which may involve any organ in the body. The principally involved systems include the skin

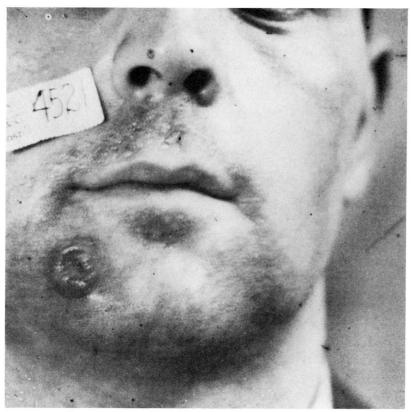

Figure 13-2. Chancre of primary syphilis in perioral region.

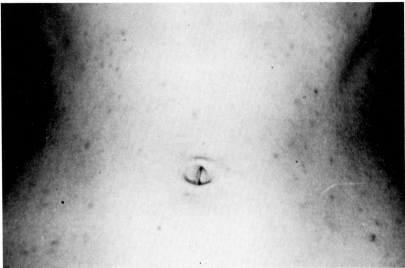

Figure 13-3. Maculopapular rash of secondary syphilis.

with benign gummatous lesions, the nervous system, and the cardiovascular system, the most serious being the latter two.

The benign gumma is a granulomatous solitary lesion with induration and local destruction occurring singly or in multiple locations with variable size. These heal asymmetrically leaving a thin atrophic noncontractile scar. Less commonly, gumma of the bone may cause fractures or joint destruction.

Neurosyphilis may be symptomatic or asymptomatic. Patients without any clinical manifestations but abnormal CSF studies such as pleocytosis, elevated protein, decreased glucose, or positive VDRL have asymptomatic neurosyphilis. The clinical signs and symptoms of neurosyphilis are nonspecific. These include seizures, stroke, general paresis, dementia, optic atrophy, and pupillary abnormalities. Here again nonspecific serologic testing may be nonreactive in up to 39% of cases.[7] A case has also been reported of a patient with nonreactive VDRL *and* FTA-ABS in which the fluorescent antibody stain was positive for *Treponema pallidum* from biopsy of arachnoid tissue.[8]

Cardiovascular syphilis may result in necrosis of the elastic tissue of the major arteries with subsequent aneurysm formation. Often the ascending aorta is involved, and distortion of adjacent structures results in aortic regurgitation and coronary artery stenosis.

Ocular Manifestations

Many different parts of the eye may be involved in secondary or tertiary syphilis (Table 13-1). These manifestations range from no or mild involvement to severe vision-threatening complications. Most manifestations are

TABLE 13-1[9]
Ocular Manifestations of Syphilis

LIDS	**IRIS AND CILIARY BODY**
Chancre	Roseolae
Gumma	Papules
Tarsitis	Gumma
Ulcerative blepharitis	**PUPILS**
CONJUNCTIVE	Light-near dissociation
Chancre	**LENS**
Papular syphilides	Capsular rupture and necrotizing
Gumma	cortical inflammation—
ORBIT	congenital syphilis
Periostitis	Dislocation
Gumma	**OPTIC NERVE**
CORNEA	Neuritis
Interstitial keratitis	Perineuritis
Ulcers	Neuroretinitis
Deep, punctate keratitis	Gumma
Keratitis profunda	**MOTILITY DYSFUNCTION**
Keratitis punctate profunda	Oculomotor, abducens, trochlear
Keratitis pustuliformis profunda	paresis—associated with basilar
Keratitis linearis migrans	meningitis
Gumma	Periodic alternating nystagmus
SCLERA	**RETINA AND VITREOUS**
Episcleritis	Chorioretinitis—pseudoretinitis
Scleritis	pigmentosa, salt and pepper
Gumma	fundus
ANTERIOR CHAMBER	Perivasculitis
HYPOPYON	Central retinal artery/vein
	occlusion
	Cystoid macular edema
	Vitritis

nonspecific and a complete careful history must be obtained as well as other general symptoms investigated. A high index of suspicion must be maintained when these nonspecific problems are encountered. The ocular manifestations may present acutely with active inflammation in the younger sexually active person or as a chronic problem in an older patient who has not been treated or inadequately treated.[9]

Rarely syphilis may cause a mild conjunctivitis, scleroconjunctivitis with more severe inflammation, or tarsitis. If the inflammation occurs adjacent to the cornea, keratitis may occur. Mucous patches of the conjunctiva have been described and on examination often contain treponemal organisms.

Syphilitic periostis may cause orbital inflammation. Most often this involves the upper rim of the orbit and is accompanied by severe pain. Although rarely an isolated finding, syphilitic periostitis often occurs concomitantly with other ocular abnormalities such as proptosis, extraocular muscle palsies, and retrobulbar neuritis. Extension into the cranial cavity, causing cavernous sinus thrombosis or meningitis, may be life-threatening.

Cornea. The most important corneal involvement in syphilis is interstitial keratitis. Congenital syphilis causes 90% of cases of interstitial keratitis and acquired syphilis 4%, with a mixture of infectious processes accounting for the remaining 6%.[10]

Interstitial keratitis occurs in 40% of patients with congenital syphilis.[11] There is a higher incidence in females than males. It has been reported as occurring anywhere from birth to the fourth decade, although 85% occurs between ages five and twenty-five.[10] Clinically it is typically a bilateral process as opposed to the acquired form which is frequently unilateral. In the acute phase symptoms include photophobia, pain and epiphora. The corneal endothelium becomes hazy and opacifications appear in the deep stroma. Corneal edema follows with bedewing of the epithelium. The cornea becomes vascularized in the deep stroma and an iritis often is present. As the inflammation subsides and recovery begins, the corneal endothelium and epithelium clear, leaving the deep stromal opacifications and "ghost vessels." The diagnosis of interstitial keratitis is often made in this later "recovered" stage in the adult with deep stromal opacifications and ghost vessels. A history of some ocular inflammation as a child should be sought as well as other stigmata of congenital syphilis. These include frontal bossing, nasal bridge abnormalities, high-arched palate, Hutchinson's teeth, deafness, and sparse outer eyebrows. Other ocular abnormalities, including salt and pepper chorioretinitis, vascular sheathing (Figure 13-4), and retinal pigment deposits, are present in 40% of patients with interstitial keratitis.[9] Of note, however, pupils are usually normal in congenital syphilis and do not show light/near dissociation. It is also important to realize that patients with interstitial keratitis from congenital syphilis have nonreactive VDRLs and reactive specific serologies (FTA-ABS).[10]

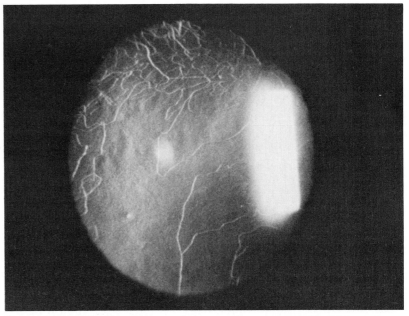

Figure 13-4. Interstitial keratitis: corneal ghost vessels seen on retro-illumination.

Corneal involvement in acquired syphilis may take other more atypical forms. Adults may present with unilateral keratitis involving the central cornea with associated uveitis with or without corneal vascularization. There may be grayish nodules in the middle or deep stroma with uveitis but no vascularization. A hypopyon may develop. A linear opacity may develop and progress across the cornea in the deep stroma and underlying endothelium. More rarely a corneal marginal ulcer or posterior abscess may occur. It is extremely rare for a true gumma of the cornea to develop.

Uveitis. Moore reported in 1931 that 4.6% of patients with secondary syphilis develop uveitis and 9.3% of patients with recurrent secondary syphilis develop an associated iritis.[12] One of several different types may occur. Roseola of the iris appears early in secondary syphilis. This represents engorgement of the vascular loops normally present in the middle third of the iris and appears as red spots which disappear within a few days. Single or multiple papules may develop at the pupillary or ciliary borders. These may persist for weeks and often leave an atrophic spot on the iris. A clinically silent, low-grade iritis has also been reported which is transient and may be self-limiting.[13] A fibrinous iritis may be observed in early or late secondary syphilis. Because it has no distinguishing clinical features, an etiologic diagnosis is based on history, accompanying systemic findings, and serologic tests. Treponemal organisms have been isolated from the anterior chamber fluid.[14,15] A severe diffuse iridocyclitis may also occur. Posterior synechiae, cataract, and secondary glaucoma are potential complications. True gamma of the iris and ciliary body may also develop even during secondary syphilis.

Chorioretinitis. The retina and choroid may be involved in either congenital or acquired syphilis (Figure 13-5). The most common manifestation in congenital syphilis is the "salt and pepper" fundus. This is caused by foci of inflammation which undergo fibrosis and scar formation with gliosis, depigmentation, pigment clumping and often bilateral chorioretinal atrophy. The lesions are usually peripheral. Less frequently, a circumscribed chorioretinitis with areas of hyperpigmentation and atrophy is seen. There may be associated attacks of interstitial keratitis. Rarely vascular narrowing and sheathing accompany retinal changes, presenting a clinical picture indistinguishable from classical retinitis pigmentosa.

Acquired syphilitic chorioretinitis occurs in the secondary or tertiary stage. A diffuse chorioretinitis is characterized initially by a hazy vitreous (Figure 13-6), retinal exudates most often in the posterior pole, and occasionally generalized retinal edema. With progression there is clumping of retinal pigment along vessels and any areas of inflammation. Areas of choroidal atrophy often surround the disc. The retinal vessels become sheathed in fibrous tissue. Recurrence is common. Rarely there may be either an isolated choroiditis or retinitis. Diffuse syphilitic neuroretinitis involves retinal edema, retinal vasculitis, papillitis and associated vitreous inflammation.[16]

Isolated retinal vasculitis without associated chorioretinitis in syphilis is rare. Neovascularization extending into the vitreous occurs but is likewise

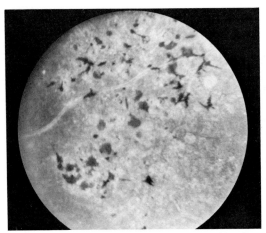

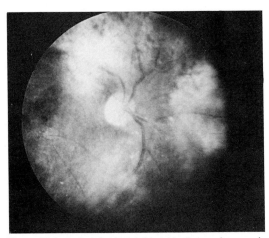

Figure 13-5. Chorioretinitis and vascular sheathing in a patient with congenital syphilis.

Figure 13-6. Active chorioretinitis with vitreous haze, retinal exudates and edema.

unusual. Nonrhegmatogenous retinal detachment with uveal effusion has been reported with treponemes found in the subretinal fluid.[17] Gumma may extend from the ciliary body to the choroid or rarely arise from the choroid itself.

Optic Nerve. Optic nerve involvement in syphilis takes several forms. The first is perioptic neuritis in which the meningeal sheath surrounding the optic nerve is inflamed without involvement of the nerve itself (Figure 13-7).[18,19] This occurs most often as an extension of meningitis in secondary syphilis. There is pain on ocular movement, but visual acuity remains normal. The discs appear swollen, but opening pressure on spinal tap is normal.

Optic neuritis may occur in congenital or acquired syphilis although it is rare in the former. Visual acuity is variably reduced with assorted visual field defects typical of those found in optic neuropathies. On ophthalmoscopy, the optic nerve is swollen. Prognosis is good with appropriate treatment, however secondary optic atrophy may develop. Retrobulbar neuritis is rarely an isolated finding in syphilis but may occur associated with orbital periostitis, chorioretinitis, and meningitis. Gumma of the optic nerve is rare.

True papilledema may also occur in syphilis when associated with increased intracranial pressure. This is seen most frequently in syphilitic meningitis, however gumma may rarely cause obstructive hydrocephalus. Syphilitic meningitis may cause a myriad of ocular abnormalities with variable presentations. Pupils may be unequal and poorly reactive to light. A syphilitic arteritis may be present causing a homonymous hemianopsia and hemiplegia. In basilar meningitis, cranial nerve palsies are often present with single or multiple, unilateral or bilateral abnormalities. The third nerve is the most commonly affected with usually incomplete paralysis of function. The pupil is often dilated and ptosis may be present. Deafness may develop and, although it is most common in the congenital form, may also be acquired in the late secondary or tertiary stages.

Neurosyphilis. The classical forms of neurosyphilis include tabes dorsalis and general paresis of the insane. These are rarely seen today in their full form because treatment during the early stages of the disease has produced atypical clinical presentations.[20] The following is a description of the *forme fruste*, recognizing that today's patient with neurosyphilis will more typically present with any one or a combination of the symptoms and signs described.

Tabes dorsalis is a degenerative process of the posterior columns and selected cranial nerves with prominent involvement of ocular structures. It occurs 10-20 years after the primary lesion and is slowly progressive. Patients complain of pain in the limbs, face, or abdomen, hypesthesias, and loss of balance and position sense. The earliest evidence of tabes is often a pupillary abnormality. Initially they are unequal and sluggish to light, sometimes developing into the classic Argyll Robertson pupil. Iris atrophy may be present and is often segmental. Multiple extraocular muscle palsies may occur and are frequently transient. Ptosis may occur and is often bilateral.

Primary optic atrophy of unknown etiology occurs in 10% of patients with tabes. Although disc pallor may precede loss of vision, loss of vision is

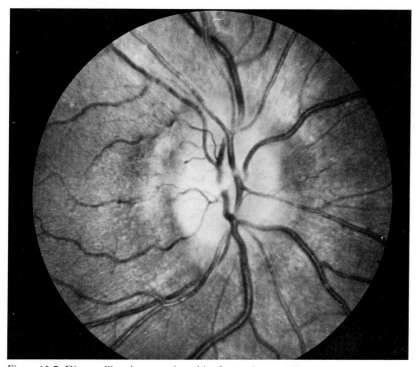

Figure 13-7. Disc swelling due to perineuritis of secondary syphilis.

usually severe or complete. The process may be slowly progressive or rapid. Involvement of one eye may precede the other but ultimately both are affected. Visual field changes include: peripheral constriction, altitudinal defects, central or cecocentral scotomas with or without peripheral field involvement and arcuate defects. Tabetic optic atrophy causing progressive visual loss is a diagnosis of *exclusion*, made after a compressive prechiasmal lesion has been excluded.[8] Other manifestations of posterior column dysfunction include: loss of position and vibration sensation, ataxia, loss of knee and ankle jerks, and loss of bladder control.

General paresis of the insane results from degeneration of the cerebral cortex. There is a chronic, slowly progressive mental deterioration initially manifest as apathy, depression, and forgetfulness, progressing to a frank organic psychosis. Other findings include: Argyll Robertson pupils, tremors of the lids, lips and tongue, optic atrophy, and extraocular muscle palsies. Hemiplegia, aphasia, and convulsions may occur. As previously stated, a patient today with neurosyphilis is much more likely to present with the incidental findings of pupillary abnormalities or optic atrophy, or any combination of the signs and symptoms described previously.

Treatment

Adequate treatment of syphilis at any stage remains controversial despite guidelines from the U.S. Public Health Service. Optimal therapeutic levels and dose schedules have not been established due to variability of tissue levels of penicillin and the relatively long dividing time of the treponemal organism. There are documented cases of treatment failure in all stages of the disease.[9,17,21-24] Recommendations for primary, secondary, and early latent syphilis of less than one year's duration is benzathine penicillin G 2.4 million units in a single dose. Alternative therapy, for patients with penicillin allergy, includes tetracycline hydrochloride 2 g daily for 15 days or erythromycin base, stearate, or ethyl succinate 2 g daily for 15 days.[25]

Patients with syphilis for more than one year's duration except neurosyphilis should receive 2.4 million units IM once a week for three successive weeks. Also patients with syphilis of long duration or late latent syphilis should undergo spinal fluid examination to look for asymptomatic neurosyphilis. If the CSF is normal, they should be treated as recommended above. If abnormal, they should receive treatment for neurosyphilis.

Previously recommended treatment for tertiary syphilis included benzathine penicillin G 2.4 million units for three weeks or aqueous procaine penicillin G 600,000 units for ten days. Because these dose regimens do not achieve adequate CSF levels,[23,26] the Centers for Disease Control have added the following for the treatment of neurosyphilis:[25] aqueous penicillin G 12-24 million units per day intravenously for ten days followed by benzathine penicillin G 2.4 million units IM weekly for three doses or aqueous penicillin G procaine 2.4 million units IM daily plus probenecid

500 mg orally every six hours for ten days followed by benzathine penicillin G 2.4 million units IM weekly for three doses.

Treatment of patients with the ocular syndromes of syphilis remains confusing. In the patient with active infection such as anterior and posterior uveitis, optic neuritis, perineuritis or neuroretinitis, CSF should be examined and followed if reactive. Regardless of the results, many are recommending treating these patients with high dose intravenous penicillin therapy.[4,9,14,22] If reactive, the CSF VDRL should be reexamined six months after treatment.

In patients with changes typical of chronic ocular syphilis, if the process appears inactive in its chorioretinal changes, optic atrophy, and old interstitial keratitis, treatment is more controversial. If the VDRL is nonreactive and there is a history of previous treatment, Sutphin, et al,[4] recommend neither additional antibiotic therapy nor lumbar puncture. A lumbar puncture is performed if there is no previous history of treatment. Others[8,21] have recommended CSF examination for any patient with syphilitic ocular disease to rule out neurosyphilis which may be asymptomatic or inadequately treated. If the CSF is normal and there is a prior history of treatment, the patient may simply be observed. If the CSF is abnormal or any progression of ocular signs and symptoms occurs, treatment with high dose intravenous penicillin is recommended.

Summary

Ocular syphilis remains challenging to diagnose because of its many nonspecific, varied and changing presentations. Diagnosis is aided by awareness of the multiple ocular manifestations of acute and chronic syphilis and obtaining a specific treponemal serologic test (FTA-ABS or MHA-TP). Remember that the VDRL and other nonspecific serologic tests may be nonreactive in 30% of patients with late syphilis.[6] Therefore, a nonreactive VDRL does not exclude the diagnosis of late syphilis. Specific serologic tests (FTA-ABS, MHA-TP) rarely, if ever, become nonreactive and are true indications that the patient has had syphilis. Such tests should be ordered if syphilis is suspected clinically. Treatment also remains challenging as evidenced by the lack of clear, well-accepted, successful therapeutic guidelines. Greater awareness of the problems pertaining to syphilis and further studies of these problems are still needed.

References
1. US Dept of Health and Human Services: Sexually Transmitted Disease (STD) Statistical Letter, Year 1981. Atlanta: Centers for Disease Control, 1982.
2. Seeley RL, Sarkar M, Smith JL: The borderline fluorescent treponemal antibody absorption test reactor. Arch Ophthalmol 87:16, 1972.
3. Shore RN: Hemagglutination tests and related advances in serodiagnosis of syphilis. Arch Dermatol 109:854, 1974.
4. Sutphin JE, Matoba AY, Wilhelmus KR, Jones DB: Decision making in ocular syphilis. Poster, Amer Acad Ophthal, Nov 1983.
5. Texas Dept of Health: Interpretation of Serologic Tests for Syphilis. Stock No. 6-115, March 1980.

6. Holmes KK: Syphilis. *In:* Harrison's *Principles of Internal Medicine*, GW Thorn, RD Adams, E Braunwald, KJ Isselbacher, RG Petersdord (eds). New York: McGraw-Hill, 1981, pp 716-726.
7. Harner RE, Smith JL, Israel CW: The FTA-ABS test in late syphilis: a serological study in 1,985 cases. *J Amer Ophth Assoc* 203:545, 1968.
8. Smith JL, Israel CW: Optic atrophy and neurosyphilis. Ann Rev Med 22:103, 1971.
9. Spoor TC, Wynn PJ, Hartel WC, Bryan CS: Ocular syphilis, acute and chronic. J Clin Neuro-Ophthalmol 3:197-203, 1983.
10. Smith LL: Testing for congenital syphilis in interstitial keratitis. Am J Ophthalmol 72(4):816, 1974.
11. Walsh FB: *In: Clinical Neuro-Ophthalmology.* Baltimore: The Williams and Wilkins Company, p 546, 1957.
12. Moore JE: Syphilitic iritis. Am J Ophthalmol 14:110-126, 1931.
13. Zwink FB, Dunlop EMC: Clinically silent anterior uveitis in secondary syphilis. Trans Ophthal Soc UK 96:148, 1976.
14. Belin MW, Baltch AL, Hay PB: Secondary syphilitic uveitis. Am J Ophthalmol 92:210-214, 1981.
15. Schmidt H, Goldschmidt E: Demonstration of motile treponemes in the aqueous humour in secondary syphilis. Brit J Vener Dis 48:400, 1972.
16. Duke-Elder S, Dobree JH: Diseases of the Retina. In: Duke-Elder: *System of Ophthalmology*, Duke-Elder S (ed). Vol 10, St. Louis: C.V. Mosby, 1967, pp 253-254.
17. DeLuise VP, Clark SW III, Smith JL: Syphilitic retinal detachment and uveal effusion. Am J Ophthalmol 94:757-761, 1982.
18. Rush JA, Ryna EJ: Syphilitic optic perineuritis. Am J Ophthalmol 91:404, 1981.
19. Kline LB, Jackson WB: Syphilitic optic perineuritis and uveitis. Neuro-Ophthalmol. Focus. 1980. JL Smith (ed). New York: Masson Publishing USA, 1980, pp 77-84.
20. Hooshmand H, Escobar MR, Kopf SW: Neurosyphilis, a study of 241 patients. J Amer Med Assoc 219:726, 1972.
21. Yobs AR, Rockwell DH, Clark JW Jr: Treponemal survival in humans after penicillin therapy, a preliminary report. Brit J Vener Dis 40:248, 1964.
22. Folk JC, Weingeist TA, Corbett JJ, Lobes LA, Watzke RC: Syphilitic neuroretinitis. Am J Ophthalmol 95:480-486, 1983.
23. Smith JL: Spirochetes in Late Seronegative Syphilis, Penicillin Notwithstanding. Springfield: Charles C. Thomas, 1969, pp 287-293.
24. Cohen MS, Gibson G, Clarte MD: Lissauer form of paretic neurosyphilis: Forgotten but not gone. Ann Neurol 11:219, 1982.
25. US Dept Health and Human Services. Sexually Transmitted Diseases, Treatment Guidelines 1982. Morbid Mortal Wkly Rep 31(suppl.):51S Atlanta: Center for Disease Control, Aug 20, 1982.
26. Ducas J, Robson HG: Cerebrospinal fluid penicillin levels during therapy for latent syphilis. J Amer Med Assoc 246:2583, 1981.

Chapter 14

Ocular and Adnexal Trauma

Mark E. Hammer, MD, FACS
Thomas C. Spoor, MD, FACS

OCULAR AND ADNEXAL TRAUMA

Introduction

Ocular and adnexal trauma is all too common. Ocular injuries due to BB's, firecrackers and foreign bodies continue to deprive too many children of their vision. Prevention is the key to management. Efforts with public education into the hazards of BB's, fireworks and their lack of redeeming social value should be encouraged. Legislators should be encouraged, cajoled and threatened to pass appropriate restrictive legislation limiting the sale and distribution of these hazardous products. Public education and appropriate legislation should publicize the role of safety glasses in preventing ocular injuries at both work and play. Until that aquarian time, ocular trauma and its management will continue to plague the ophthalmologist.

Management of ocular and adnexal trauma has been extensively reviewed elsewhere.[1,2] This chapter will review the management of ocular and adnexal trauma for the triaging ophthalmologist hoping to avoid errors of commission and omission. Such errors will be minimized if one thinks anatomically and functionally when evaluating ocular and adnexal trauma. Take the example of markedly decreased acuity in an otherwise normal appearing eye. If the patient also has a closed head injury, the suspicion of a traumatic optic neuropathy should be confirmed by appropriate neuro-ophthalmologic and radiologic evaluation. Conversely, intracranial involvement should be ruled out when evaluating orbital injuries because of the proximity of the anterior cranial fossa to the orbital roof and the middle cranial fossa to the orbital apex. Additionally, occult injury to the globe should always be suspected when evaluating apparent adnexal injury.

Documenting visual acuity is of paramount importance when evaluating trauma to the eye and adnexa. Medically, it tells you how well the eye is functioning. Poor visual acuity is disconcerting in a normal-appearing eye. This will prompt a more compulsive evaluation to determine the reason for the decreased vision. The legal implications of documenting visual function prior to treatment are obvious. Excepting immediate first aid for caustic ocular burns, visual acuity should be determined initially when evaluating and treating any ocular or adnexal injury.

History

History is often overlooked in ophthalmology, especially in the emergency room setting. It is important to determine the what and where of any injury.

"*What* were you doing and what were you using when you injured your eye?" You would expect totally different ocular injuries to occur if a patient were scraping rust from under his car (superficial corneal foreign body or abrasion) as opposed to striking metal on metal (intraocular metallic foreign body).

"*Where* were you when your eye was injured?" A corneal abrasion caused by vegetable matter (suspect fungal keratitis) may potentially require very different treatment and follow-up than an abrasion caused by a sheet of paper.

General health should be assessed. Does the patient have any illness or allergy that may alter your planned treatment? What treatment has already been administered and when?

Lids

Treatment of the injured eyelid should be preceded by a thorough evaluation of the visual function and the underlying globe. Occult perforations or injury to the globe may occur in conjunction with apparently minor lid lacerations (dart, scissors, etc.).[1] There is no substitute for a complete and thorough ocular exam even when evaluating "obviously simple" lid lacerations.[2] Conversely, the globe may be totally spared in the presence of very severe lid lacerations (Figure 14-1).

Treatment of lid lacerations is essentially surgical and extensively reviewed elsewhere.[3-6] Canalicular lacerations should be suspected with any injury to the medial lid or canthus. If doubt exists, the canaliculi should be probed or irrigated with a fluorescein solution to detect subtle lacerations. Upper canalicular lacerations deserve the same compulsive repair as lower ones, for they are functional in 50% of the population.[3,7]

Lid and canalicular lacerations need not be repaired with the same urgency as an open globe. No harm is done by waiting 12-24 hours for safer anesthesia, a rested surgeon, and optimal operating room conditions.[3] It is important to initially repair these lacerations properly. A few extra moments during the initial procedure will save the patient secondary or tertiary procedures (Figure 14-2). No harm is done by referring a complicated lid laceration for more expert primary repair, even if it is delayed 24-48 hours.

Orbital Trauma

Orbital trauma can be classified as penetrating or concussive. Both can cause visual loss and extraocular motility dysfunction. Penetrating orbital injuries may be caused by either sharp implements, i.e., knives, or projectiles such as BB's and bullets.

Visual loss or motility dysfunction usually occurs at the moment of injury via transection of the optic nerve or cranial nerves, respectively. Visual

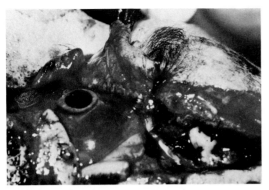 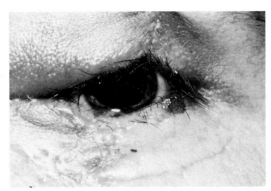

Figure 14-1. Severe lid and facial lacerations caused by a motorboat propeller. Globe is totally spared, visual acuity 20/20. Arrow points to frontal gray matter indicating intracranial involvement.

Figure 14-2. Posttraumatic notching of upper lid.

acuity should be documented upon initial evaluation. Long-term visual and motility dysfunction may occur secondary to compression of nerves by hemorrhaging orbital vessels or edematous tissue. Severe orbital hemorrhage may cause occlusion of the central retinal artery.

When evaluating penetrating or contusive orbital injury, occult penetration of or contusive injury to the globe should be ruled out. Such injuries may be subtle or quite obvious. Penetrating injuries should be ruled out by indirect ophthalmoscopy (under anesthesia if necessary) or surgical exploration. Contusive injuries to the globe (Table 14-1) may be detected by slit lamp exam and indirect ophthalmoscopy.

TABLE 14-1.
SEQUELAE OF CONTUSIVE OCULAR INJURY

CORNEA
  abrasion
  blood Staining
  edema

LENS
  cataract
  subluxation

VITREOUS
  hemorrhage

RETINA
  edema
  hemorrhage
    preretinal
    intraretinal
    subhyaloid

Detachment
  holes

IRIS
  recession
  dialysis

GLAUCOMA
  recession
  ghost cell
  RBC
  hypotony

CHOROID
  effusion
  tears
  hemorrhage

Ophthalmologists are often not adept at detecting occult intracranial injury. Because the orbit is separated from the anterior cranial fossa by a thin orbital roof, intracranial involvement should be suspected with any superior orbital injury (Figure 14-1). Appropriate diagnostic tests should be sought. Plain x-rays or CT scans may demonstrate intracranial air (pneumocephalus), a sure sign that the cranial cavity has been violated (Figure 14-3). The deep orbit is contiguous with the middle cranial fossa. Therefore, intracranial involvement should also be suspected in any patient with a deep, penetrating orbital injury. Intracranial involvement will alter your surgical approach, requiring neurosurgical consultation. Unrecognized intracranial injury may result in CSF leaks, meningitis, or cerebral abscess formation. In summary, remember the relationship of the orbit to the anterior and middle cranial fossa. Suspect intracranial involvement. Obtain the appropriate x-rays, CT scans, and neurosurgical consultation when evaluating an orbital injury.

BB and Pellet Injuries. BB and pellet injuries are all too common. Damage to ocular and orbital structures usually occurs at the time of injury. Fortunately, they are often compatible with good visual function. Surgical intervention is rarely beneficial or necessary. If the globe is penetrated by either of these projectiles, the prognosis for useful vision is dismal.[8]

Initial evaluation should include documentation of visual acuity and the presence or absence of an afferent pupillary defect. Slit lamp examination, tonometry, and dilated fundus examination should then be performed. An orbital CT scan will localize the pellet in the orbit, demonstrate its rela-

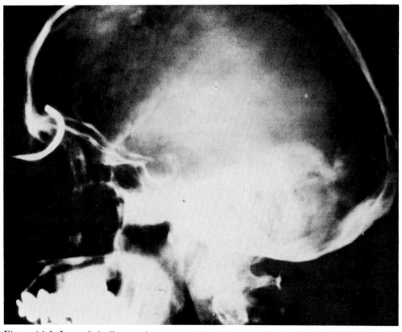

Figure 14-3. Lateral skull x-ray demonstrates involvement of anterior cranial fossa by orbital foreign body.

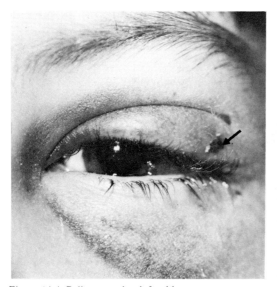 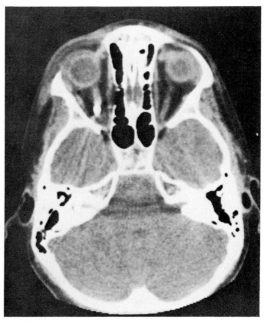

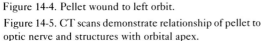
Figure 14-4. Pellet wound to left orbit.

Figure 14-5. CT scans demonstrate relationship of pellet to optic nerve and structures with orbital apex.

tionship to the optic nerve and globe, and rule out intracranial penetration. Associated ocular injuries such as hyphema are then treated appropriately. An antibiotic of choice is administered to prevent orbital infection from either the projectile or adjacent sinus. The patient is followed for evidence of infection or fistula formation.

Case 1. A nine-year-old boy was shot in the orbit with a pellet gun (Figure 14-4). A moderate orbital hemorrhage and limitation of ocular abduction was present. Visual acuity was 20/40. No afferent or inverse Gunn pupil was present. Anterior segment and intraocular pressure were normal. Fundus examination demonstrated mild macular edema and peripheral hemorrhage and edema. Computed tomography localized the pellet at the orbital apex (Figure 14-5). He was treated with oral dicloxacillin. After two weeks, visual acuity had improved to 20/15. The orbital swelling and motility defect had resolved.

Case 2. A seven-year-old boy was shot with a BB which lodged in his lateral orbit, adjacent to his globe. Visual acuity and ocular exam were normal except for peripheral retinal hemorrhage. After four weeks of observation, the peripheral retina appeared atrophic. Visual acuity decreased to 20/25 due to hypotony and macular folds. The BB was removed from the belly of the lateral rectus (Figure 14-6) with restoration of ocular pressure and normalization of acuity. Three years post-injury the patient is asymptomatic.

The pellet in Case 1 was causing no ocular dysfunction, was unreactive, and was located in a surgically difficult area. It was best left alone. Case 2

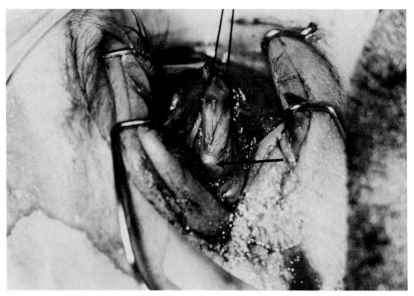

Figure 14-6. BB lodged in belly of lateral rectus muscle exposed at surgery.

was managed conservatively until vision deteriorated. The BB then had to be removed since it was interfering with normal ocular function.

Bullet injuries to the orbit may be treated much like BB or pellet injuries. The prognosis is much more guarded since the mass and velocity of the projectile are much greater. Severe ocular injury, intracranial penetration, and extensive orbital damage are more common. The principles of management are similar. Document visual function and ocular injury; then localize the projectile to rule out intracranial involvement.

Blunt Orbital Trauma—Orbital Hemorrhage. Visual loss after blunt orbital trauma may result from a traumatic optic neuropathy or central retinal artery occlusion caused by severe orbital hemorrhage and elevated pressure. Decreased acuity in the presence of an orbital hemorrhage demands an explanation. First, look for an afferent pupillary defect via the swinging flashlight test. If concurrent ocular or orbital injury has resulted in an ipsilateral fixed and dilated pupil, afferent visual dysfunction may be detected by demonstrating an inverse Gunn pupil. Shine a bright light upon the involved, dilated pupil for several seconds (Figure 14-7A). Observe the normal pupil as you shift the light from the involved to uninvolved eye. If the normal pupil then constricts (Figure 14-7B), you have an afferent defect on the side of the dilated pupil.

When the light was shined in the involved eye, the midbrain received decreased input due to the conduction defect. Subsequently, the consensual reaction caused the uninvolved (normal) pupil to dilate. As the light is shifted to the normal eye, the dilated normal pupil constricts in response to the direct pupillary light reaction. The dilated, involved pupil remains dilated, because it cannot constrict due to traumatic iridplegia or efferent injury.

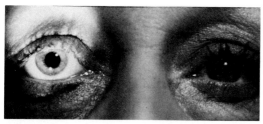
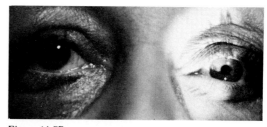

Figure 14-7A   Figure 14-7B

Figure 14-7A & B. Inverse Gunn pupil. Right eye is amaurotic due to optic nerve injury, pupil dilated due to ciliary ganglion injury. Light in blind right eye causes left pupil to dilate via consensual reaction. When light shifted to normal, left pupil constricted due to normal direct response.

Impending or real central retinal artery (CRA) occlusions accompanying orbital hemorrhage allow no time for consultations or referrals. If fundus exam reveals pulsations in the CRA, the intraocular pressure is at or above diastolic blood pressure. If it reaches systolic pressure, a CRA occlusion will follow. The patient with CRA pulsations needs to be observed carefully and efforts made to reduce intraorbital pressure. This is most expeditiously done by immediate lateral canthotomy, allowing expansion of the orbit contents and reduction of pressure. Observe the fundus. If the central retinal artery is now perfusing, you have bought time for further evaluation. A large, localized hemorrhage may be demonstrated by ultrasonography and aspirated with a 22 gauge needle. If ultrasound is not available, the orbital septum may be penetrated in each quadrant with a #11 Bard-Parker blade in an attempt to drain an expanding hematoma. An expanding hemorrhage that cannot be drained or controlled by these measures may necessitate emergent orbital decompression by removing the medial wall and floor of the orbit. This allows orbital contents and hemorrhage to expand into the ethmoid and maxillary sinuses, decreasing intraorbital pressure and allowing the central retinal artery to perfuse.

Traumatic Optic Neuropathy. Blunt trauma to the orbit or facial bones may cause visual loss due to optic nerve avulsion, infarction or compression by an optic nerve sheath hematoma, edema, or a bone fragment. A potentially reversible optic neuropathy may result from spasm of the nutrient vessels. Conventional teaching stressed the importance of the temporal course of visual loss. If the patient noted loss of vision immediately after injury, avulsion or infarction was presumed and no treatment rendered. A history of slowly progressive visual loss after blunt orbital or cranial trauma prompted a vigorous neuroradiologic search for an optic canal fracture and subsequent transcranial or transethmoidal decompression. Some authors have claimed impressive results and restoration of vision.[9,10] These patients are often intoxicated or seriously injured and unresponsive. A visual acuity and accurate history of visual loss is difficult to obtain. Fortunately one can detect the presence of an optic neuropathy and quantitate it to some extent by examining the pupils for the presence of an afferent pupillary defect or an inverse, afferent pupil. We suggest immediate treatment of traumatic optic neuropathies with massive doses of intravenous corticosteroids, i.e., Solu-medrol 250 mg every six hours after an initial dose of 500 mg, or Decadron greater than 1 mg/kg/day as initial treatment for 12-24 hours.[11] During this time, the patient may become more cooperative. A better visual acuity and history of visual loss can be obtained. Neuroradiological evaluation of the optic canals with high quality computed tomography and polytomography with Rhese and base views may demonstrate an intracanalicular fracture. Subsequent transcranial or transethmoidal decompression may then be beneficial. The prognosis for regaining useful vision is guarded, but excellent results have been reported.[10,12]

A syndrome of post-traumatic venous stasis retinopathy and an enlarged optic nerve has recently been described.[13] These patients present with gradual progressive loss of vision after blunt facial or cranial trauma. Disc edema, engorged retinal vessels, and retinal hemorrhage are seen in the fundus. Computed tomography demonstrates enlargement of the optic nerve sheath. In this clinical setting, surgical decompression of the optic nerve through a medial orbitotomy and incision of the sheath may result in a dramatic return of vision and normalization of the fundus.

Central Retinal Artery Occlusion. There is no good treatment for central retina artery (CRA) occlusions. Treatment goals are to dilate the retinal arterioles and rapidly lower intraocular pressure in an attempt to dislodge embolic material. This strategy may dilate an occluded arteriole or direct an embolus peripherally minimizing the amount of ischemic retinal damage. If emboli are present, a carotid or cardiac source must be ruled out by appropriate tests and consultation. If no emboli are seen, an arteritic etiology should be considered.

Immediate treatment is necessary. Hayreh[14] has demonstrated irreversible damage to the monkey retina after 100 minutes of arteriolar occlusion. There are anecdotal reports of restored vision up to 24 hours after occlusion. These occlusions may not be complete. The following treatment regimen may be beneficial: immediate sublingual nitroglycerine (available in all emergency rooms) and inhalation of 5% carbon dioxide and 95% oxygen to dilate the retinal vessels. If there is no immediate restoration of arteriolar flow, anterior chamber paracentesis may be done at the slit lamp. Penetrate the globe at the limbus with a 30 gauge needle on a tuberculin syringe and withdraw aqueous. This maneuver rapidly decompresses the eye, lowering intraocular pressure. If the central retinal artery remains occluded, we have cannulated the supraorbital artery and infused 20 mg of papaverine followed by heparinized saline. This rapidly and dramatically dilates the retinal vessels and may be done under local anesthesia. This procedure has successfully restored retinal perfusion and vision in some cases.[15,16]

Orbital Fractures

Treatment of orbital fractures is controversial, but the evaluation is not.

Regardless of which specialist does the surgery, the patient should have the benefit of an ophthalmologic evaluation, even if the facial injury is remote from the eye. Over 60% of patients with mid-face fractures have ocular injuries.[17] Ophthalmologic evaluation should document visual acuity, associated ocular or adnexal injury, and motility defect. Decreased acuity without obvious ocular damage indicates a traumatic optic neuropathy. Evidence of extension of the orbital fracture to the apex or optic canal should be sought.

Le Fort fractures involve the maxilla and may (Le Fort II & III) or may not (Le Fort I) involve the orbit. Le Fort II fractures involve the maxilla, nasal bones, and medial orbital floors. There may be a concomitant ocular injury. Patients with mid-facial fractures often develop epiphora due to nasolacrimal duct obstruction eventually requiring dacryocystorhinostomy. Le Fort III fractures are extensive and result in separation of the maxilla from the skull with rather extensive orbital involvement. These fractures are commonly associated with ocular as well as intracranial injuries. Extension of the fracture to the orbital apex and optic canal may cause marked visual loss secondary to a traumatic optic neuropathy.

Simple fractures of the zygoma are often missed by the ophthalmologist evaluating periorbital trauma. They can be detected by comparing the contours of both malar eminences for symmetry. More extensive fractures also involve the lateral and inferior orbital rim. They are detected by palpating a step-off of the orbital rim. Patients are exquisitely tender over this fracture site. Inferior rim fractures are invariably accompanied by medial orbital floor fractures. Extraocular muscle entrapment in these fractures is uncommon.[6]

Orbital roof fractures may involve the frontal sinus and anterior cranial fossa with associated intracranial injury. CSF leaks and ptosis with upgaze palsy secondary to injuries to the superior division of the oculomotor nerve can occur. Extension of the fracture along the base of the skull may produce a carotid cavernous fistula or CSF leak.

Blunt trauma to the orbit may cause fracture of the floor or medial wall, leaving the rims intact.[18,19] The medial orbital wall (lamina papyracea) is very thin and easily fractured. These fractures may be asymptomatic, presenting with mild epistaxis and orbital emphysema. Observation is the only treatment necessary. Oral antibiotics may help prevent orbital infection. The medial rectus may be incarcerated in the fracture site. These patients complain of diplopia and have restricted ocular abduction. Surgical reduction is necessary. More anterior medial orbital fractures may damage the nasolacrimal duct or lacrimal sac, causing epiphora. These patients eventually require a dacryocystorhinostomy to obviate their symptoms.

Blowout fractures of the orbital floor are common sequelae to blunt orbital trauma. Indications for surgical intervention range from almost none[20] to their presence on x-ray. The latter may do better, for many never required surgery. Management is controversial. All agree that visual acuity should be documented prior to treatment and any concomitant ocular injuries (e.g., hyphema) should be detected and treated. Reasonable indications for surgery include diplopia with entrapment of orbital contents (extraocular muscle or septa) in fracture site and cosmetically significant

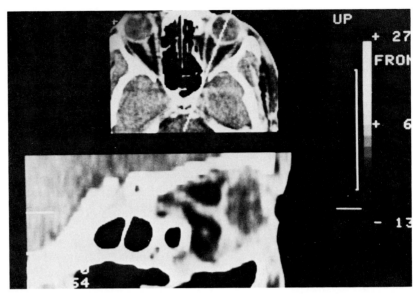

Figure 14-8. CT scan and oblique reconstruction demonstrating posterior orbital floor fracture with entrapment of inferior rectus.

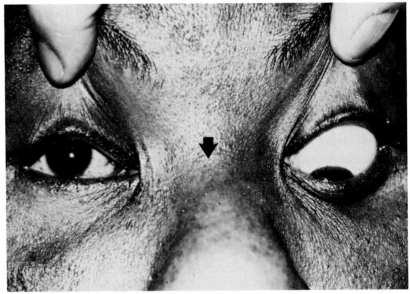

Figure 14-9. Restricted downgaze in patient with posterior orbital floor fracture (CT in Figure 14-8).

enophthalmos. Prior to surgery, the fracture site may be exquisitely localized by CT scanning with appropriate oblique and coronal reconstruction. The relationship of the inferior rectus and optic nerve to the fracture site can be determined, as can the anterior or posterior location of the fracture (Figure 14-8). A patient with a posterior orbital floor fracture may be hypertropic with restricted downgaze (Figure 14-9). A patient with an anterior floor fracture may be hypotropic with upgaze restriction. Optimal timing of surgery is within the first two weeks. Patients should *not* be operated upon until orbital swelling and hemorrhage have subsided, ocular injury, e.g., hyphema, has resolved, and optic nerve injury or extraocular motility deficit stabilized. If the involved eye is the patient's only sighted eye, surgery is contraindicated. Surgical techniques have been extensively described elsewhere[1,3,6] and will not be repeated here.

Chemical Burns

Chemical burns to the eye may be relatively innocuous, causing mild irritation, or severe, causing painful loss of vision. The severity of a chemical burn depends upon the nature of the agent (acid or alkali), the amount instilled, the concentration or pH of the solution, exposure time, and associated cations.

Acid causes less ocular damage than alkali since it coagulates the epithelial surface forming a relative barrier to further penetration. Additionally, corneal stroma naturally buffers solutions with a pH less than 4.0. Alkali rapidly penetrates all corneal layers, disrupting cells and collagen, allowing continued penetration of alkali into the anterior chamber. Strong alkalies cause ischemic coagulation and necrosis of cornea and sclera with subsequent opacification and softening. The pH in the anterior chamber is rapidly elevated. Coagulation of aqueous, trabecular and lenticular proteins may cause glaucoma and cataract formation.

Some clinically significant acids and their common source are listed in Table 14-2. Due to tissue coagulation and buffering, ocular damage is done within the first few hours after exposure. The exceptions are hydrofluoric acid and acids containing heavy metals. These may rapidly penetrate the cornea, damage the endothelium, and subsequently opacify it.[1] Treatment

---

TABLE 14-2.
CLINICALLY SIGNIFICANT ACIDS

ACID	SOURCES/USES
Sulfuric (H_2SO_4)	Battery acid
	Oil of vitriol
Sulfur dioxide (SO_2)	refrigerant
Sulfurous (HSO_3)	bleach
	fruit preservative
Nitric (HNO_3)	
Hydrochloric (HCl)	cleaning solutions (tile)
Muriatic	
Acetic (CH_3COOH)	vinegar (4-10%)
	glacial acetic acid
Chromic (Cr_2O_3)	chrome plating
Hydrofluoric (HF)	etching glass, silicone
	refining uranium
	frosting glass

TABLE 14-3.
CLINICALLY SIGNIFICANT ALKALIES

ALKALI	SOURCES/USES
Ammonia (NH_3)	household ammonia (cleaning agent)
Ammonium hydroxide (NH_4OH)	fertilizers, refrigerant
Sodium hydroxide (NaOH)	lye
	drain cleaner (i.e. Drano)
Potassium hydroxide (KOH)	potash
Calcium hydroxide ($Ca(OH)_2$)	lime, quick lime
	plaster, mortar, cement
	whitewash
Magnesium hydroxide ($Mg(OH)_2$)	sparklers and flares

of acid burns is *immediate* copious irrigation. Irrigation immediately is more important than whether one irrigates with water or saline. Use whatever is available and not toxic to the eye. If particulate matter is involved, check the cul-de-sacs during irrigation. Treat with appropriate topical antibiotics and cycloplegia.

Alkali burns at their best are bad and are usually awful. Table 14-3 describes some clinically significant alkalies in order of their ability to penetrate the eye. Ammonia, soluble in both water and lipid, rapidly penetrates corneal epithelium and stroma causing the worst ocular injuries. Sodium hydroxide (lye) is the most common cause of ocular alkali burns, due to its availability and use as a drain cleaner (Drano, Liquid Plumber). Calcium hydroxide is a component of plaster, cement, mortar and white-wash, substances not commonly thought of as alkali. Fortunately it penetrates the eye poorly. Take care to remove all particulate matter from eyes exposed to these materials.

The sequelae and long-term treatment of ocular alkali burns is beyond the scope of this chapter. The cornerstone of treatment is immediate irrigation with any available nontoxic liquid, usually water. More irrigation is better than less, but 30 minutes usually suffices. The pH in the cul-de-sac can be checked as an endpoint of treatment. If in doubt, irrigate more. Search for and remove particulate matter. Inspect fornices and sweep with a wet Q-tip if necessary. Paracentesis and irrigation of the anterior chamber with a sterile phosphate buffer has been shown to reduce the pH of the aqueous in severe alkali burns.[1] Its role is not yet clearly established. Topical antibiotics and cycloplegics should be used. Intraocular pressure is controlled with carbonic anhydrase inhibitors and timolol as necessary or if the intraocular pressure cannot be measured. Topical steroids are thought to be relatively safe for the first 7-10 days after injury, even if the epithelium is not intact. If the epithelium is not intact, topical steroids should be discontinued after the first week so as not to inhibit the reparative process and abet ulceration. If the epithelium is intact, topical steroids may be continued after the first week.

Soft contact lenses with high oxygen permeability may aid epithelial healing and are fit immediately or as soon as feasible after injury. To prevent corneal ulceration, include the timely use and discontinuation of topical steroids, collagenase inhibitors and topical and systemic ascorbate. H-acetylcysteine (Mucomyst) is a commercially available collagenase inhibitor that may be started immediately and administered topically every four hours. Methoxyprogesterone is currently being evaluated as an inhibitor of collagenase synthesis. Clinical trials presently in progress are evaluating topical and systemic ascorbate as an aid to collagen synthesis.

Blunt Ocular Trauma

Blunt Injuries to the Anterior Globe. Eyes ruptured after blunt ocular trauma are rarely salvageable; but an attempt should be made to repair them primarily. Lesser contusive injuries may cause a variety of ocular damage (Table 14-1).

Traumatic Hyphema. Traumatic hyphemae are a common sequelae to blunt ocular trauma. Blood in the anterior chamber may cause systemic manifestations including nausea, vomiting, disorientation, and lethargy. These signs can mimic signs of elevated intracranial pressure secondary to a closed head injury. Our non-ophthalmologist colleagues should be alerted to this when sharing in the care of a patient with a traumatic hyphema. Mechanisms of visual dysfunction following traumatic hyphema may be preventable or non-preventable. Non-preventable mechanisms are those occurring at the time of initial injury, i.e., all the sequelae to blunt ocular trauma (Table 14-1). There is little to do for these injuries until the hyphema has reabsorbed and the eye quieted. They should, however, be documented prior to discharge. Preventable causes of visual dysfunction are the sequelae to blood in the anterior chamber. These include corneal blood staining and glaucoma. Secondary glaucoma may result from plugging of the trabecular meshwork by RBCs, sickled RBCs, or ghost cells.[21-24] There is no unanimity of opinion[25,26] and few well-controlled studies[27-29] concerning the treatment of traumatic hyphema. Treatment should allow blood to reabsorb from the anterior chamber as rapidly as possible and minimize rebleeding.

Six to thirty-eight percent of traumatic hyphemas will rebleed between the second and fifth day.[27,29,30] What influences rebleeding and how may it be prevented? The size of the initial hyphema has little to do with its tendency to rebleed. Small hyphemas are just as likely to rebleed as large hyphemas.[27] Ingestion of aspirin greatly enhances the chances of rebleeding.[31,32] Although few physicians would prescribe aspirin for patients with traumatic hyphema, aspirin may be an ingredient in other pain medications, e.g., Percodan, and prescribed by the unwary physician. A compendium of aspirin-containing products is available.[33] Aspirin may also be ingested by the patient prior to seeking medical treatment. These patients have a very high rate of recurrent hemorrhage (58%) in a small series.[34]

The stereotype high-risk hyphema patient would be a chronic aspirin ingestor with sickle cell trait and an "8-ball" hyphema. Complete or "8-

ball" hyphemas have a worse prognosis than smaller hyphemas. Intraocular pressures are more difficult to control and pressure rises are higher. Patients with sickle cell trait have a greater risk of rebleeding and hemorrhagic complications.[22,23] Sickle cell screening should be obtained in any black patient with a traumatic hyphema. Such high-risk patients require more aggressive management than those with uncomplicated hyphema. Platelet transfusions may be given to treat aspirin ingestion.[34] Uncontrolled intraocular pressures or early corneal blood staining should prompt early surgical treatment.[22,23] Surgical approaches include simple irrigation/aspiration, peripheral iridectomy,[35] removal of clot with vitrectomy instrumentation, irrigation/aspiration through a trabeculectomy incision, and manual expression of the clot through a large incision. All these techniques have their advocates. The appropriate technique is that with which the operating surgeon feels most comfortable. These eyes are not easy to operate on. They are inflamed and bleed profusely. Visual differentiation of iris and fibrin clot is often difficult. We advocate the least amount of surgery that will allow control of intraocular pressure and reabsorption of blood while minimizing the risk of rebleeding.

The vast majority of hyphema patients do not require surgery. Hyphema management is primarily a medical problem of preventing rebleeding and controlling intraocular pressure. Many regimens and medications have been tried (few in a randomized, controlled manner) and all have their vocative advocates.[25,26] Most agree that bed rest, patching, shielding the involved eye, sedation as necessary, and avoidance of aspirin are acceptable treatment. Many medications, both topical and systemic, have been advocated to either prevent rebleeding or hasten absorption of blood. Cycloplegics, miotics, topical and systemic steroids, estrogens and aminocaproic acid (Amicar) all have their advocates. Only Amicar has been shown in double-blind controlled studies to be more effective than placebo in preventing secondary hemorrhage in traumatic hyphema.[28,29,36] Treatment with systemic Prednisone (40 mg/day) has been observed to markedly minimize rebleeding,[37,38] but this has not been convincingly documented or confirmed by a double-blind controlled study.[27] Both systemic steroids and Amicar may have significant side-effects.[25,26,39] We have noted rebleeding with both agents. Neither agent is a panacea.

Treatment goals of traumatic hyphema require minimizing manipulation to prevent rebleeding and to let the blood reabsorb. We hospitalize all hyphemas, be they microscopic or "8-ball," for a minimum of five days or until the hyphema has resorbed. Visual acuity, size of hyphema, intraocular pressure and any obvious ocular damage are documented. The eye is patched and shielded. The patient is placed at bed rest with bathroom privileges. The head of the bed is elevated to 30 degrees. Appropriate sedation and antiemetics are administered as required. We try to avoid topical medications to minimize manipulation of the injured eye. Medications administered twice daily are preferred. They can be administered by the ophthalmologist himself at least daily during ocular examination. If the patient was previously dilated or cycloplegia is necessary for comfort, we administer atropine 1% bid to avoid motion of the iris. Corneal abrasions are treated with antibiotic ointment instilled after daily examination. Elevated intraocular pressure is treated with Timoptic ¼% or ½% bid Diamox 500 mg sequels bid are added as necessary to maintain pressure in the normal range. Intraocular pressure not responding to this regimen is treated with hyperosmotics, e.g., oral glycerol or intravenous mannitol. If pressures remain unresponsive or corneal blood staining appears, the clot is evacuated surgically. Total or "8-ball" hyphemas are likely to be unresponsive to medical control of intraocular pressure and require surgical intervention.

Our treatment of uncomplicated hyphema is hospitalization, bed rest with bathroom privileges, patching and shielding the involved eye, elevation of head of bed to 30 degrees, sedation, antibiotics and laxatives as necessary, and strict avoidance of aspirin-containing compounds. No topical medications are routinely used. Recently we have added Amicar 100 mg/kg/q4h to a maximum dose of 30 mg/24 hours for five days without any untoward side-effects.[28,29] Nausea is treated with an antiemetic of choice (Compazine 10 mg). We examine patients daily to detect rebleeding, which in our experience is almost always accompanied by pain. A hyphema patient complaining of pain should be re-examined expeditiously. If the eye has rebled, the intraocular pressure should be determined and, if elevated, treated. We have observed markedly elevated intraocular pressures (60-80 mm Hg) occurring immediately after a secondary hemorrhage. These patients have not responded to medical management and subsequently required surgery to control their intraocular pressure. Intraocular pressures should be determined by applanation. Patients are hospitalized for at least five days or until their hyphemas have completely resorbed. Prior to discharge patients are dilated for indirect ophthalmoscopy. Activity is restricted for two additional weeks. On a follow-up visit at two weeks, gonioscopy and peripheral retinal examination are performed. Yearly ophthalmologic examinations are advised to detect late onset angle recession glaucoma.

Blunt Injuries to the Posterior Globe.

Blunt injury to the posterior segment may be transmitted with little anterior segment trauma. Traumatic maculopathy can be extremely disabling. In the acute stage, subretinal hemorrhage, retinal edema, and a macular hole can be seen in the central macular area (Figure 14-10). In the chronic stage, light pigment stippling is apparent on ophthalmoscopy (Figure 14-11). Fluorescein angiography is helpful in demonstrating the degree of macular and foveal involvement of the retinal pigment epithelium (Figure 14-12). Peripapillary choroidal ruptures are often associated with a macular hemorrhage. A crescentic papillo-centric break in Bruch's membrane will be seen in the chronic phase (Figure 14-13). Often this is observed acutely by a subretinal hemorrhage (Figure 14-10). Blunt trauma probably causes similar changes in the peripheral retina much more frequently (Figure 14-14). Since the peripheral visual deficits are not evaluated acutely, they are much less frequently detected. The same acute changes of retinal hemorrhage, retinal edema, and, more rarely, jagged retinal breaks are apparent. After several weeks, white choroidal ruptures, pigment stippling, retinal pigmented epithelial hyperplasia, and RPE depigmentation are seen. In the chronic phase, subretinal neovascular membranes originating from the

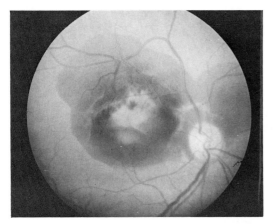

Figure 14-10. Subretinal and retinal hemorrhage in the macula from blunt trauma transmitted from the anterior segment.

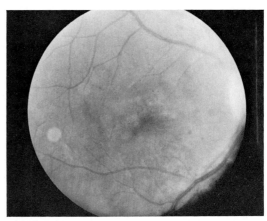

Figure 14-11. Pigment stippling in the macula from old contusive injury.

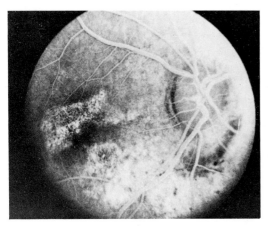

Figure 14-12. Fluorescein angiography accentuates retinal pigmented epithelial (RPE) injury from old contusive injury.

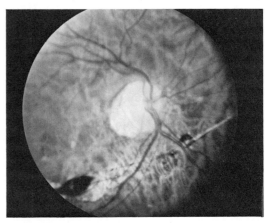

Figure 14-13. Crescentic papilla-centric break in Bruch's membrane seen after contusive injury.

breaks in Bruch's membrane can occur. Treatment with laser photocoagulation is probably indicated if the subretinal neovascular membrane threatens the foveal region.[40]

In an extremely severe contusive injury of the globe, such as that seen after a bullet passing through the orbit without rupturing the globe, large choroidal hemorrhages and edema may be seen. Here the retina is lifted high above its usual position on the convex surface of a choroidal hemorrhage. Occasionally, small to moderate amounts of vitreous hemorrhage are present without an apparent tear or hole in the retina. This occurs by rupture of retinal vessels due to the acute shearing action of a shock wave passing through the globe at the time of the injury. The choroidal hemorrhage and edema as well as the vitreous hemorrhage will resolve with appropriate treatment of the periorbital injuries.

Peripheral retinal tears can occur acutely when there is substantial blunt trauma to the globe, such as being struck by a wooden broom or axe handle or by a squash or tennis ball. Since these tears mainly occur at the level of the ora serrata, indirect ophthalmoscopy with scleral depression is usually required for their detection and confirmation. Frequently, these eyes will have a hyphema which is a contraindication to scleral depression, acutely. Additionally, the lids and periorbital tissue may be swollen and tender, making scleral depression difficult if not impossible. These patients should, therefore, be followed closely with indirect ophthalmoscopy without scleral depression for a week or two. At two weeks it is safer and more comfortable to scleral depress and perform a complete examination of the peripheral retina. Retinal tears and detachment can also occur at sites of peripheral retinal atrophy from old or new contusive trauma.[41] Therefore, it is important to inform patients with peripheral blunt trauma that they need to be followed indefinitely at regular intervals with indirect ophthalmoscopy to detect retinal tears and detachment. They should also be informed of the signs and symptoms of detachment, so they will promptly seek medical care in the event of this late complication.

Blunt, contusive trauma can also result in scleral rupture. Defection of occult scleral lacerations or intraocular foreign bodies may be aided by demonstrating intraocular air on computed tomography. Usually, this

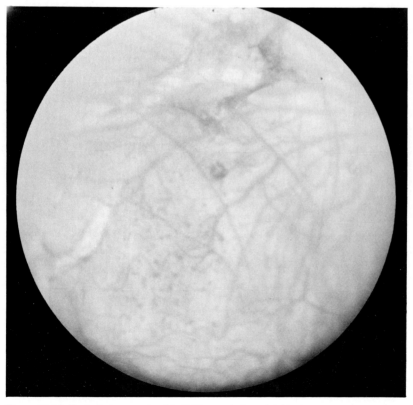

Figure 14-14. Retinal pigmented epithelial hyperplasia and depigmentation after peripheral retinal contusive injury.

occurs where the sclera is thinnest, just posterior to the insertion of the four recti muscles. The sclera is also thin in an equatorially-oriented circle connecting the posterior aspect of the insertion sites of the four recti muscles. Contusive, choroidal ruptures will therefore often extend equatorially along this circle. Massive, subconjunctival hemorrhage and swelling usually accompany this event. Intraocular and vitreous hemorrhage are usually present. These findings are often obscured by a hyphema. Computed tomography and careful ultrasonography may support the suspicion of an occult scleral rupture, if there has been a loss of ocular volume. If you have a strong suspicion that the globe is ruptured, it is better to err on the side of exploring the globe. A careful limbal peritomy is performed. The sclera anterior to the ora serrata is explored initially. Then explore the sclera posteriorly in all four quadrants. Finally, explore beneath the four rectus muscles.

The Open Globe

Penetrating Ocular Injuries and the Open Globe. A laceration of the globe is a relative emergency and should be promptly repaired. A recent review, however, demonstrated little difference in eventual visual outcome in eyes immediately repaired and when repair was delayed for 24 hours.[42] Management includes prevention of infection and surgical repair of the laceration with restoration of the integrity of the globe. We routinely utilize broad spectrum intravenous antibiotics preoperatively and continue them for 48-72 hours postoperatively. Intravenous administration is necessary to achieve blood levels sufficiently high to be effective. Such levels cannot be obtained with oral antibiotics. Antibiotic prophylaxis for longer than 48-72 hours has little therapeutic benefit and selects for resistant organisms.

Various antibiotic regimens are appropriate as long as broad spectrum coverage is attained. Anaerobes should be covered if suspected by history. Our typical intravenous antibiotic regimen would be:

Aminoglycoside (Garamycin) 80 mg q8h

Cephalosporin (Ancef) 1 gm q4h

Clindamycin (Cleocin) 300 mg tid if anaerobes suspected

Periocular antibiotics are administered at the conclusion of surgery.

Garamycin 20 mg

Ancef 150 mg

Cleocin 30 mg (if anaerobes suspected)

Postoperatively, intravenous antibiotics are continued for 48-72 hours and a broad spectrum topical antibiotic (Garamycin) is applied every 4 hours.

Surgical Repair. All degrees of difficulty are encountered when repairing a lacerated or ruptured globe. Specific surgical techniques are discussed later in this chapter, but certain principles should be stressed now. General anesthesia should be utilized. Your anesthesia team should be reminded that you are dealing with a potentially or obviously open globe. Intubation should be atraumatic. Depolarizing agents causing tetanic contractions (succinylcholine) with possible extrusion of intraocular contents should be avoided. Prep the eye yourself to ensure gentle handling. When in doubt, explore! If you suspect an occult laceration or rupture of the globe, and if you cannot rule it out after your examination, explore the globe under general anesthesia. If there is a question of an occult intraocular foreign body, repair the laceration and re-evaluate postoperatively.

Complete indirect ophthalmoscopy may be precluded by media opacities. High resolution computed tomography with 1½ to 2 mm overlapping sections through the globe may then detect an occult foreign body. We believe that the scan should be obtained after primary wound closure. A better study is obtained with closed globe and you don't risk extrusion of the ocular contents through the laceration site as a result of heavy-handed or misguided manipulations. When an intraocular foreign body is detected, appropriate surgery or referral is expedited.

Sympathetic Ophthalmia. The dreaded sequela to the traumatized eye is sympathetic ophthalmia, a bilateral, granulomatous, panuveitis following ocular trauma or surgery. It may occur from ten days to many years after the inciting injury, eighty percent of cases occurring within three months.[43] Its incidence has declined dramatically since its recognition and now complicates about 0.1% of ocular injuries in the United States. It is now sufficiently rare that many younger ophthalmologists may never see a case. However, any perforating injury to the eye and some contusive injuries may incite sympathetic ophthalmia,[43,44,45] especially in cases where iris or ciliary body has prolapsed. Incidences of sympathetic ophthalmia as high as 3-5% have been reported in trauma cases when the traumatized eye suffered uveal prolapse and was not enucleated.[45] Early enucleation prevents sympathetic ophthalmia. We believe an attempt should be made to repair all ruptured or lacerated globes primarily. Postoperatively, the patient is re-evaluated when awake and alert. The visual status and integrity of the globe are determined by examination, and ultrasonography if necessary. If the eye is blind and disorganized beyond surgical restoration, it should be enucleated to prevent sympathetic ophthalmia. Early enucleation within 8-10 days of injury is preferable. Enucleation within two weeks of injury almost always prevents the development of sympathetic ophthalmia.[45]

Penetrating Injuries to the Posterior Globe.

Penetrating injuries which appear to involve only the anterior segment may involve the retina and vitreous primarily and more frequently secondarily. A dart injury which appeared to involve only the peri-limbal sclera, sparing the lens (Figure 14-15A), actually perforated the entire vitreous depth, penetrating the retina posteriorly near the optic nerve (Figure 14-15B). Vitreous fibrosis extending from the anterior wound eventually necessitated lensectomy and vitrectomy to interrupt the anterior posterior fibrous traction (Figure 14-15C). Epi-retinal fibrosis from the posterior scar, however, resulted in distortion and localized detachment of the central foveolar region (Figure 14-15D). More frequently, a sharp perforation of the anterior segment by a needle-like object will traverse the cornea, iris, and lens. Repair of the cornea, removal of the cataractous lens, and anterior vitrectomy will restore

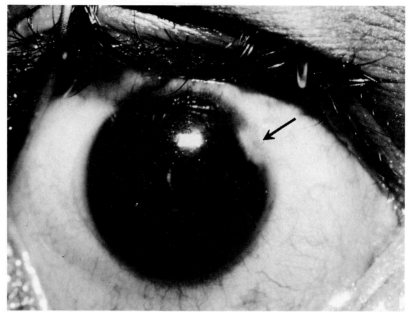

Figure 14-15A

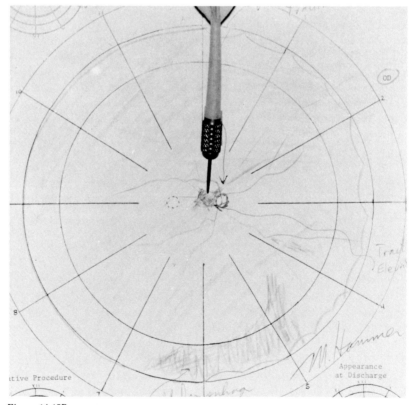

Figure 14-15B

Figure 14-15A. Perilimbal site of anterior dart penetration. (➤) Arrow. Figure 14-15B. This retinal drawing shows the posterior perforation of the dart.

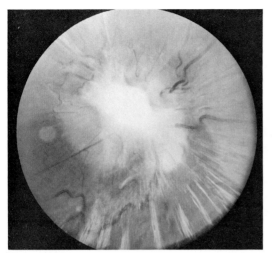
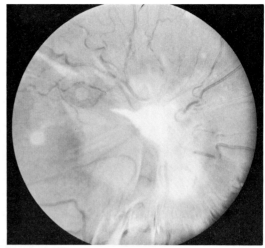

Figure 14-15C   Figure 14-15D

Figure 14-15C. Tenting of the posterior retina from epiretinal and anterior-posterior vitreo-retinal traction. Figure 14-15D. Postoperative epi-retinal distortion from fibrosis at posterior dart perforation site.

the anterior segment function. A peripheral, chorioretinal scar will often be seen where the object either penetrated or touched the peripheral retina. No additional therapy is usually required if an adequate anterior vitrectomy has been performed. These lesions should be observed on a regular and indefinite basis postoperatively, as they can progress to a retinal tear with retinal detachment.

Secondary involvement of the retina occurs if vitreous has been incarcerated in a corneal wound. Fibrosis along the vitreous fibrils with subsequent contraction results in a retinal tear at the posterior vitreous base. This leads to a rhegmatogenous retinal detachment. Such cases can also progress to severe proliferative vitreo-retinopathy with preretinal and subretinal fibrosis and traction detachment (Figure 14-16A). Advanced vitreous techniques involving preretinal and subretinal fibrous membrane dissection, intraocular gas fluid exchange, and scleral buckling are indicated (Figure 14-16B).

In posterior lacerations of the globe, the cornea, anterior chamber, iris, and lens may all be relatively uninvolved. There is a potential for seeing the internal aspect of a posterior perforation with the indirect ophthalmoscope. If the fundus can be examined merely by using a dilating drop without manipulation or pressure on the globe, the examination will be very helpful for planning treatment of posterior segment involvement. At the very least orbital x-rays are required to detect an occult intraocular foreign body. If there is a moderate suspicion of an intraocular foreign body, a high resolution CT scan should be obtained. X-ray and CT scan may be delayed until after surgery when expeditious. Broad spectrum intravenous antibiotics should be started immediately. Topical antibiotic drops should not be given at this time due to their toxicity to the exposed intraocular contents.

Surgical Technique. The patient is then taken promptly to the operating room where closure of the scleral laceration is performed. The anesthe-

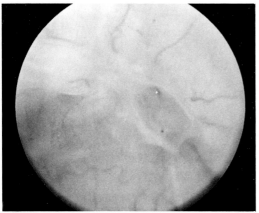
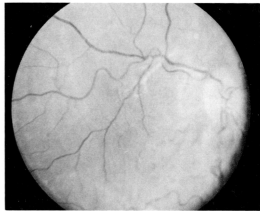

Figure 14-16A   Figure 14-16B

Figure 14-16A. Total retinal detachment with advanced proliferative retinopathy after perforation of anterior segment.
Figure 14-16B. Postoperative retinal reattachment of Figure 14-18A after preretinal and subretinal fibrous membrane
dissection, intraocular gas-fluid exchange, and scleral buckling.

siologist is instructed not to use rapid depolarizing agents such as succinylcholine since this will result in further extrusion of intraocular
contents from massive contracture of the lid and extraocular muscles.
Careful lid retraction is best achieved with 4-0 silk sutures placed through
the lid margins. Dissection of the conjunctiva, episclera, and Tenon's tissue
overlying the most anterior part of the scleral wound is then performed
using sharp dissection. As soon as the scleral edges of both sides of the
laceration are visualized from the most anterior part of the scleral laceration, a suture is placed through both sides of the scleral laceration to
approximate it. It is important during the procedure not to place any undue
pressure on the globe. If the laceration appears to be relatively wide and
difficult to approximate, a larger suture such as 5-0 mersaline is used. If the
laceration is relatively small and easy to approximate, a finer suture such as
8-0 monofilament nylon may be used. A sharp spatula needle with a swaged
suture finds easy scleral passage, and is less likely to result in further
compression or distortion of the globe. After the anterior part of the
laceration is closed with widely spaced sutures, the posterior or further
extent of the laceration is exposed by careful dissection of overlying tissues.
The exposed portion of the laceration is closed as noted above. This
process is repeated until the entire laceration has been closed with relatively widely spaced sutures. It is not uncommon for these lacerations to
extend beneath the rectus muscles. When necessary for atraumatic closure
of the globe, the rectus muscle is cut from its insertion and tagged with a
suitable suture such as 7-0 chromic catgut. Once the entire extent of the
wound has been closed with relatively widely spaced sutures, additional
sutures of 8-0 nylon should be placed between the previously placed
sutures. Attempts should be made to place these sutures through almost
full-thickness sclera without injuring the choroid or the retina. One suture
should be placed approximately every millimeter along the entire length of

the scleral laceration. The scleral laceration should appear to be reasonably well approximated. Some of the initial sutures usually have to be removed when the final extent of the wound is discovered. Stellate lacerations often are approximated incorrectly by the initial few sutures. During the closure process, copious and continuing hemorrhage is often encountered. This requires able assistance including frequent and ample irrigation with balanced salt solution, careful sponging with cellulose sponges, and delicate retraction. Prolapsed vitreous should be excised with the Vannas scissors and cellulose sponges. Exposed choroidal and retinal tissue should be reposited, unless it is obviously necrotic or too far out of the wound to be atraumatically reposited.

In the event of a small peripheral scleral laceration involving a small retinal perforation and a small amount of vitreous hemorrhage, scleral closure alone may suffice. If the wound is larger with probable retinal incarceration, retino-cryopexy and a local scleral buckle are performed in anticipation of delayed vitreo-retinal traction. The wound should then be carefully watched for development of vitreous traction and fibrous ingrowth. Many of these wounds will stabilize and not require further treatment with retention of excellent visual acuity. Some, however, will develop progressive vitreo-retinal fibrosis with subsequent retinal detachment often progressing to proliferative vitreo-retinopathy. If a shallow peripheral retinal detachment does develop, it may be treated initially with a scleral buckle. If there is obvious, rapid detachment with extensive traction or if there is a recurrent traction detachment after scleral buckling, posterior vitrectomy is indicated. The obvious goal of the vitrectomy is to interrupt vitreo-retinal and epi-retinal traction. There is usually fibrous proliferation along the anterior hyaloid face which is adherent to or directly apposed to the posterior lens capsule. If the lens is cataractous, it should be removed so that this membrane can be completely excised, peripherally. There is controversy as to whether or not a clear lens should be removed in this situation. The sacrifice of a clear lens is justified by the urgent requirement of complete removal and peripheral trimming of the anterior hyaloid face.[46] Vitreo-retinal traction between the ciliary body and peripheral retina is also much more likely to be thoroughly relieved after a lensectomy.

If a posterior scleral laceration results in sufficient hemorrhage to prevent indirect ophthalmoscopy (especially if the laceration site is not visible), a posterior vitrectomy is indicated. This is justified by the high incidence of total retinal detachment complicated by proliferative vitreo-retinopathy in such cases. It is felt that early posterior vitrectomy improves the prognosis in these cases. There is controversy as to the exact timing of vitrectomy. One study indicates that posterior vitrectomy at the time of the repair of the initial scleral laceration gives the best long-term results.[47] It is more widely believed that secondary posterior vitrectomy performed between three and fourteen days after the initial repair is preferable.[48,49] If the posterior laceration is caused by a sharp object with little contusive injury, earlier vitrectomy is preferred. If there is substantial periorbital and ocular contusion, a later vitrectomy time is selected so that choroidal hemorrhage and edema will have subsided.

Corneal opacities and irregularities from the original trauma can make routine posterior pars plana vitrectomy difficult or impossible. A specially-designed keratoprosthesis can be inserted in an 8.0 mm corneal trephine incision to improve posterior segment visualization.[50] Pars plana vitrectomy is then performed (Figure 14-17A and B). The keratoprosthesis is replaced with a corneal donor button after the posterior vitrectomy.

The ophthalmologist will occasionally encounter iatrogenic posterior perforations of the globe. The most common is perforation of the globe during placement of the scleral suture during muscle surgery. Withdrawal of the suture and placement of a small amount of cryopexy around the perforation site is usually adequate treatment. The patient is followed postoperatively to make sure that delayed retinal detachment does not occur. Much less frequently intraocular injection may occur during injection of a periorbital medication. In the case of an intraocular depo-steroid injection this can easily occur when periocular steroids are injected in a patient with rheumatoid scleritis (Figure 14-18). Immediate pars plana vitrectomy is indicated. The preservatives and other toxic substances in this medication will cause retinal necrosis. If the substance is promptly removed from retinal contact, some retinal viability may be retained. In one case the retina became necrotic, developed large tears and total retinal detachment when removal of this substance was delayed. It is seldom necessary to repair the perforation site itself, unless profound hypotony is present. In the case of the patient with scleromalacia secondary to rheumatoid scleritis, a rupture of the globe occurred on the opposite side of the globe from the injection site. The globe is thought to have ruptured at a point weakened by rheumatoid scleritis when the intraocular pressure was acutely elevated by intraocular injection of the steroid (Figure 14-18). In this patient repair of the sclera was required.

Posterior Segment Intraocular Foreign Bodies. The detection of an intraocular foreign body is a problem in the general emergency

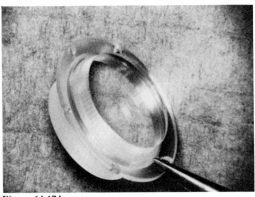
Figure 14-17A

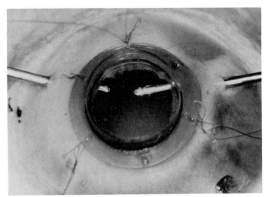
Figure 14-17B

Figure 14-17A. A specially-designed keratoprosthesis for closed vitrectomy combined with penetrating keratoplasty in patients with corneal opacities who require posterior vitrectomy. Figure 14-17B. Keratoprosthesis with pars plana vitrectomy instruments in place.

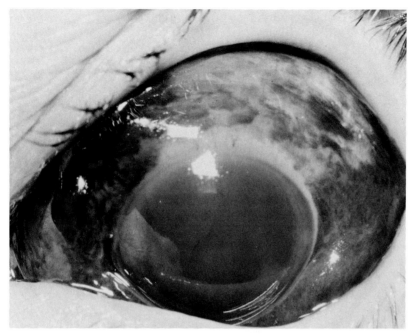

Figure 14-18. Scleral rupture at a point weakened by rheumatoid scleritis on the opposite site of the iatrogenic intraocular injection site.

room. In one case a disgruntled lover disintegrated his lower jaw with a shotgun in full view of his young lady. She was immediately examined in the emergency room where numerous small lacerations were seen about her face (Figure 14-19A). She complained of irritation of her left eye. Her visual acuity was completely normal at that time. No other abnormality was noted. She was treated with topical antibiotic drops. Three days later she returned to a different emergency room complaining of an acute decrease in her visual acuity. A hypopyon was noted in the anterior chamber of the left eye at that time. On slit lamp evaluation a small self-sealing corneal perforation approximately one millimeter long was seen in the peripheral cornea (Figure 14-19B). The lens was still completely clear. A small, opaque object was seen in the vitreous. Computed tomography confirmed a bone or tooth density foreign body in the anterior peripheral vitreous (Figure 14-19C). Prompt, pars plana vitrectomy, removal of the intraocular bone fragment, and antibiotic irrigation of the posterior segment resulted in recovery of phakic 20/20 vision in this eye (Figure 14-19D).

Whenever there is the remotest possibility of an intraocular foreign body, posterior anterior, lateral, and Water's view of the orbital contents should be obtained. If the suspicion of an intraocular foreign body is slightly greater or if there has been a perforation of the globe, a high resolution CT scan should be obtained. It is important to request closely spaced, overlapping cuts usually of two millimeters or less through the orbital region. The CT scan has a better ability to detect intraocular foreign bodies than the ordinary skull films. The CT scan has brought to the general hospital the sophistication of detection and localization of intra-

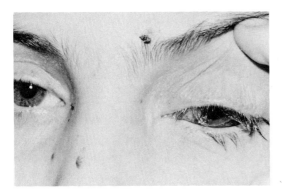

Figure 14-19A

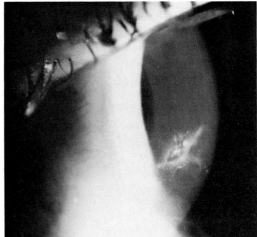

Figure 14-19B

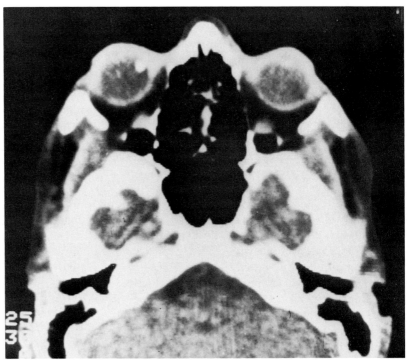

Figure 14-19C

Figure 14-19A. Multiple punctate facial lacerations of witness to attempted suicide with a shotgun. Figure 14-19B. Small, self-sealing peripheral corneal laceration caused by bone or tooth fragment. Figure 14-19C. Computed tomography confirming bone density foreign body in the anterior peripheral vitreous.

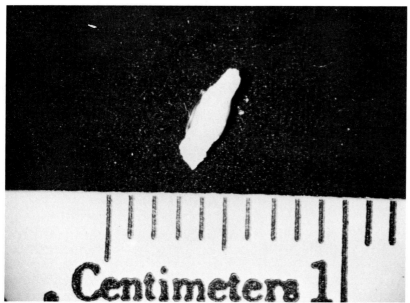

Figure 14-19D

Figure 14-19D. Bone fragment removed from vitreous with vitrectomy techniques.

ocular foreign bodies formerly available only in a few eye centers. The decision of whether or not to remove an intraocular foreign body is usually clear but occasionally is difficult. Iron foreign bodies which are not of the rust-resistant type and copper-containing foreign bodies except for marine brass usually require prompt removal. The composition of the intraocular foreign body can be deduced from the conditions of the initial accident. A cupric or brassy appearance or the early appearance of brownish rust or greenish corrosion on the foreign body can be helpful. For the magnetic foreign bodies a weak magnetic field is applied by holding an electromagnet at some distance from the eye. Magnetically-induced movement is seen with the indirect ophthalmoscope. If the foreign body is not directly visible with the indirect ophthalmoscope, induced movement can be detected using B-scan ultrasonography for visualization.

A very small ferrous or cupric foreign body may be present in the peripheral part of the eye with retention of good visual acuity initially. Is it worth undertaking vitrectomy and foreign body extraction in an eye with a visual acuity of 20/40 or better to prevent the possibility of future onset of toxic metallosis of the retina? It is reasonable to follow this patient with serial electroretinography. If the A-wave amplitude increases abnormally, early toxic retinal metallosis is present, especially if there is an accompanying decreased B-wave amplitude.[51] This is a definite indication for prompt extraction of the foreign body. The electroretinographic and retinal toxic changes are reversible if the foreign body is removed at this stage.

Glass, plastic, ceramic, stone, and other apparently nontoxic substances are tolerated as intraocular foreign bodies indefinitely. Certain special glasses, however, contain metal salts which promote an inflammatory reaction in the eye and are toxic to the retina. This has been specifically demonstrated for photo-gray glass.[52] In a rabbit model, copper, silver, cobalt, nickel, and halides contained in this glass promoted an abnormal amount of vitreous inflammatory response.[53] Such chemical activity justifies early extraction of these toxic foreign bodies.

A 10-year-old boy was shooting BB pellets at a concrete sewer pipe. A ricochetting BB struck his photo-gray glasses resulting in a laceration of the cornea (Figure 14-20A & B). After primary repair of the cornea, a large traumatic iris coloboma and moderately advanced cataract were present. Computed tomography (Figure 14-20C & D) showed a discoid intraocular foreign body matching in shape and size the entire missing fracture cone from the photo-gray glasses. Prompt lensectomy, vitrectomy, and removal of the nine millimeter photo-gray glass fracture-cone was performed. No postoperative fragments were noted in the eye on x-ray study. With a contact lens refraction, 20/20 visual acuity was recovered.

When a small, intraocular foreign body of unknown but suspected benign composition is retained in the eye with relatively good visual acuity, the decision to observe rather than remove the foreign body is warranted. It is prudent to follow such a patient with serial electroretinography until you are convinced that there are no progressive changes of retinal toxicity from the foreign body. Polymethylmethacrylate anterior and posterior chamber lenses occasionally will dislocate into the vitreous cavity. If the intraocular lens becomes fixed to the wall of the eye in an area away from the visual axis, it is not necessary to remove the intraocular lens. Close follow-up with the indirect ophthalmoscope is warranted to detect the possibility of retinal tears and subsequent detachment. If an intraocular lens with sharp edges or of substantial size does not become fixed to the wall of the peripheral retina, extraction is necessary. The justification for extraction is that continued trauma to the retina will result in retinal tears and detachment or in an accumulation of blunt trauma to the fovea resulting in decreased visual acuity.

Surgical Technique. There are a variety of techniques for the actual

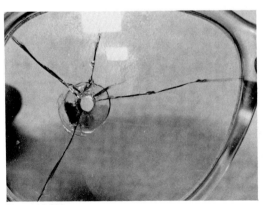

Figure 14-20A

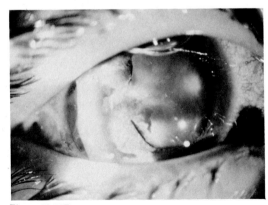

Figure 14-20B

Figure 14-20A. Photo-gray lens shattered by ricocheting BB. Figure 14-20B. Corneal laceration closed at time of original injury.

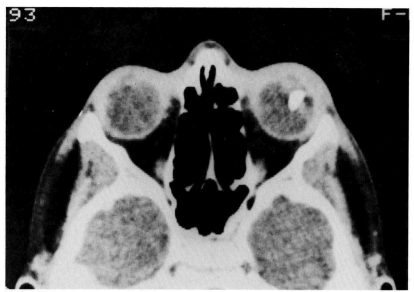

Figure 14-20C

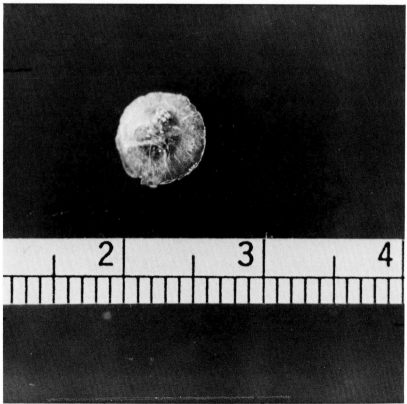

Figure 14-20D

Figure 14-20C. Computed tomography showing a discoid intraocular foreign body matching in size and shape the entire missing fracture cone from the photo-gray glasses. Figure 14-20D. Top view of glass foreign body.

removal of intraocular foreign bodies. The enormous number of variables involved in the creation of the wound, in the composition and position of the intraocular foreign body, and in the equipment on hand for removal of the foreign body make each one of these cases nearly unique. In the case of a magnetic intraocular foreign body, there is substantial literature discussing the techniques of magnetic extraction through the pars plana for vitreous foreign bodies and through a scleral and retinal incision directly overlying the foreign body when it was adherent to the retinal surface.[54] The recent development of sophisticated pars plana vitrectomy and vitreo-retinal membrane dissection techniques has supplanted the earlier magnetic extraction technique. The development of diamond-studded intraocular foreign body forceps and rare earth magnets formed to a 20 gauge needle diameter have assisted in delicate manipulation and controlled removal of intraocular foreign bodies. The ability of the surgeon to control the removal trajectory of an intraocular foreign body is an important advantage to the pars plana vitrectomy approach. Magnetic extraction through the pars plana of a partially-tethered magnetic foreign body could result in unanticipated damage to the lens and retina. Magnetic extraction of a small fibrosed foreign body on the retinal surface through a lamellar scleral flap was often unsuccessful and could result in localized vitreo-retinal incarceration and distortion of the retina. Nevertheless, one series did not show a clear advantage of pars plana extraction with vitrectomy techniques over the older direct posterior extraction techniques.[54] In the case of nonmagnetic foreign bodies, the vitrectomy technique and newer intraocular foreign body forceps have been a clear boon to extraction of these foreign bodies. Diamond-studded foreign body forceps have been particularly valuable in the removal of hard, irregular, glass-like foreign bodies or round, smooth metallic foreign bodies which previously were difficult to grasp and even more difficult to maintain a stable grip upon.[55]

An eleven-year-old girl sustained an anterior scleral laceration and intraocular foreign body after a bottle rocket blew up inside a coke bottle. The intraocular foreign body was estimated to be 12 millimeters by 4 millimeters by 5 millimeters. It had an approximately rhomboidal, prismatic shape and was composed of clear, white glass with numerous sharp edges (Figure 14-21A). The peripheral laceration was through the ciliary body and pars plana region. It was closed the day of admission. The foreign body settled to the inferior aspect of the globe as the patient was placed in the sitting, upright position. Her visual acuity remained 20/20. The lens was clear and completely uninvolved by the injury. Over the following week the foreign body became fibrosed down and suspended above the retinal surface by fibrous bands. The patient was discharged home and followed with instructions not to participate in active sports and to restrict her activities accordingly. She did well and retained 20/20 vision for a year-and-a-half at which time an inferior retinal detachment was noted. Scleral buckling was performed with initial retinal reattachment. One month later the retina redetached with progressive proliferative vitreo-retinopathy (Figure 14-21B & C). Vitrectomy with extraction of the intraocular foreign body was performed. Although the lens remained clear and compatible with 20/20 vision, it was decided to remove the lens so that limbal extraction of this

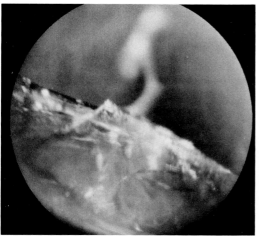
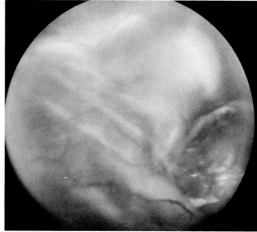

Figure 14-21A   Figure 14-21B

Figure 14-21A. Superior edge of a large irregular intraocular glass foreign body. Figure 14-21B. Retinal detachment around intraocular foreign body.

large, intraocular foreign body would be performed. The foreign body was removed without complication (Figure 14-21D). Air-fluid exchange and revision of the scleral buckle was performed. Postoperatively, the best visual acuity with contact lens refraction was 20/40. The patient, however, was never able to comfortably wear or retain a contact lens in the eye.

Primary removal of an intraocular foreign body through the initial scleral laceration is seldom indicated, unless the foreign body is actually protruding through the wound and can be easily grasped. Usually, the sclera is closed primarily by techniques described above. The intraocular foreign body is then removed at a later date after more complete studies have been performed. A reasonable argument for immediate extraction of an intraocular foreign body known to be composed of iron or copper can be made, since these foreign bodies will often be effectively encapsulated by fibrous tissue within 36 hours of the injury. Iron-containing foreign bodies are particularly prone to firm encapsulation. After dissection of the capsule by vitrectomy technique, there are often residual, fibrous strands which appear to grow directly from the foreign body. These act as microscopic tethers to the motion of a foreign body that is loosely grasped by forceps or manipulated with a magnet. Although smaller foreign bodies can be safely removed through the pars plana, larger, irregularly-shaped foreign bodies are preferably removed through the limbus even if the sacrifice of a clear lens is required. When the limbus is to be widely opened during a pars plana vitrectomy, a double Fleiringa ring should be sewn on at the beginning of the case. This will keep the globe from collapsing when vitrectomy instruments are inserted through the pars plana even if the limbal wound is incompletely closed. If an electromagnet or permanent magnet is to be used for extraction or manipulation of the foreign body, the use of a nonmagnetic lid speculum or lid sutures as well as nonmagnetic forceps and other instruments is advised. If nonmagnetic forceps are not available, the

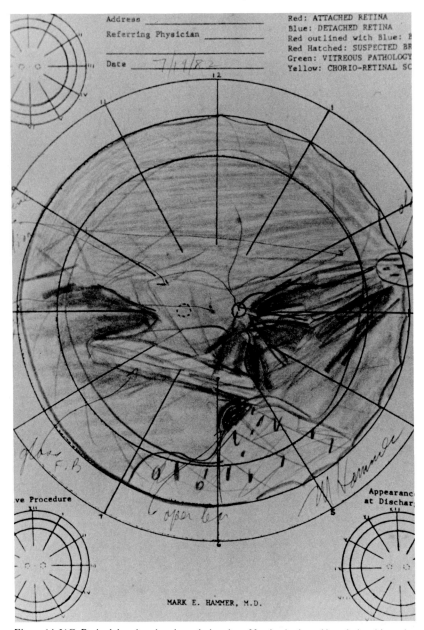

Figure 14-21C. Retinal drawing showing relative size of foreign body and its relationship to the retinal detachment.

pars plana wound may be gaped open with sutures (Figure 14-22A). These sutures are placed in the edges of the scleral wound and used to gape the wound during extraction of the metallic foreign body with the magnet (Figure 14-22B).

Prevention of endophthalmitis is another important consideration (see Chapter 15). Broad spectrum intravenous antibiotics are usually started prior to surgery. The status of tetanus immunization is also checked at this

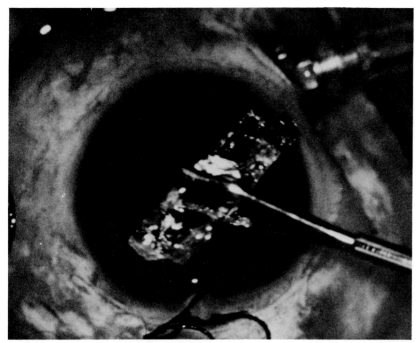

Figure 14-21D. Glass foreign body securely grasped with diamond studded forceps at the time of limbal extraction.

time. Periocular and topical antibiotics are ordinarily begun after the globe has been closed. High velocity, metallic, intraocular foreign bodies are often said to be self-sterilizing. This, however, is not always the case.

A 25-year-old man noted sudden pain and loss of vision in his right eye while working in a sawmill. He recalled rubbing his eye with his hand which was very dirty. On later inspection his hands appeared to be indelibly

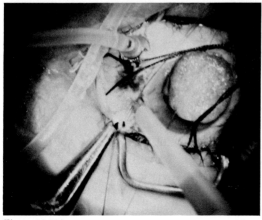

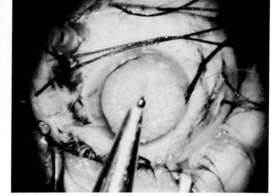

Figure 14-22A   Figure 14-22B

Figure 14-22A. Sclerotomy is gaped open with sutures during magnetic foreign body extraction. Figure 14-22B. Small iron foreign body clinging to tip of magnet immediately after pars plana extraction.

blackened with a combination of mud, grease, and other grime chronically present around the sawmill. An x-ray demonstrated a metallic intraocular foreign body. This was removed through the pars plana with a magnet (Figure 26A). The patient was treated with intravenous and subconjunctival antibiotics. Between 36 and 48 hours complete loss of vision and increasing pain was noted in the eye. After 48 hours the anterior segment was completely opaque, and there was an inferior corneal ulcer. An attempt at pars plana aspiration of the intraocular contents through an 18 gauge needle yielded only hemorrhagic, purulent material. Gram positive cocci were noted on a gram-stain of this material. The patient was begun on periocular and systemic chloramphenicol. At 72 hours the cornea had completely disintegrated, and intraocular contents were spontaneously extruded (Figure 14-23). Evisceration was performed at this time. The culture subsequently confirmed Bacillus cereus. The rapid destruction of the eye by Bacillus cereus has been reported.[56] This organism must be anticipated whenever ocular injury occurs in a dirty environment. Once Bacillus cereus is established, the vision is rarely saved. Soil contamination, a low velocity metallic foreign body, and penetrating injury involving the vitreous is a combination warranting systemic and periocular clindamycin, gentamycin and semisynthetic penicillin or cephalosporin injection. If the signs and symptoms of endophthalmitis ensue, vitrectomy combined with intraocular clindamycin injection is warranted.

The routine use of small doses of intravitreally-injected gentamycin in traumatically-induced scleral wounds has been suggested but has not been widely advocated.[57,58] Clinical experience has shown that 100 to 200 micrograms of gentamycin injected in 1/10 cc of balanced salt solution in the mid-vitreous cavity slowly through a pars plana incision is safe. Additionally, the ocular penetration of many of the popular combinations of "shotgun" systemic antibiotics is not good. Although intraocular gen-

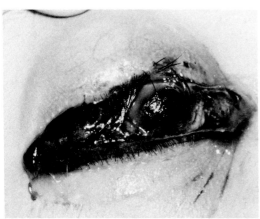

Figure 14-23A

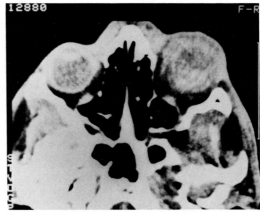

Figure 14-23B

Figure 14-23A. Corneal disintegration and extrusion of ocular contents 72 hours after Bacillus cereus inoculation by a metallic intraocular foreign body. Figure 14-23B. Computed tomography showing panophthalmitis approximately 72 hours after traumatic Bacillus cereus inoculation.

tamycin will not cover the entire spectrum of potential pathogens, it does have some activity against most of the more common organisms which cause exogenous endophthalmitis. For all the above reasons the use of prophylactic intravitreal gentamycin in perforating posterior segment trauma is reasonable.

Summary

The essentials of management of ocular trauma include documentation of visual acuity, a complete history and examination, and appropriate medical management and timely surgical intervention. Restoring the integrity of the globe, prevention of infection, clarification of ocular media and return of visual function are the treatment goals. Prevention of injury, through appropriate legislation and public education, is the treatment of choice. *(Editor)*

References
1. Paton D, Goldberg MD: Management of Ocular Injuries. Philadelphia: 1976.
2. Runyan RE: Concussive and Penetrating Injuries of the Globe and Optic Nerve. St. Louis: Mosby, 1975.
3. Callahan MA, Callahan A: Ophthalmic Plastic and Orbital Surgery. Birmingham: Aesculiapius Publishing Co., 1979.
4. Iliff CE, Iliff WJ, Iliff NT: Oculoplastic Surgery. Philadelphia: W.B. Saunders, 1979.
5. Soll DB: Management of Complications in Ophthalmic Plastic Surgery. Birmingham: Aesculapius Publishing Co., 1976.
6. McCord C: Oculoplastic Surgery. New Haven: Raven Press, 1983.
7. Jones LT, Wobis JS: Surgery of the Eyelids and Lacrimal System. Birmingham: Aesculapius Publishing Co., 1976.
8. DeJuan E, Sternberg P Jr., Michels RG: Penetrating Ocular Injuries: types of injuries and results. Ophthalmology, 90:1301-1317, 1983.
9. Fukado Y: Results of 350 Cases of Surgical Decompression of the Optic Nerve. Trans Fourth Asia-Pac Congress Ophthalmol 4:96-99, 1972.
10. Kennerdell JW, Amsbaugh GA, Myers EM: A Transantral-ethmoidal Decompression of Optic Canal Fracture. Arch Ophthalmol, 94:1040-1043, 1976.
11. Anderson RL, Pane WP, Gross CE: Optic Nerve Blindness Following Blunt Forehead Trauma. Ophthalmology, 89:445-455, 1982.
12. Sofferman RA: Spheno-ethmoidal Approach to the Optic Nerve. Laryngoscope 41:184-196, 1982.
13. Hupp SL, Buckley EG, Byrne SG, Tenzel RR, Glasner JS, Schatz NS: Post-Traumatic Venous Obstruction Retinopathy Associated with Enlarged Optic Nerve Sheath. Arch Ophthalmol, 102:254-256, 1984.
14. Hayreh SS, Kolder HE, Weingeist TA: Central Retinal Artery Occlusion and Retinal Tolerance Time. Ophthalmol, 87:75-78, 1980.
15. Varley EWB, Holt-Wilson AO, Watson PG: Acute Retinal Artery Occlusion Following Reduction of a Fractured Zyome and Its Successful Treatment. Brit J Oral Surgery, 6:31-36, 1968.
16. Younge BR, Rosenblum RJ: Treatment of Acute Central Retinal Artery Occlusion. Mayo Clin Proc, 53:408-410, 1978.
17. Holt JE, Holt GR, Glodsett JM: Ocular Injuries Sustained During Blunt Facial Trauma. Ophthalmology, 90:14-18, 1983.
18. Converse JM, Smith B, Obear MF, Wood-Smith D: Orbital Blow-Out Fractures: A Ten-Year Survey. Plast Reconstruct Surg, 39:20-36, 1967.
19. Smith B, Regan WR: Blow-Out Fracture of the Orbit. Mechanism and Correction of Internal Orbital Fracture. Am J Ophthalmol 44:733, 1957.

20. Putterman AM, Stevens T, Urist MJ: Non-surgical Management of Blow-Out Fractures of the Orbital Floor. Am J Ophthalmol, 77:232, 1974.

21. Wilensky JT: Blood Induced Secondary Glaucoma. Ann Ophthalmol, 1659-1662, 1979.

22. Goldberg MF: Sickled Erythrocytes, Hyphema and Secondary Glaucoma. Ophthal Surg, 10:17, 1979.

23. Goldberg MF: Diagnosis and Treatment of Secondary Glaucoma After Hyphema in Sickle Cell Patients. Am J Ophthalmol, 87:43, 1979.

24. Campbell DG, Simmons RJ, Grant WM: Ghost Cells As A Cause Of Glaucoma. Am J Ophthalmol, 81:441, 1976.

25. Romano P: Systemic Steroids or Aminocaproic Acid in The Management of Traumatic Hyphema?—Yes. Arch Ophthalmol 102:180-190, 1984.

26. Jampol LM, Goldberg M: In Reply. Arch Ophthalmol 102:190, 1984.

27. Spoor TC, Hammer M, Belloso H: Traumatic Hyphema: Failure of Steroids To Alter Its Course: A Double-Blind Prospective Study. Arch Ophthalmol, 98:116-119, 1980.

28. McCetrick JJ, Jampol LJ, Goldberg MF, et al: Aminocaproic Acid Decreases Secondary Hemorrhage After Traumatic Hyphema. Arch Ophthalmol 101:1031-1033, 1983.

29. Crouch ER, Frenkel M: Aminocaproic Acid in the Treatment of Traumatic Hyphema. Am J Ophthalmol, 81:355-360, 1976.

30. Rakusin W: Traumatic Hyphema. Am J Ophthalmol, 74:284-297, 1972.

31. Crawford JS, Lewandowski RL, Chan W: The Effect of Aspirin on Rebleeding in Traumatic Hyphema. Am J Ophthalmol, 80:543, 1975.

32. Gorn RA: The Detrimental Effect of Aspirin on Hyphema Rebleed. Ann Ophthalmol 11:351, 1979.

33. Leist ER, Barnwell JG: Products Containing Aspirin. New Engl J Med 291:710, 1974.

34. Gangley JP, Geiger JM, Clement JR, Rigby PG, Levey GJ: Aspirin and Recurrent Hyphema After Blunt Ocular Trauma. Am J Ophthalmol 96:797-801, 1979.

35. Parrish R, Bernardino V: Iridectomy in the Surgical Management of Eight-Ball Hyphema. Arch Ophthalmol 100:435-437, 1982.

36. Goldberg MF: Antifibrinolytic Agents in the Management of Traumatic Hyphema. Arch Ophthalmol 101:1029-1030, 1983.

37. Yasuna E: Management of Traumatic Hyphema. Arch Ophthalmol, 91:190-191, 1974.

38. Rynne MV, Romano P: Systemic Corticosteroids in the Treatment of Traumatic Hyphema. J Ped Ophthalmol Strabismus 17:141-143, 1980.

39. Fujikawa LS, Meisler DM, Mozik RA: Hyperosmolar Hyperglycemic Non-ketotic Coma: A Complication of Short-Term Systemic Corticosteroid Use. Ophthalmol 90:1239-1242, 1983.

40. Schatz H: Laser Treatment of Fundus Diseases, a comprehensive text and composite slide collection. San Anselmo, California: Pacific Medical Press, 1980, p 104.

41. Gottlieb F: Compensibility in Traumatic Retinal Detachment, Proceedings of the Conference on Subretinal Space, H Zauberman (ed), Documenta Ophthalmologica Proceedings Series, Vol 25, The Hague: Dr. W. Junk, b.v., 1981, pp 93-211.

42. Barr CC: Prognostic Factors in Corneoscleral Laceration. Arch Ophthalmol 101:919-924, 1983.

43. Aronson SB, Elliot JH: Ocular Inflammation. St. Louis: C.V. Mosby, 1972.

44. Hogan MJ, Zimmerman LE: Ophthalmic Pathology, 2nd ed. Philadelphia: W.B. Saunders, 1962, p 376.

45. Friedlaender MH, Allansmith MR: Ocular Manifestations of Immune Disease in Pathobiology of Ocular Disease. New York: Marcel Dekker, Inc., 1982, p 170.

46. Charles S: Vitreous Microsurgery. Baltimore: Williams and Wilkins, 1981, p 124.

47. Coleman DJ: Early Vitrectomy in the Management of the Severely Traumatized Eye. Am J Ophthalmol 93:543-558, 1982.

48. Charles S: Vitreous Microsurgery. Baltimore: Williams and Wilkins, 1981, pp 143-154.

49. Michels RG: Vitreous Surgery, San Francisco: American Academy of Ophthalmology Manuals Program, 1981, pp 78-82.

50. Hammer ME: Plano Fundus Lens for Penetrating Keratoplasty and Closed Vitrectomy. Ocutome Newsletter, Vol 5, No 3, 1980.

51. Knave B: Electroretinography in Eyes with Retained Intraocular Metallic Foreign Bodies. Acta Ophthalmol (Suppl) 100, 1969.
52. Keeney AH: New Hazards of Penetrating Wounds of the Eye. Tr Am Ophthalmol Soc, Vol 74, pp 331-340, 1976.
53. Percival SPB: Late Complications from Posterior Segment Intraocular Foreign Bodies with Particular Reference to Retinal Detachments. Br J Ophthalmol 56:462-468, 1972.
54. Machemer R: Diamond-coated all-purpose foreign body forceps. Am J Ophthalmol 91:267, 1981.
55. O'Day DM, Smith RS, Gregg CR: The Problem of Bacillus Species Infection with Special Emphasis on the Virulence of Bacillus cereus.
56. Peyman GA, Carroll CP, Raichand M: Post-traumatic Endophthalmitis. Arch Ophthalmol 87:320-329, 1980.
57. Brinton GA, Toppin TM, et al: Post-traumatic Endophthalmitis. Arch Ophthalmol, 102:457-550, 1984.

Chapter 15

Endophthalmitis

M. Gilbert Grand, MD

ENDOPHTHALMITIS

Introduction

Endophthalmitis represents an ophthalmic catastrophe that must be managed as a true emergency. To the present time, the issue of which of the alternative forms of management of patients with endophthalmitis is best remains speculative. Well-designed, statistically-controlled prospective randomized studies have not been undertaken. The reasons for this include the fact that there are multiple variables among patients with endophthalmitis, namely the type of organism, the duration of infection prior to identification, and the interval before initiation of treatment after establishment of the diagnosis. Accordingly, there are some aspects in the management of endophthalmitis that do not lend themselves to hard and fast rules. Nevertheless, clinical experience has shown us that there are some issues which are reasonably clear and these will be presented from a somewhat dogmatic point of view. The purpose of this chapter is to provide a rational plan that can be used in the midst of crisis to deal with patients with endophthalmitis (Figure 15-1).

Historical Perspective

Vitrectomy surgery has provided the ophthalmologist with the opportunity to reconsider the management of a number of diseases including

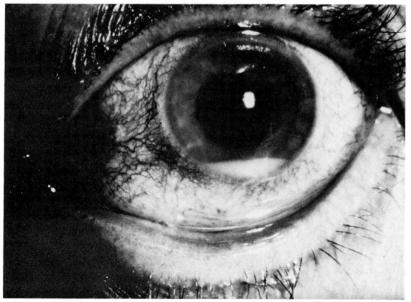

Figure 15-1. Clinical findings of endophthalmitis include ptosis, marked conjunctival reaction, hazy cornea, hypopyon, and loss of red reflex. This photograph depicts a typical presentation of endophthalmitis with these findings.

endophthalmitis. Previous methods for treatment of bacterial endophthalmitis using systemic and periocular medications have only been moderately successful. A minority of eyes treated by such means have retained useful vision but many eyes ultimately have become phthisical and required enucleation.[1,2] Poor results in the treatment of endophthalmitis are due to a multiplicity of factors including sensitivity of ocular tissue to inflammation and toxins, resistance to antibiotics, and poor penetration of antibiotics into the vitreous. The impermeability of the blood retinal barrier, presumably due to tight junctions of vascular endothelial cells or retinal pigment epithelial cells, results in low concentrations of antibiotic in the vitreous itself.[3] While other factors play an important role in the failure of therapy in the management of endophthalmitis, it is this inability to achieve a sufficient level of antibiotics for bacteriocidal effect within the vitreous that appears to be the major cause of failure. The use of intraocular antibiotics has been discussed for approximately 40 years, intravitreal Penicillin having been evaluated by von Sallmann in 1945[4] and subsequently by Leopold.[5] For a variety of reasons, including the potential toxicity of intraocular antibiotics, the use of intravitreal antibiotics did not gain widespread acceptance. However, considerable data has been obtained showing appropriate doses of antibiotics can be administered intravitreally effectively without obvious toxicity.[3]

The advent of advanced microsurgical techniques applied to the vitreous has allowed an increased level of surgical confidence in vitrectomy. The use of intravitreal antibiotics with or without adjunctive vitrectomy surgery now provides a logical means to approach endophthalmitis.

Etiology

Endophthalmitis can be defined as any severe intraocular inflammation. While it may be caused by infectious agents, it may also represent a reaction to toxic substances, necrotic tumors, noninfectious uveitis, or infarction of intraocular tissue.

Endophthalmitis can be subdivided into two etiologic types: endogenous and exogenous. Endogenous endophthalmitis is the result of disseminated infectious agents in debilitated or immune deficient patients. It can be seen in patients who are experiencing a bacteremia or septicemia, or in patients who abuse drugs by means of the intravenous route. Physicians should remember that endogenous endophthalmitis may occur in patients who are receiving intravenous nutrition. In such patients, cultures of indwelling catheter lines may be critical in determining the etiologic organism responsible for endophthalmitis.

Exogenous endophthalmitis refers to patients who develop endophthalmitis following penetration or perforation of the globe, typically relative to intraocular trauma or surgery. In patients with exogenous endophthalmitis after surgery, the inoculum of infection may occur due to contaminated solutions, airborne dissemination, spread from periocular infection, or may be related to prolonged surgical procedures, particularly those in which there may be devitalized tissue or the use of implanted materials. An immune compromised host may be more vulnerable to such exogenous infections as well as to endogenous infection.

Infectious forms of endophthalmitis are caused by gram positive or gram negative bacterial organisms, fungal organisms, and parasites. It is critically important to recognize that *all* organisms, those commonly known as pathogens, as well as those known as nonpathogens, can cause endophthalmitis.[6] In most reported series, staphylococcal organisms are the most common etiologic agent of infectious endophthalmitis.[3] In recent years, there has been an increased tendency toward gram negative and fungal infections. Of the fungal infections, Candida remains the most common causative organism.[3]

Aseptic endophthalmitis, also known as sterile endophthalmitis, is generally described as a mild, slowly progressive disease with less severe signs and symptoms than infectious endophthalmitis. Furthermore, aseptic endophthalmitis is, in general, responsive to corticosteroid therapy. However, a true endophthalmitis caused by a low virulence organism can easily mimic an aseptic endophthalmitis. The treatment of aseptic endophthalmitis includes cycloplegics, topical corticosteroids and sometimes systemic corticosteroids. However, it is critically important to be certain that the diagnosis of aseptic endophthalmitis is, in fact, correct. Clinical judgment in this instance is extraordinarily important. It is, however, equally important for the physician to recognize that he can be mistaken and that, in their early phases, low virulence organisms can mimic an aseptic endophthalmitis. Therefore, close follow-up is critical and if the patient does not respond adequately to treatment, or if the inflammatory response worsens, one must presume the inflammation is of infectious origin and act accordingly.

Establishing the Diagnosis

Patients with endophthalmitis typically present with symptoms of pain and marked reduction in visual acuity. The most common signs associated with endophthalmitis are a reduction in the corneal reflex, an unusual degree of periocular swelling and chemosis, hyperemia of the conjunctiva, anterior segment reaction including hypopyon, debris in the vitreous, reduction in the red reflex, and clouding of the media. Additionally, frank pus in a conjunctival bleb, or surrounding sutures from a surgical or traumatic wound may be indicators of endophthalmitis.

The ophthalmologist should be suspicious of endophthalmitis in any patient who presents with intraocular inflammation greater than that expected from any antecedent surgical or traumatic event. In patients with no antecedent surgical or traumatic history, the physician should attempt to elicit a history that would suggest a predilection for endogenous dissemination of infection. Whereas fulminate endophthalmitis is readily recognized, early stages present a dilemma in diagnosis when trying to separate aseptic from septic inflammation. Perhaps the single most important admonition is that, when faced with this differential diagnosis, the attending physician should be suspicious of an occult endophthalmitis and conduct frequent examinations. While it is not possible to make strict rules as to how frequently such a patient should be seen when faced with this diagnostic dilemma, it seems prudent that the patient should be evaluated more than once within a given 24-hour period.

In a review by Bohigian and Olk, it was shown that many cases initially thought to be sterile or aseptic endophthalmitis were, in fact, infectious endophthalmitis.[7] Of 51 culture positive cases reviewed, 15 cases (29.4%) were initially thought to be sterile. This emphasizes the difficulty in the differentiation between aseptic and septic endophthalmitis and the importance of careful evaluation of such patients at frequent intervals.

When in doubt, assume that the patient has a true infectious endophthalmitis. Successful treatment of endophthalmitis depends upon early diagnosis, prompt treatment, and the virulence of the organism. Of these factors, the physician has no control over the type of organism involved and, therefore, can only influence the outcome of an infection by means of assuring early diagnosis and the prompt initiation of therapy.

A *critical step in the management of endophthalmitis is obtaining a specimen of the vitreous.* Additional information may be obtained by means of culturing the anterior chamber, conjunctiva, or the margins of a traumatic or surgical wound. However, culturing the vitreous should be the ophthalmologist's prime goal. Specimens of intraocular fluid should be obtained in the operating room. This minimizes the risk of contamination of the globe with a new agent, reduces the risk of growing contaminants, and allows management of potential problems such as wound dehiscence. Obviously, in those instances where access to an operating room is limited or will require substantial delay, specimens should be obtained under sterile conditions in the best facility available, such as a treatment area.

The technique for obtaining a specimen is as follows: Lid and conjunctival cultures should be obtained prior to the use of any topical anesthetic as these may contain inhibitors of bacterial growth. Whereas a 25-gauge needle may be used for obtaining a specimen of aqueous, in general, a larger caliber needle will be required for vitreous aspiration, such as a 22-gauge needle. Anterior chamber taps can be obtained using a tuberculin syringe with a sharp 25-gauge needle passed via the limbus into the vitreous chamber or via a keratotomy. The microvitreoretinal (MVR) blade used for making sclerotomy incisions at the time of vitrectomy may be passed partially through the cornea until the tip appears in the anterior chamber. This allows subsequent passage with a needle, using very minimal force and avoiding distortion on the globe or surgical wound. In phakic patients, the vitreous aspiration can be obtained by means of a sclerotomy over the pars plana approximately 4 mm posterior to the limbus. Alternatively, in aphakic or pseudophakic patients, access to the vitreous can be achieved either by means of a pars plana sclerotomy, or in selected patients, via the limbus passing the point of the needle into the posterior segment through the pupil. *At the time of vitreous aspiration, intravitreal antibiotics should be administered via the same puncture sites.*

It is recommended that the physician himself carry the specimen directly to the laboratory and instruct the technicians in the desired plating of the specimen. In general, vitreous should be plated on blood agar as well as chocolate agar, thioglycolate and Sabouraud's media that contains no inhibitors. If limited material is present, a liquid medium should be chosen, and if growth occurs, further subculturing can be obtained. Glass slides should be prepared for subsequent staining with Gram's, Giemsa, or silver stains. Unfortunately, the results of smears are not diagnostic and one cannot base therapeutic decisions on the result of a smear. Smears may be positive in only approximately 50% of culture positive eyes.[8] Therefore, one cannot base a decision on the presence or absence of infection, or the type of etiologic agent causing infection on the information obtained by smear.

One should consider passing the specimen through a milipor filter or using centrifugation to concentrate the specimen prior to plating. In patients suspected of fungal endophthalmitis, an initial vitrectomy may best obtain an adequate specimen. One may be particularly concerned that fungal organisms would be adherent to vitreous fibrils rather than free floating in liquid vitreous, and thus might not be harvested by means of aspiration of liquid vitreous alone. The determination of fungal endophthalmitis can be made on the basis of culture. Additionally, a histologic evaluation of a specimen centrifuged and processed for pathologic evaluation may be useful. Whereas KOH smears were used in the past, currently many pathologists prefer to evaluate smears stained with PAS or GMS (modified Grocotts methenamine silver) to determine the presence of fungal organisms.[8]

Management

Three alternatives can be employed in the management of endophthalmitis. These are:

1. The use of systemic and periocular medications alone.
2. The use of intravitreal injection of antibiotics in combination with periocular and systemic medications.
3. The use of vitrectomy with intravitreal injection, in addition to the concomitant administration of periocular and systemic medications.

Timing of Therapeutic Intervention. Whether the physician chooses to aspirate a vitreous specimen and inject intravitreal antibiotics as his initial procedure, or to perform a primary vitrectomy with the injection of intravitreal antibiotics, the timing of such intervention is of paramount importance. *In every case, one should obtain a vitreous specimen and inject antibiotics as soon as the diagnosis of endophthalmitis is suspected.* In general, I recommend the use of antibiotics by means of multiple routes in the management of infectious endophthalmitis. Patients should be treated with topical antibiotics, systemic antibiotics and subconjunctival antibiotics, as well as intravitreal antibiotics. Cycloplegics will greatly reduce ciliary body spasm and associated discomfort. Whereas narcotics may be necessary at the time of the immediate presentation of endophthalmitis, it is my clinical experience that discomfort associated with endophthalmitis diminishes remarkably following the initiation of intravitreal antibiotics or vitrectomy.

Intravitreal antibiotics can be administered by two basic routes. Some authors recommend the use of an antibiotic in the vitreous infusion line.[9] This would be contraindicated in patients in whom vitrectomy is being performed to obtain a specimen for culture, in which case the use of antibiotics in the infusion line might inhibit growth of organisms. Alternatively, one can obtain the specimen and then add antibiotics to the infusion fluid. I prefer to administer intravitreal antibiotics at the completion of the vitreous tap or vitrectomy procedure. Table 15-1 shows dosages for intravitreal antibiotics.[10] Usually, such medications are diluted to 0.1 ml. volume. The injection is then administered intravitreally into the anterior portion of the central vitreous. It is recommended that the bevel of the needle be pointed toward the anterior chamber to avoid a "jet stream" effect on the retina. A minor inflammatory response in patients in whom endophthalmitis is suspected may be treated by means of intravitreal antibiotic at the time of aspiration only without vitrectomy. The physician should be reminded not to wait for the results of culture and sensitivity, but instead to treat with a broad spectrum of antibiotics administered in intravitreal, subconjunctival, intravenous, and topical routes. Until final cultures are obtained, it is recommended that initial therapy include antibiotics designed to cover a wide range of potential organisms. Table 15-2

TABLE 15-1.
ANTIBIOTIC DOSAGE FOR INTRAVITREAL INJECTION[1]

Antibiotic	Dosage/0.1 ml	Diluent[2]
Amikacin	400 mcg*	Normal Saline
Amphotericin B	1-5 mcg*	Sterile Water
Ampicillin	5 mg	Sterile Water
Carbenicillin	2 mg	Sterile Water
Cefazolin	2.25 mg	Sterile Water
Chloramphenicol	2 mg	Sterile Water
Clindamycin	1 mg	Normal Saline
Erythromycin	500 mcg*	Normal Saline
Gentamicin	100-400 mcg*	Normal Saline
Kanamycin	500 mcg*	Normal Saline
Methicillin	2 mg	Normal Saline
Oxacillin	500 mcg*	Normal Saline
Tobramycin	500 mcg*	Normal Saline
Vancomycin	0.5-1 mg	Normal Saline

*This dosage is micrograms.
Antibiotic doses for intravitreal injection are prepared immediately prior to use in no more than 0.1 ml final volume.

1. Modified from Jules Stein Eye Institute Pharmaceutical Notes, Vol. 2, No. 11, May, 1982.
2. Use diluent without preservatives.

shows three alternative regimens of antibiotic usage.[11] Alterations would obviously depend on a patient's age, health, and allergic status. However, the physician should be advised to consult each hospital's infectious disease control service to determine the sensitivities of organisms recently cultured and to use this list of sensitivities as a guide in the selection of antibiotics.

It is most important to remember the possibility of potential allergic or systemic reactions to antibiotic usage. After obtaining a final culture, the type of antibiotic can be altered according to the organism sensitivities. This allows change from broad spectrum to more specific coverage. Additionally, one should be alert to the potential for systemic toxicity such as ototoxicity or renal toxicity that may be associated with antibiotic usage, and to alter dosages accordingly.

Re-injection of Antibiotics. in general, infections cause by Staphylococcus epidermidis can often be cured by means of a single intravitreal injection, as well as systemic antibiotics. Infections caused by all other organisms should be carefully monitored and the potential re-injection of antibiotics should be considered. The half-life of intravitreal Gentamicin in phakic, aphakic, infected or noninfected eyes is approximately 48 hours.[8] Vitreous levels of Ancef (cefazolin) may exceed the mean inhibitory concentration for five days after intravitreal administration.[12] In general, I consider re-injection of antibiotics in patients with infections other than Staphylococcus epidermidis at 48 hours unless the patient is having a prompt response to therapy. At the time of re-injection, a new culture should be obtained to be certain that, at the time of the initial procedure, a new infectious organism was not inoculated into the globe. The culture and reinjection can be performed with topical anesthesia only, passing a needle through a previously placed keratotomy site made at the time of the

---

TABLE 15-2.
BROAD ANTIBACTERIAL COVERAGE FOR INITIAL TREATMENT OF ENDOPHTHALMITIS[1]

	Alternative One	Alternative Two	Alternative Three[2]
Topical	Gentamicin[3] and Vancomycin	Gentamicin and Cefazolin	Gentamicin and Bacitracin
Subconjunctival	Gentamicin[3] and Vancomycin	Gentamicin and Cefazolin	Gentamicin and Methicillin
Intravenous	Gentamicin[3] and Vancomycin	Gentamicin and Cefazolin	Gentamicin and Methicillin and Penicillin G

1. Modified from Bohigian George M: Handbook of External Diseases of the Eye.
2. Current therapy for patients with definite and severe Penicillin hypersensitivity, e.g., hypotension, anaphylactoid reaction.
3. Tobramycin may be substituted for Gentamicin.

primary vitrectomy. A keratotomy performed at the time of the initial procedure is, therefore, useful as a route for intracameral injection upon completion of the procedure and additionally as a route to obtain a repeat culture and reinject antibiotics at intervals in the course of the postoperative management of the patient.

Potential toxicity of antibiotics used in the intravitreal fashion is difficult to determine. It is difficult to know if reduction in retinal function or changes in the appearance of the pigment epithelium is due to a given dose of antibiotics, a "jet stream" effect, or the varying effects of toxicity of the antibiotic versus the toxicity of the infectious organism. Furthermore, a dosage level that may be toxic in one individual may be safe in others.

Vitrectomy. A physician has three alternatives when considering the potential use of vitrectomy in the management of patients with endophthalmitis, as follows:

- Vitrectomy may be performed initially to make the diagnosis, as well as to aid in therapy.
- A second alternative would be to obtain a suitable aspiration of vitreous for culture and to perform vitrectomy depending on the results of that culture, such as, the growth of an organism documenting a true infection or the virulence of the offending organism.
- The third alternative is to manage the infection by means of intravitreal antibiotics and systemic medications and to use vitrectomy for the management of late complications such as organization of the vitreous.

The decision to perform a primary vitrectomy is most difficult. Some physicians believe that vitreous aspiration via a needle and syringe is hazardous in that vitreous fibrils may be aspirated resulting in traction on the peripheral retina and potentially causing retinal breaks. The decision for these physicians to perform a primary vitrectomy with state-of-the-art vitreous cutters seems reasonable. An alternative approach is to perform a vitreous aspiration or vitrectomy depending on the degree of vitreous involvement. That is, those patients with minimal vitreous debris might be managed by means of initial culture and intravitreal injection of antibiotics, whereas those patients with severe vitreous opacities precluding an adequate view of the retina would be treated by means of primary vitrectomy.

My current indications for vitrectomy are as follows:

- Patients who present with profound visual loss such as light perception or hand motions.
- Should the initial vitreous aspiration grow organisms that are considered "virulent," vitrectomy should be considered. Most physicians consider all organisms other than Staphylococcus epidermidis is this virulent category.
- One should consider vitrectomy in patients who are treated initially with intravitreal antibiotics but who become clinically worse despite therapy.
- The presence of frank pus in the vitreous should be considered an indication for vitrectomy.
- Patients suspected of having fungal endophthalmitis should be con-

sidered for primary vitrectomy to maximize the potential to detect a fungal organism.

- Vitrectomy should be considered in traumatically injured eye with endophthalmitis. Vitrectomy in this instance allows culture of the vitreous, intravitreal antibiotic administration, and additionally allows detection of any occult intraocular injury involving the posterior segment. Furthermore, vitrectomy in this setting allows the removal of exogenous biologic material such as vegetable matter.

Technical Aspects of Vitrectomy. Vitrectomy can be performed using either local or general anesthesia. The advantage of general anesthesia is the avoidance of a retrobulbar block in an eye that is severely inflamed. In such eyes, adequate anesthesia may be difficult to obtain. Furthermore, one avoids the potential hazards of a retrobulbar hemorrhage in an eye with a recent wound that might result in undue intraocular pressure with resultant dehiscence of the wound. A disadvantage of general anesthesia is the fact that a patient presenting with endophthalmitis requires immediate treatment and may not be in suitable physical condition or in adequate systemic health to tolerate general anesthesia and may require more delay than local anesthesia. Aspiration of vitreous and/or aqueous can usually be obtained painlessly with local anesthesia such as topical medications or local infiltration. The risk of local anesthetic such as a retrobulbar block includes the unpredictability of the degree of anesthesia and the potential for wound rupture. In general, if an aspiration of anterior chamber and vitreous fluids is all that is required, this can be obtained with regional infiltration. If a vitrectomy procedure itself is required, one should consider retrobulbar block or general anesthesia.

There are many technical problems associated with vitrectomy, particularly in patients who have endophthalmitis. Physicians who are not familiar with vitrectomy techniques should not attempt vitrectomy in patients suspected of endophthalmitis. The particular technical problems associated with pars plana vitrectomy in patients with endophthalmitis include:

- Increased difficulty in visualization of the intraocular contents due to a number of factors including corneal edema, layering of debris on the endothelium, debris on the intraocular lens, membranes in the pupillary space, or membranes on both anterior and posterior surfaces of an intraocular lens.
- An unusual degree of bleeding may occur from sclerotomies, as well as from the iris.
- Scleral necrosis may occur making wounds leaky during a procedure and difficult to close at the completion of surgery.
- The surgeon should recognize that vitreous organization in patients with infectious endophthalmitis is often of a rather marked degree. Layers of vitreous membranes frequently occur extending posteriorly through the vitreous cavity, all the way to the surface of the retina. Such vitreous layers are analogous to the layers of an onion, with the most posterior layer in intimate contact with the internal limiting membrane of the retina.

369

- It is important to recognize that in such patients the retina is extremely friable and any manipulation of the retina or attempts to "peel" membranes from its surface will likely result in retinal breaks and ultimate detachment.

Technical considerations in performing vitrectomy include the use of a moderate or a long infusion cannula. Using the Ocutome System, a 4 or 6 mm infusion cannula is recommended and infusion ports of similar lengths with other systems should be considered. The technical aspects of vitrectomy include the fact that the anterior segment must frequently be cleared prior to proceeding to work in the posterior segment. In eyes that are aphakic, a typical pars plana approach can be used. However, in eyes that are pseudophakic with an anterior chamber lens or a posterior chamber lens, it may be difficult to reach the anterior chamber by means of the pars plana. Eyes with a Medallion type lens sutured to the iris frequently allow access between the iris sphincter and the intraocular lens for an approach to the anterior segment. In cleaning the anterior segment, one must recognize that there is frequently a membranous coating of debris that extends over the iris into the angle. While in some patients this may readily be lavaged, in others this membrane has to be physically stripped from the angle and will deliver itself very much like a crepe. Attendant with stripping of this membranous debris is often the accompaniment of punctate hemorrhages from the surface of the iris. Remember that only a core vitrectomy may be accomplished. In cases with "onion layering" organization of the vitreous, do not attempt to clear all the way to the retina. If white purulent debris is seen lying on the retinal surface, it would be wise to avoid manipulating it, such as with picks or suction devices, as such manipulation will undoubtedly result in retinal breaks and detachment.

Unfortunately, there is no published, well-designed study providing adequate data to establish the potential indications for vitrectomy or its efficacy in the management of endophthalmitis. Results of various treatment modalities are difficult to assess because there is tremendous variation among patients in regard to the magnitude of inoculum, the virulence of the infectious organism, delays in diagnosis, and underlying host factors. Whereas many patients with endophthalmitis who have been treated by means of vitrectomy have had less uniformly good results, such poor responses to treatment may be due to the exquisite sensitivity of the eye to inflammation and the poor penetration of antibiotics in the eye. Experimentally, staphylococcus aureus can be cured up to 18 hours following the administration of an inoculum by means of periocular and systemic medications alone. Such infections can be cured up to 24 hours with the additional use of intravitreal medication. Between 24 and 48 hours, such infections can be cured by means of vitrectomy, in addition to antibiotics.[13] Forster has shown the cure rate in endophthalmitis after cataract surgery is the same in those patients in whom antibiotic was injected into the vitreous as in those patients who underwent vitrectomy as well as intravitreal injection.[8] However, to date, a control study has not been performed, and vitrectomy is usually performed in those cases that have the clinically most severe presentation and worst prognosis. While the potential benefit of vitrectomy has not yet been demonstrated, it has been reasonably well established that the penetration of antibiotics into the vitreous by means of systemic routes is generally inadequate to achieve inhibitory levels. Therefore, in all cases of infectious endophthalmitis, I favor the use of intravitreal antibiotics.

Special Considerations

Intraocular Lens. Infections in tissue that contains prosthetic material have often been difficult to control, and removal of the prosthetic material has frequently been required. The intraocular lens may be an exception to this principle. It has been known for many years that in the presence of endophthalmitis, the intraocular lens can often be left in place and the endophthalmitis cured by means of standard techniques of vitrectomy and intravitreal antibiotic administration. In general, when faced with endophthalmitis in a pseudophakic eye, I treat the endophthalmitis as if the eye were aphakic, leaving the intraocular lens untouched. It should be recognized, however, that the presence of an intraocular lens can make management difficult from the standpoint of visualization. Frequently a membranous deposit of inflammatory debris occurs on both the anterior and posterior surfaces of the intraocular lens. At the time of vitrectomy this membranous material is cut free from the anterior and posterior surfaces of the intraocular lens to allow visualization of the vitreous cavity and posterior segment.

An instance in which I consider removal of an intraocular lens is the suspected presence of fungal endophthalmitis. This is due to a theoretical risk that fungal elements may become incorporated into the lens. In patients with a wound rupture in which the intraocular lens may be dislocated, it is frequently easier to remove the intraocular lens and repair the wound without making attempts to reposition the lens. Additionally, in those patients requiring vitrectomy who have an anterior segment that has become totally opacified precluding pars plana vitrectomy, an open sky vitrectomy may be required. In this uncommon instance, I would advocate removal of the intraocular lens.

Suture Infection. At the time of vitrectomy, if a suture appears to be the focus of infection with purulence surrounding the suture, it is prudent to remove that suture and repair the wound with new sutures in adjacent healthy cornea or sclera.

Opaque Cornea. Those patients presenting with endophthalmitis and a totally opaque cornea can frequently be managed by means of vitrectomy. Whereas external illumination frequently does not allow visualization of the intraocular contents, endo-illumination such as used during vitrectomy procedures often will provide an improved visualization of intraocular structures. Frequently, the clinical appearance of the anterior segment is such that one suspects the cornea will not allow adequate visualization. However, the surgeon may be surprised to find that after completing a washout of the anterior segment, a pars plana vitrectomy can be accomplished with visualization through the cornea. However, in cases in which the cornea is so opaque that visualization cannot be accomplished, the patient should be managed by means of aspiration of vitreous and aqueous for culture with concomitant injection of antibiotics. Alternatively, an open sky vitrectomy, sometimes analogous to an incision and drainage of an abscess, can be performed. While this may not allow total clearing of the media, it will greatly reduce the magnitude of the infection, removing the large portion of the infective inoculum, washing toxic waste from the eye and allowing the instillation of antibiotics.

Filter Blebs. Patients who have filter bleb infections present a unique situation. It is frequently assumed that the presence of pus in the filtering bleb is an isolated phenomenon and does not indicate infection elsewhere within the eye. In general, however, if a culture of the anterior chamber is positive, in that same patient the vitreous would also prove culture positive. Therefore, when faced with this situation, the surgeon should be advised to culture the vitreous as well as the anterior chamber and to inject antibiotics in both compartments. Additional use of vitrectomy would depend on the previously outlined guidelines. For reasons that remain unclear, it appears that streptococcal organisms and Homophilus influenzae are very frequent sources of infection in filter bleb infections. Consequently, the attending surgeon should be aware and prepare to culture for these organisms. Furthermore, antibiotic usage in such patients should include coverage for these two organisms until sensitivities are available. It should be recognized that streptococcus is an extremely virulent organism within the eye, and prompt attention to the possibility of a streptococcal endophthalmitis should be paid.

Trauma. In instances where an eye has suffered penetrating trauma and the question of infection is raised, the attending surgeon should recognize that infections do occur in a significant proportion of such patients. If at all in doubt in such instances, the surgeon would be admonished to presume that the eye is infected until proven otherwise and to treat the eye as if an endophthalmitis exists. It is of great importance in this situation to recognize the variation and types of organisms that may grow from traumatically injured eyes. Furthermore, one should pay close attention to the possibility of clostridial infections. The status of the patient's tetanus immunization should be ascertained. Consultation with infectious disease experts may be useful, and appropriate measures such as the use of tetanus toxoid or hypertetanus immune globulin should be considered.

Use of Corticosteroids

The use of corticosteroids remains controversial in the management of patients with endophthalmitis. Traditionally, it was taught that corticosteroids were contraindicated. However, corticosteroids have proven useful in a number of ocular inflammatory diseases. In endophthalmitis, the degree of inflammation and response to infection is severe and consequently eyes may be cured of infection only to be blind due to inflammation and its consequences. Peyman has shown dexamethasone can be administered intravitreally without toxicity.[3] It has been my practice to treat patients with intravitreal dexamethasone (400 mcg) as well as with periocular dexamethasone. Depending on a patient's health, the use of systemic corticosteroids may also be advisable in the immediate postoperative period. Patient's with ulcer disease or diabetes may not tolerate systemic administration of corticosteroids and may instead be treated with periocular corticosteroids. The purpose of such steroid administration is to reduce the inflammatory response to infection and reduce the secondary organization of the vitreous that may occur. However, if you intend to use steroids in the management of endophthalmitis, it is critical to have adequate and appropriate antibiotic coverage. It may be prudent to delay steroid administration until one is confident that the infecting organism is sensitive to the antibiotics being used and that the infection is responding clinically.

Summary

Endophthalmitis remains an ophthalmic catastrophe and a true emergency. A high index of suspicion must be maintained when evaluating postoperative patients. When in doubt, assume that the patient has a true infectious endophthalmitis. Obtaining a specimen of vitreous for culture and administration of appropriate intravitreal antibiotics are critical for effective treatment. This should be done in every case of suspected endophthalmitis. Vitrectomy now has a major role in the management of endophthalmitis and is technically more difficult in the infected eye.

Special considerations in the management of endophthalmitis include: the presence of an intraocular lens, suture infection, corneal opacities, filtering blebs, and a history of penetrating trauma. The prognosis for endophthalmitis remains poor, but is improving with prompt, aggressive treatment.

(Editor)

References
1. Allen HE, Mangiaracine AB: Bacterial endophthalmitis after cataract extraction: A study of 22 infections in 20,000 operations. Arch Ophth 72:454, 1964.
2. Hughes WF Jr., Owens WC: Postoperative complications of cataract extraction. Arch Ophth 38:577, 1947.
3. Peyman GA, Sanders DR: Advances in uveal surgery, vitreous surgery and the treatment of endophthalmitis. Appleton-Century-Crofts, 1975.
4. von Sallmann L, Meyer K, DiGrandi J: Experimental study on Penicillin treatment of ectogenous infections of vitreous. Arch Ophth 32:179, 1944.
5. Leopold IH: Intravitreal penetration of Penicillin and Penicillin therapy of infections of the vitreous. Arch Ophth 33:211, 1945.
6. Jaffe NS: Cataract surgery and its complications. Second Edition, CV Mosby, 1976.
7. Bohigian GM, Olk RJ: Endophthalmitis: A six year review at Barnes Hospital. ACTA Ophthalmol 24:573-576, 1983.

8. Forster RK, Abbott RL, Gelender H: Management of infectious endophthalmitis. Ophthalmology 87:313-319, 1980.

9. Peyman GA, Raichand M, Bennett TO: Management of endophthalmitis with pars plana vitrectomy. BJO 64:472-475, 1980.

10. Gardner SK: Antibiotic doses for intravitreal injection. Jules Stein Eye Institute Pharmaceutical Notes, Vol 2, No 11, May 1982.

11. Bohigian GM: Handbook of external diseases of the eye. Alcon Laboratories, 1980.

12. Civiletto SE, Fisher JP: Toxicity, efficacy, and clearance of intravitreal cefazolin. Invest Ophthal Vis Science (supplement) April 1979; 132.

13. Cottingham AJ, Forster RD: Vitrectomy in endophthalmitis. Arch Ophth 94:2078-2081, 1976.

Chapter 16

Understanding Antibiotics

Clifford C. Dacso, MD, MPH
Patrick E. Nolan, MD

UNDERSTANDING ANTIBIOTICS

Introduction

Ophthalmic infections are unique in that the kinetics of antibiotics and their penetration into the sanctuary of the eye become of paramount importance. Choice of antimicrobials in eye infections can therefore not be made solely on antimicrobial susceptibility patterns. In the case of fungal and viral infections of the eye and adnexa, the choice of agent becomes even more confounding since susceptibility testing for these infectious agents are not commonly available.

The purpose of this discussion is not to outline treatment strategies, as these are discussed under the rubric of the specific disorders, (Chapter 15) but rather to demonstrate the appropriate thought patterns of pharmacology and microbiology when applied to infections of the eye. Three variables enter into this decision making: first, is the observed infection caused by the isolated organism? Second, does the drug kill the bug? Third, can the drug get to the bug?

The first of these variables is the fulfillment of the well-known Koch-Henle postulates, which establish the causal relationship between the microorganism and the observed pathology. The isolation of this causal organism is of utmost importance and must be pursued with great ardor by the physician whenever possible. Empiric antimicrobial therapy is specifically to be eschewed whenever possible. Clinical syndromes are, generally, not sufficiently distinctive to allow the clinicians to establish an etiologic diagnosis by observation alone. A typical scenario of empiric antibiotics involves the infection which was diagnosed clinically and the patient begun on antibiotics. In 48 hours the patient's condition has deteriorated without evidence to support the agent or agents chosen. The clinician is then faced with the unpleasant choice of adding or changing empiric agents since culture at this time, well into therapy, may be misleading at best. The most effective method of circumventing this problem is to obtain appropriate cultures whenever possible prior to the initiation of antimicrobial chemotherapy. Clinical syndromes certainly do exist in which cultures cannot be obtained or may be misleading. Ophthalmic infections present more of these situations than those of other disciplines and those treating infections of the eye are commonly guided by clinical appearances alone.

Antimicrobial Susceptibility Testing

When cultural material is available, the second variable, antimicrobial susceptibility, comes into play. There are two major techniques used in conventional clinical laboratories to ascertain the ability of an antimicrobial agent to inhibit the growth of a bacterium. The first is the method of Bauer and Kirby described in the mid-1960's. In this method a standardized inoculum of bacteria is applied to a plate of nutrient agar of specified composition and specified size. On top of this "lawn" of inoculum is placed a disc of filter paper impregnated with a defined amount of antibiotic. This plate, with the discs applied, is incubated for 18-24 hours at the end of which zones of inhibition of growth of varying diameters are present surrounding the discs. These are then measured using either a micrometer or template. The diameter of the zone of inhibition determines whether the organism is sensitive (S), resistant (R), or indeterminate (I). This method is highly reproducible and well accepted as a benchmark in clinical medicine. Its major drawbacks are its inability to quantitate the degree of sensitivity or resistance and its inability to supply data on killing as opposed to inhibition.

A second method of antimicrobial susceptibility testing which has, of late, found increasing acceptance among clinical laboratories is the determination of the minimum inhibitory concentration (MIC) or that smallest concentration of antibiotic in medium capable of inhibiting growth of the organism. This method does again require a pure growth of the organism, typically an overnight broth. The inoculum is applied to serial dilutions of antibiotic in medium and incubated. Growth of the organism is commonly assessed by observing the turbidity of the broth. This technique has the advantage of being amenable to automation and that laboratory media may be prepared in advance and frozen. Results of the test are expressed not as simply "sensitive" or "resistant" but rather as the concentration in micrograms per milliliter of antibiotic required to inhibit growth.

Although the same thought process is used to choose antimicrobial therapy regardless of the method of susceptibility testing used, the MIC method seems to provoke more confusion as a result of the volume of information supplied. In order to know whether or not a given drug is effective one therefore needs not only the MIC but also the concentration of antibiotic attainable at the site of infection. In fact, the method gives little more information than the Bauer-Kirby technique since the "cutpoints" or zone diameters describing "sensitive" or "resistant" are determined by the minimum inhibitory concentration of the antibiotic.

A major limitation of both the MIC and Bauer-Kirby methods of susceptibility testing is their inability to determine bactericidal activity. Based on data generated by these two tests, it is impossible to distinguish bactericidal (antibiotics which kill) from bacteriostatic (agents which simply inhibit growth). In most clinical situations this is a meaningless distinction since if bactericidal proliferation is halted the normal host defenses such as polymorphonuclear leukocytes, natural killer cell activity, complement, and humoral immunity destroy the bacteria. There are clinical situations in which host defenses are less active and in these the distinction between bacteriostatic and bactericidal activity is more important. These are situations such as corticosteroid therapy, underlying immunosuppressive illness such as Hodgkin's lymphoma or the acquired immune deficiency syndrome (AIDS) and immunosuppressive medication. Additionally there are avascular areas such as heart valves, cornea and vitreous, infections of which rely more on antibiotics for cure.

Finally, as most ophthalmologists know, pharmacology studies on eye infections are commonly performed on lower animals. Even nonhuman primates are used sparingly. Thus, studies must be interpreted with even more caution than that accorded to most scientific investigation.

With the exception of the external structures of the eye, systemically administered antimicrobials are of little use other than to maintain a concentration gradient favoring the infected site. Alterations in the corneal and scleral barriers are seen in the inflammatory conditions but both lipo- and hydrophilicity are required for intraocular penetration by drugs. Preferred routes of administration and drugs of above are not within the province of this chapter.

Antibiotics can be broadly classified by their spectra of activity. Within each category is a number of "me-too" drugs which supply little or no advantage in terms of coverage. Thus, in the ensuing discussion these will be grouped together.

Antibiotic Toxicities

All antibiotics share certain toxicities and have some general limitations to their use over and above the specific characteristic toxicities of each agent. Virtually all antibiotics and some antineoplastic agents have been implicated in the pathogenesis of pseudomembranous enterocolitis. This is a disorder commonly associated with abdominal pain, diarrhea, fever, and leukocytes in the stool. Diagnosis is established by demonstration of the causative organism, Clostridium difficile, in the stool along with its toxin. The diagnosis may be suspected in the presence of fecal leukocytes or sigmoidoscopic exam showing the characteristic pseudomembranes. Although initially associated with clindamycin the disease is now generally considered to be a sequela of all antibiotics. Treatment is initiated with either vancomyin orally or, in milder cases, with metronidazole orally or even cholestyramine.

All antibiotics have the capacity for promoting superinfection. The mechanism by which they do this is by no means clear. Alteration of the normal flora plays a part in the genesis of superinfection. With broader spectrum agents superinfection takes place with progressively more resistant organisms. Some antibiotics may have direct immunosuppressive properties which increase their propensity for causing superinfection. Superinfection is best treated, as in the case of most infections, by prevention. The best prevention is the selection of the narrowest spectrum agent capable of eliminating the observed infection.

Another general toxicity of antibiotic administration is intravenous infusion related sepsis. This entity potentially afflicts all intravenous infusions and its risk is directly proportional to the duration of the intravenous catheterization. Although not a side-effect directly attributable to drug effects, it is a consequence of intravenous drug administration. Once again the best therapy for infusion related sepsis is prevention. Intravenous catheters should be changed no less frequently than every seventy-two hours, regardless of whether or not the IV site appears inflamed. Infusion related sepsis should be suspected in those patients who appear septic with no obvious source or reason. Most commonly, this disease responds to discontinuation of the catheter. Antibiotic therapy is rarely required unless metastatic infection has supervened.

As a general rule, antibiotic prescribing obeys the law of unintended consequences. Careful attention to susceptibility testing data and the use of the narrowest spectrum drug possible will minimize the invocation of this universal principle. Finally, untested combinations of antibiotics are to be avoided as they are likely to have surprising and possibly deleterious actions.

The Penicillins

The penicillins are among the most frequently used antibiotics. The β-aminopenicillanic acid nucleus is a structure combining β-lactam and thiazolidine rings. Resistance to the original penicillins emerged via production of penicillinase by staphylococci. This enzyme opens the β-lactam ring to form inactive penicilloic acids. Semisynthetic penicillins change the acyl side chain on the β-lactam ring to either: (1) confer steric hindrance to opening of the β-lactam ring by penicillinase-producing organisms, or (2) confer an extended spectrum of activity to include various gram-negative organisms.

Penicillins inhibit bacterial cell wall synthesis by interfering in the third stage of the biosynthesis of peptidoglycan, a complex macromolecule providing rigid mechanical stability to the cell wall.

Pencillin G. Penicillin G is a benzylpenicillin, that is a benzyl side chain attached to the β-aminopenicillamic acid nucleus. Most species of streptococcus are highly sensitive to this drug although the enterococcus requires the addition of an aminoglycoside to be effective. It is more effective than the semisynthetic penicillins against non-penicillinase-producing Staphylococcus aureus and Neisseria gonorrhoeae and it is the drug of choice for Neisseria meningitidis, Treponema pallidum and most anaerobic organisms excluding penicillinase-producing strains such as Bacteroides fragilis, and some other bacteroides strains with high-grade resistance.

Penicillinase-resistant Penicillins. Methicillin, nafcillin, oxacillin, cloxacillin and dicloxacillin are semisynthetic penicillins with acyl side chains that prevent opening of the β-lactam ring by penicillinase. They are agents of first choice in staphylococcal infections caused by penicillinase-producing organisms, which account for 70-90% of all staphylococcal isolates.

These penicillins are not usually employed in topical ophthalmic therapy because of the availability of older agents without β-lactam rings in which topical, but not systemic, therapy is safe. Adequate anterior chamber concentration can be obtained with methicillin. Intravitreal administration is also possible. Because of increased association with interstitial nephritis, methicillin is used less often than nafcillin or oxacillin in parenteral form.

The mechanism for the emergence of "methicillin-resistant" staphylococci appears to be the failure to bind penicillin-binding proteins in the bacterial cell wall rather than circumvention of the stability to β-lactamase.

Ampicillin and Amoxicillin. These are aminobenzyl-penicillins that have activity against gram-negative organisms conferred by the addition of the amino group. This makes them less effective than penicillin G against pneumococci and most streptococci, Neisseria organisms and clostridia, but adds activity against Proteus, Shigella, non-typhi Salmonella, non-penicillinase-producing Haemophilus influenzae and greater in vivo activity against enterococci. Like all penicillins, anterior chamber or vitreous concentrations are poor following topical or systemic therapy. Amoxicillin has superior gastrointestinal absorption and higher blood levels compared to ampicillin. Because of older, effective agents for topical use against gram-negative organisms and because of lack of activity against Pseudomonas, these drugs are seldom indicated in bacterial ocular infections.

Anti-pseudomonal Penicillins. Carbenicillin, ticarcillin, azlocillin, mezlocillin and piperacillin have acyl-amino side chains that confer a spectrum of activity to include Pseudomonas aeruginosa.

Their major benefit is stability to the beta lactamase of Pseudomonas aeruginosa. This does not imply stability to staphylococcal beta lactamase by which the antipseudomonal penicillins are hydrolyzed. The unique side-effects are hypokalemia from presentation of a non-absorbable sodium to the distal tubule, platelet aggregation inhibition, and volume overload. Like all penicillins, hypersensitivity is a major limiting factor.

The Cephalosporins

Because of their ease of administration, relative lack of toxicity, and aggressive marketing, cephalosporins are the most commonly prescribed hospital antimicrobial agents. They are rarely the drugs of first choice and are almost invariably expensive. They are often overused.

For convenience, cephalosporins are divided into generations and are listed in Table 16-1. All cephalosporins contain the 7-aminocephalosporanic acid nucleus. Cephalosporin C was the first compound isolated from Cephalosporium acremonium although it is not clinically useful. All cephalosporin agents are bactericidal. They are susceptible to hydrolysis by a series of beta lactamases generically called cephalosporinases. The cephamycins are similar to the cephalosporins but are derived from Streptomyces spp. Similar uncertainty exists concerning the mechanism of action of these compounds although they are clearly cell wall active and require a binding protein.

First Generation Agents. The first generation agents are all similar in antimicrobial spectrum. They are active against penicillinase producing staphylococci, streptococci excluding the enterococcus, and some Enterobacteriaceae including some E. coli, Klebsiellae, and Enterobacter spp. Pseudomonads are routinely resistant. The cephalothin disc is used generically for susceptibility of the first generation agents. Cephalothin was the first. It has a short half-life and is undetectable in serum three hours after intravenous administration. It provides good serum and tissue levels but is not effective in CNS infections and should never be used when these are suspected. It is excreted primarily by the kidney. Cefazolin has a half-life (T½) of 1.8 hrs as compared to 30 minutes with cephalothin. It is less painful given IM. Because of its longer duration of action, cefazolin may be given at longer intervals, up to eight hours for less serious infections. Cephapirin is similar to cephalothin and has advantage only when cheaper. Cephradine has an oral and parenteral form. Cephaloridine is no longer used because of its nephrotoxicity. Cephalexin is among the most expensive and, orally, the most commonly used against streptococci except the enterococcus. The majority of domiciliary acquired urinary tract Enterobacteriaceae are susceptible. It is well absorbed and achieves good urinary levels. Its T½ requires four times/day dosing. Cephradine is equivalent to cephalexin. Cephaloglycin is poorly absorbed and should not be used. Cefdaroxil has the same spectrum of activity but because of its long T½ can be used twice a day. Cefaclor is similar to cephalexin but has activity against H. influenzae.

Second Generation Agents. Cefamandole has increased activity against some hospital acquired Enterobacteriaceae and separate disc testing must be performed. Pseudomonads are resistant. Most N. gonorrheae are susceptible as are most H. influenzae, both ampicillin sensitive and ampicillin resistant strains. The drug does not achieve therapeutic CNS levels. Its kinetics are similar to cephalothin. Anaerobic gram negative organisms are not susceptible at attainable levels. An additional side-effect with cefamandole has been vitamin K responsive bleeding with prolonged use.

Cefoxitin is a cephamycin antibiotic with expanded gram negative spectrum. It is less active *versus* gram positives than the first generation agents and is less active than cefamandole against mutually susceptible strains. This is generally not clinically significant. It is effective against 80% of B. fragilis strains. In critically ill patients, cefoxitin should not be used as a single agent nor should it be employed with known B. fragilis sepsis. The dosage must be reduced with renal failure. Ceforanide is a second generation agent with a T½ which allows every twelve hour dosing. Cefonicid has a T½ of four hours and thus extended dosing is also possible.

Third Generation Agents. In general the third generation agents have extended gram negative spectra but have lost significant gram positive activity. With the exception of cefsulodin they have no appreciable anti-pseudomonal activity. Nor do they have activity against enterococci. Because of their broad spectra of activity, the third generation agents promote superinfection with enterococci, pseudomonas, yeasts, and resistant organisms such as acinetobacter spp. and non-aeruginosa pseudomonads. They almost universally achieve therapeutic levels in the central nervous system. Each agent must be tested separately for *in vitro* activity.

Side-Effects of the Cephalosporins. The incidence of primary allergic phenomena is approximately 5%. In patients with immediate type hypersensitivity reactions to the penicillins, cephalosporins must be avoided. In patients with other allergies to penicillin, the incidence of cross allergenicity is 5-15%.

There are some data that some cephalosporins are synergistically nephrotoxic with the aminoglycosides. This is controversial.

Positive Coombs tests are common in patients on high dose cephalosporins, but overt hemolysis is rare.

Hypoprothrombinemia with clinical bleeding is most commonly seen with cefamandole and moxalactam but all of the classes have the potential for causing this.

Vancomycin

Vancomycin was introduced in 1956 because of emerging resistance of staphylococci to penicillin therapy. It was subsequently supplanted by methicillin and analogues. Recently it has seen a resurgence of use for several indications.

It is a derivative of Streptomyces orientalis and is structurally unrelated to any other class of antibiotic. It inhibits biosynthesis of cell wall phospholipids and peptidoglycan polymers. It also inhibits the synthesis of RNA and injures protoplasts by altering their cytoplasmic membranes. It is active only against gram positive bacteria. Against some enterococci it is only bacteriostatic, so an aminoglycoside aminocyclitol is commonly added for bactericidal activity. Since it does not depend on penicillin binding proteins for effect, it works against methicillin-resistant staphylococci including S. aureus and S. epidermidis.

Vancomycin is unabsorbed orally and achieves very high stool concentrations, making it an ideal agent for luminal gram positive pathogens such as C. difficile. Intravenously it achieves good serum levels and penetrates the synovium, ascitic, peritoneal and pericardial fluids. Vancomycin penetrates the inflamed meninges.

The drug is excreted primarily by the kidneys and thus dose must be reduced in the context of renal failure. Its toxicity is primarily to the ear. Very high serum levels (>80 micrograms/ml) are associated with ototoxicity. Nephrotoxicity is rare and is in the form of interstitial nephritis. Both ototoxicity and nephrotoxicity are additive in the presence of aminoglycosides. The "vancomycin reaction" is a red truncal rash appearing during rapid infusion of the drug. It disappears with slowing of the infusion and does not connote allergy. Fever and chills, formerly a hallmark of vancomycin therapy, are rarely seen with the new purer preparations. In anephric or anuric patients the effective duration of action of the drug is one week, making it the ideal agent for the treatment of dialysis associated gram positive infections.

Erythromycin

Erythromycin is a macrolide antibiotic produced by the actinomycete Streptomyces erythreus. It is composed of a macrocyclic lactone ring (macrolide) attached to two sugar moieties. It binds to the 50S ribosomal subunit to inhibit bacterial protein synthesis.

Erythromycin is very effective against most gram positive organisms including many staphylococci and virtually all non-enterococcal streptococci. Some anaerobes and gram negatives are susceptible as well. It is bacteriostatic and some staphylococci are naturally resistant. Mycoplasmae, Legionellae, T. pallidum and ureaplasmae are usually sensitive.

Given orally its major side-effect is gastrointestinal upset. The estolate form has been associated with cholestasis. Parenterally the drug causes pain on injection which limits its use.

Tetracyclines

The tetracyclines have a nucleus which consists of four fused rings giving rise to their name.

They have a very broad spectrum of activity including many gram-positive, gram-negative, aerobic and anaerobic bacteria. Their special place is in activity against organisms not sensitive to other antibiotics such as rickettsiae, mycoplasma and chlamydia.

They act to inhibit bacterial protein synthesis by binding to the 30S ribosomes subunit.

Adverse effects include proximal gastrointestinal irritation and epigastric burning and distress, nausea and vomiting, as well as distal side-effects of irritative diarrheas and candidal colonization. Hepatotoxicity and nephrotoxicity are much less common. Tetracycline should not be administered to children, or pregnant or nursing women because of its effects on bones and teeth.

Neomycin

Neomycin is an aminoglycoside antibiotic first described in 1949 which is available now only for topical use.

Its spectrum of activity includes many gram-negative bacteria with the exception of Pseudomonas aeruginosa and anaerobic Bacteroides spp. Staphylococci are highly sensitive to these drugs but all streptococci and the gram-positive bacilli are relatively resistant. Staphylococcus strains resistant to neomycin as well as bacitracin (often combined in topical applications) have been described.

Neomycin and other aminoglycoside antibiotics interfere with bacterial protein synthesis by binding to the 30S subunit of bacterial ribosomes, resulting in a miscoding of mRNA codons and the production of faulty bacterial proteins.

Ototoxicity, nephrotoxicity, neuromuscular blockade, staphylococcal enterocolitis, gastrointestinal side-effects and contact dermatitis are well described and preclude common oral or parenteral use.

Neomycin sulfate solution is supplied in a concentration of 30 to 50 mg/ml and is effective treatment for conjunctivitis caused by susceptible organisms. It is toxic to the corneal epithelium if used frequently.

Polymyxin B

Polymyxin B is a polypeptide antibiotic first isolated in 1947 from Bacillus polymyxa. It is not generally available commercially in a pure form. Its activity and dosage are usually measured in units. One milligram of pure polymyxin B is equivalent to 10,000 units.

Polymyxin B is highly active against many important gram-negative bacteria including Pseudomonas aeruginosa and Haemophilus influenzae; gram positive organisms are all resistant.

Polymyxin B binds to and damages the bacterial cytoplasmic membrane of susceptible gram-negative bacteria, leading to leakage of intracellular components. Nephrotoxicity, neurotoxicity and hypersensitivity reactions preclude systemic use of this antibiotic.

Polymyxin B sulfate is often combined with neomycin and bacitracin because the latter two are ineffective against Pseudomonas aeruginosa. The development of bacterial resistance to this drug is uncommon. It is an effective topical preparation in conjunctivitis caused by susceptible organisms. It is available in solution at a concentration of 20,000 U/ml.

Sulfacetamide

Sulfacetamide is a "short-acting" sulfonamide antibiotic whose sodium salt is available as a topical agent.

The sulfonamides originally had a wide range of activity against gram-positive and gram-negative organisms, though acquired bacteria resistance has limited their broad spectrum.

The sulfonamides interfere with bacterial purine and DNA synthesis by blocking the synthesis of essential folic acid precursors. Structurally related to para-amino benzoic acid, they act by competitive blocking of the enzyme dihydrofolic acid synthetase, thus crippling the enzymatic pathways.

Hypersensitivity manifestations following topical sulfonamide therapy are well described. Stevens-Johnson syndrome has followed the use of sulfonamide eye drops.

The advantages of sulfacetamide are the very high aqueous concentrations obtainable after topical application and the non-irritating nature of the drug to the delicate linings of the eye. Preparations are available in solution and ointment from 100 to 300 mg/ml and can be applied every two hours or even more frequently. Emergence of *in vivo* resistance is the most common limiting factor.

Bacitracin

Bacitracin is a polypeptide antibiotic isolated from a strain of Bacillus species in 1943 and used systemically until about 1960. It was employed for use in severe staphylococcal infections but because of its nephrotoxicity and the availability of safer anti-staphylococcal drugs it is now restricted to topical use.

It is highly active against most gram-positive bacteria, especially Staphylococcus aureus and Group A β-hemolytic streptococci. Neisseriae, H. influenzae and T. pallidum are sensitive but other gram-negative bacilli are resistant. Acquired resistance in staphylococci is known to occur but is rare with this drug.

Bacitracin interferes with bacterial cell wall synthesis and has virtually no side-effects when used topically. It has been shown to have good penetration into the aqueous humor after topical application in rabbits. Suppurative conjunctivitis and infected corneal ulcers caused by susceptible organisms respond well to the topical application of bacitracin. The solution or suspension is available in 10,000 U/ml concentration and the ointment in 500 U/gram of suitable base. It is frequently combined with neomycin and polymyxin B in topical preparations to effect a broader range of activity.

Antiviral Agents

Because of the large number of specific viral illnesses of the eye, antiviral chemotherapy is well studied. Specific therapy is discussed under each disease.

Ara-A. This agent has a broad spectrum of activity against DNA viruses. The mechanism of action is complex but the drug appears to have selective inhibitory activity against viral DNA synthesis as opposed to cellular DNA synthesis. It is a safe drug. In ophthalmology, its major use is in Herpes simplex keratitis.

Acycloguanosine (Acyclovir). Acyclovir works by inhibiting virus polymerase after uptake into the cell by virus encoded thymidine kinase. Although very effective *in vitro*, its *in vivo* use is limited to topical and systemic administration against primary herpes genitalis and disseminated herpes infections.

Idoxuridine. By its incorporation into viral DNA, idoxuridine renders the molecule more fragile. This drug is highly effective in Herpes Simplex keratitis but is very toxic systemically and is no longer used parenterally.

Amantadine. Amantadine is useful in the prophylaxis and treatment of influenza A infection. It has no parenteral form and no specific use in ophthalmic infections. Rimantidiue is a similar drug with similar activity.

Antifungal Agents

Amphotericin B. Amphotericin B is an antifungal agent which works by binding to the sterol moiety of the fungus. It is active against a broad range of fungi and is synergistic in some cases with flucytosine. It penetrates the eye poorly upon intravenous injection and is quite toxic. The major side-effects of intravenously administered amphotericin B are hypokalemia, renal and hepatotoxicity and anemia. Subconjunctival injection of amphotericin B produces a distinct yellowish discoloration of the conjunctiva which is not reversible. Reports of pink, raised nodules appearing on the conjunctiva have appeared in the literature. These resolve upon discontinuation of the subconjunctival injection.

Flucytosine. Flucytosine is a broad spectrum antifungal which is commonly administered orally. It achieves good aqueous humor concentrations. The major limitation of flucytosine is the development of resistance during therapy. It is usually used in conjunction with amphotericin B. Flucytosine may depress the bone marrow and cause nausea and vomiting. The effects are exacerbated by azotemia since the drug is primarily excreted by the kidney.

Imidazole Derivatives. These agents, miconazole, clotrimazole, and ketoconazole, have broad antifungal activities. Clotrimazole is used primarily for vaginal candidiasis. Miconazole is effective topically and parenterally for candidiasis, however amphotericin B remains the drug of choice for severe infections. Ketoconazole can be given orally and is effective against a broad range of fungi. It does not achieve effective levels either in the central nervous system or in the urine.

Generally, antifungal chemotherapy is complex and should be attempted only by those experienced in the use and toxicities of the available agents.

attempted only by those experienced in the use and toxicities of the available agents.

Summary

Does the bug cause the disease? Does the drug kill the bug? Can the drug get to the bug? These are important tenents in infectious disease and in the treatment of ocular infections, specifically endophthalmitis (Chapter 15) and orbital cellulitis (Chapter 2).

The ophthalmologist needs to be reminded of the importance of isolating the pathogen and obtaining sensitivities from serious ocular and orbital infections. This makes choosing the appropriate antibiotic much easier and treatment safer and more efficacious. Antibiotic administration is not benign and may have severe systemic complications. The ophthalmologist should be aware of these. The wide variety of available antibiotics are discussed and their primary and secondary activities, major drawbacks and toxicities tabulated into an easily referable table.

Additionally, the widely detailed and advertised cephalosporins are discussed in relative detail, and the efficacy, advantages and disadvantages of each "generation" of cephalosporin are explored.

APPENDIX
Primarily Gram Positive Acting Agents

Drug	1° Activity	2° Activity	Major Drawbacks	Major Toxicities
Penicillin G oral, IV, IM	Streptococcal species excluding enterococcus Treponemes Non β-lactamase producing N-gonorrheae	Non β-lactamase producing anaerobes	β-lactamase susceptibility	Hypersensitivity
Ampicillin Amoxicillin oral, IV, IM	Penicillin G + non β-lactamase producing, Haemophilus influenzae Not for treponemes Enterococcus	Some E. coli	β-lactamase susceptibility	Hypersensitivity rash
Methicillin Oxacillin Nafcillin oral, IV, IM	β-lactamase producing Staph aureus		Less effective vs non β-lactamase producing organisms than Pen.G	Hypersensitivity Interstitial nephritis (methicillin) Leucopenia (oxacillin, nafcillin)
Vancomyin oral, IV	Gram + organisms esp. methicillin resistant staph aureus Enterococcus	Clostridium difficile (orally)	Sclerosing to soft tissue. Undetectable in aqueous following IV admin.	VIII nerve, rare interstitial nephritis. Rash, no cross reactivity with penicillin.
Erythromycin oral, IV	Gram +organisms	Chlamydia, Legionella, Mycoplasma	unpredictable vs. S. aureus bacteriostatic	GI upset, hepatotoxicity
Cephalothin, IV, IM Cefazolin, IV, IM Cephepirine, IV, IM Cefalexin, oral	Gram + aerobic organisms except enterococci	Some E. coli and Klebsiella	Generally expensive	Hypersensitivity

Gram Positive and Gram Negative Acting Agents

Drug	1° Activity	2° Activity	Major Drawbacks	Major Toxicities
Tetracycline Doxycycline oral, IV	α hemolytic strep, chlamydia, gonococcus, mycoplasma, rickettsiae	Brucellosis, some anaerobes	Bacteriostatic, "spotty" spectrum vs. bacteria No CNS levels	Discolors children's teeth. Developmental disorders in fetus.
Trimethoprim-sulfamethoxazole. oral, IV	Aerobic gram negative rods except pseudomonas	Some gram positive aerobes. Nocardia	No activity vs. anaerobes, pseudomonas or enterococcus No CNS levels	Hypersensitivity is common

APPENDIX (continued)

Cefamandole IV, IM	Selected aerobic gram negatives	S. aureus and streptococci except enterococcus	No anaerobic activity, resistance may be inducible. short half-life. Unpredictable vs. Klebsiella. No predictable CNS activity	Bleeding hypersensitivity
Cefoxitin IV, IM	Selected aerobic gram negatives, anaerobic gram negatives.	Gonococcus streptococci except enterococcus	Poor vs. S. aureus, unpredictable vs. enterobacter. No CNS activity	Hypersensitivity
Chloramphenicol oral, IV, IM	Selected aerobic, anaerobic gram positive and gram negative H. Influenzae	Rickettsiae	Bacteriostatic. Spotty resistance requires susceptibility testing (e.g., Hemophilus)	Idiopathic aplastic anemia. Bone marrow suppression

Primarily Gram Negative Acting Drugs

Drug	1° Effect	2° Effect	Major Drawback	Major Toxicities
Gentamicin Tobramycin Netilmicin Amikacin IV, IM	Aerobic gram negatives	M. tuberculosis	Inactivated by low pH, poor penetration into CNS, resistant strains exist (genta > tobra, netil > amikacin), resistance transferable via plasmid	Ototoxicity nephrotoxicity
Cefotaxime Moxalactam Cefoperazone Ceftazidime Ceftizoxime Ceftriaxone* Cefsulodin* IV, IM	Multiple drug resistant gram neg aerobes, Aerobic gram negs in CNS	Gram neg anaerobes, β-lactamase + N. gonorrheae	No activity vs. enterococcus Unpredictable vs. pseudomonas Expensive, superinfection common, weak vs. gram positives	Hypersensitivity bleeding (moxalactam)
Carbenicillin Ticarcillin Azlocillin Mezlocillin Piperacillin IV, IM	Aerobic gram negative rods esp. pseudomonas aeruginosa when used with aminoglycoside	Gram negative anaerobes	Weak vs. gram +, β-lactamase susceptible, expensive. activity varies vs. pseudomonas (carb < ticar <azlo, mezlo < piperacillin)	Bleeding (antiplatelet) hypokalemia, hypersensitivity, Na+ overload
Aztreonam* IV, IM	Aerobic gram negative rods		No anaerobic or gram positive activity	Hepatotoxicity
Ciprofloxacin* Norfloxicin* oral	Aerobic gram negative rods esp. pseudomonas		Limited spectrum	Hypersensitivity

Other Agents

Drug	1° Activity	2° Activity	Major Use	Major Drawback
Bacitracin	Gram + aerobic		topical	systemically toxic
Metronidazole IV, p.o.	Gram − anaerobes	Entamoeba histolytica Trichomonas vaginalis Giardia lamblia	systemic infections	antabuse-like possibly carcinogenic
Clindamycin	Gram − anaerobes	Staph aureus S. pyogenes	systemic, topical	bacteriostatic
Sulfanilamide	Selected gram + and gram −		topical	hypersensitivity
Colistin Polymyxin B	selected gram −		topical	nephrotoxicity when absorbed or used systemically

Cephalosporin Agents By "Generation"

first generation	second generation	third generation
cephalothin (Keflin)	cefamandole (Mandol)	cefotaxime (Claforan)
cephaloridine (Loridine)	cefoxitin (Mefoxin)	moxalactam (Moxam)
cephapirine (Cefadyl)	ceforanide (Precef)	cefoperazone (Cefobid)
cefazolin (Kefzol, Ancef)	cefonocid (Monocid)	ceftizoxime (Ceftizox)
cephradine (Velosef, Anspor)		cefatzidime (Fortaz)
cephalexin (Keflex)		ceftriaxone
cefadroxil (Duricef, Ultracef)		cefsulodin
		others

*not yet available as of January, 1985

391

INDEX

Page numbers in *italics* indicate main listings.